IN THE SHADOW OF ILLNESS

IN THE SHADOW OF ILLNESS

PARENTS AND SIBLINGS OF THE
CHRONICALLY ILL CHILD

by Myra Bluebond-Langner

PRINCETON UNIVERSITY PRESS   PRINCETON, NEW JERSEY

Library of Congress Cataloging-in-Publication Data
Bluebond-Langner, Myra, 1948–
In the shadow of illness : parents and siblings of the chronically
ill child / by Myra Bluebond-Langner.
p.   cm.
Includes bibliographical references (p.   ) and index.
ISBN 0-691-02783-8 (cl : alk. paper)
1. Death—Psychological aspects—Case studies.   2. Parents of
terminally ill children—Case studies.   3. Brothers and sisters—
Death—Psychological aspects—Case studies.   4. Terminally ill
children—Family relationship—Case studies.   5. Cystic fibrosis—
Psychological aspects—Case studies.   I. Title.
BF789.D4B635   1996
155.9′16—dc20   96-6800 CIP Rev.

_____ **For the Families** _____

THEN SISYPHOS IN TORMENT I BEHELD

BEING ROUSTABOUT TO A TREMENDOUS BOULDER.

LEANING WITH BOTH ARMS BRACED AND LEGS DRIVING,

HE HEAVED IT TOWARDS A HEIGHT, AND ALMOST OVER,

BUT THEN A POWER SPUN HIM ROUND AND SENT

THE CRUEL BOULDER BOUNDING AGAIN TO THE PLAIN.

WHEREON THE MAN BENT DOWN AGAIN TO TOIL,

DRIPPING SWEAT, AND THE DUST ROSE OVERHEAD.

The Odyssey, Book IX, lines 709–16, trans. Robert Fitzgerald

Contents

List of Tables

Preface

MY INTEREST in well siblings of children with chronic, life-threatening illnesses goes back twenty-five years, to my first study of children with cancer. During the time I was preparing *The Private Worlds of Dying Children* (Princeton, 1978), I often wondered what it must be like to live with a sibling who is ill, perhaps even dying. The plight of well siblings, though beyond the scope of that project, came through loudly and clearly. I will never forget the five-year-old who, upon learning of the death of her eight-year-old-brother, said, "Good. Now can I have his toys?" Another world here needed to be explored.

In 1980 I was invited to a Cystic Fibrosis Foundation conference on the psychosocial aspects of cystic fibrosis (CF). At the time, both clinicians and parents sought a way to understand how well siblings were affected by growing up with a chronically ill child. The work to date had drawn no clear conclusions about the well siblings of children with CF or any other chronic, life-threatening disease. On the basis of what I learned at the conference, I decided that the well siblings of children with CF would be an excellent population in which to investigate the impact of chronic, life-threatening illness on well siblings.

Understanding a bit about CF makes it easy to see why one might select this population for such a study. CF is the most common fatal genetic disease in the United States today. The median age of survival is presently twenty-nine years (although it was nineteen years at the time of this study). The CF gene is recessive. At the time of conception when both parents are carriers there is a one-in-four chance that the child will have CF and a two-in-four chance that the child will be a symptomless carrier and a one-in-four chance that the child will be neither affected nor a carrier. It is estimated that one in twenty Americans carries the CF gene.

CF causes the body to produce abnormally thick mucus, which blocks passages in the lungs and becomes the nidus of recurrent bacterial infections. CF mucus also obstructs the pancreas and blocks the passage of digestive enzymes to the small intestine, thus impairing absorption of nutrients. It is often difficult for a person with CF to maintain an adequate weight.

The responsibility for treating these symptoms falls, on a daily basis, to the family. Chest physical therapy—pounding on the chest and back—is used to dislodge mucus so that it can be expectorated.[1] A session of chest physical

---

[1] At the end of this book is a glossary of clinical and technical terminology as used in the medical literature as well as in everyday speech by family members and clinicians. The glossary

therapy lasts, ideally, thirty-five to forty minutes and may be recommended from two to four times a day, depending upon the severity of the disease. Chest physical therapy is often preceded by the inhalation of bronchodilators and/or antibiotics. Inhalation of medication via a nebulizer can add anywhere from ten minutes to several hours a day to the airway-clearance routine.

Because of the involvement of the pancreas, persons with CF must take pancreatic enzymes with each meal and snack. In infancy and until the child learns to swallow a capsule, enzyme capsules are opened and the contents mixed with applesauce. Vitamin supplements are also used. As the disease progresses and children have difficulty maintaining weight, high-fat diets, high-calorie drinks, and supplements are often recommended. In some cases nocturnal nasogastric or gastrostomy feedings become necessary.

Over time pulmonary damage increases and pulmonary function decreases. Complications often develop, including hemoptysis, diabetes, and colonization with bacteria resistant to multiple antibiotics (e.g., Burkholderia cepacia [at the time of the study known as Pseudomonas cepacia]). Parents' time is further consumed by increases in home therapy as well as by more frequent trips to the hospital, often a distance from home. Surgical intervention may be required for the treatment of hemoptysis, nasal polyps, nutritional deficits, and/or for the insertion of central intravenous catheters to administer medicines.

As the patient becomes increasingly short of breath (from inadequate oxygen supply), attempts are made to improve respiratory function through the use of even more aggressive antimicrobial therapy, pulmonary toilet, and oxygen.

Death comes when the lungs have become irreversibly scarred from chronic infections and the airways are so massively distended that they pool large amounts of infected mucus, thus preventing gas exchange.

Although there is no cure for CF, new advances in lung transplantation and various drug therapies have increased the median age of survival. The current median age of twenty-nine years is an increase of ten years during the last decade. The development of gene therapy holds promise for even longer survival rates.

How do families manage under the terrible burden of this disease? Doesn't this disease take a terrible toll on these families, both collectively and individually?

Pursuing these questions, I set out to focus on well siblings and designed a study that would get at what they thought about this disease, their parents, and their ill sibling. Those with CF and their parents were to be interviewed and observed only for background.

I found that the well siblings' understanding of themselves and others is

---

is not meant to be a medical dictionary. It is intended to explain unfamiliar terms that occur in the ordinary conversation of those family members and clinicians who are quoted.

linked to their parents' responses and to their ill siblings' condition and illness experiences. I also found that I could discuss the well siblings' views of the disease and their relations to their ill siblings and parents only by placing them within the context of everyday family life. Documenting and analyzing the changes in the everyday lives of these families were necessary, for this is the context from which the knowledge and experience of the well siblings derives.

I saw that, despite the terrible burdens placed upon both body and spirit, these families appear, at least for long periods of time, very much like other families. I realized that understanding the impact of CF on well siblings does not come from searching for something wrong in their lives, nor does it come through the identification of some form of pathology or from the discovery of abnormal behavior caused by a trying situation. Rather, understanding lies in appreciating how the family, including the well sibling, goes about preserving its integrity, living life as it is, in the face of CF's intrusion.

The book is written in four parts. I begin in Part I with a discussion of some representative work to date on well siblings of children with CF and other chronic, life-threatening illnesses, and explain my own approach. I introduce two fundamental concepts of the book: first, the strategies that parents use to contain the intrusion of CF, and second the natural history of the illness. In Part II (Chapters 2–10) I present the reader with the data, with an ethnography of the everyday lives of the families and the siblings. This is done in the form of accounts by members of nine different families, who are at different points in the progression of the disease. Part III (Chapters 11–13) contains the analysis of the data. In Chapter 11 I lay out the basic context for this analysis, the major issues the parents of chronically ill children face, and the ways in which parents of children with CF deal with them over the course of the illness. In Chapter 12 I discuss the relationship between the strategies that the parents adopt and the well siblings' views of the disease and their ill siblings' condition. In Chapter 13 I examine the role that the parents' strategies and the well siblings' views play in how these siblings conduct their relationships with their parents and ill siblings. I also consider how the well siblings and other members of the family perceive the well siblings' position in the family—their rights, privileges, duties, and responsibilities. The Afterword addresses the clinical implications of the analysis.

Acknowledgments

THIS BOOK has been a long time in coming; ten years from the day I started my fieldwork until I delivered the manuscript to Princeton University Press. Dick, my husband, and Rachel and Jessica, our daughters, have been there from the beginning. Rachel and Jessica have grown up with this project, and I think that in no small way been shaped by it—by the process of research and writing as well as through the people that they have met at St. Christopher's Hospital for Children. Dick provided much-needed support and encouragement as well as advice at every stage. He remains my best and toughest critic. While I am quite certain that this book would have been far better if I had taken more of his advice, I also know that then it would not have been mine. In the end I must and do take full responsibility for it.

I am also fortunate in having several close friends and colleagues who took time from their own busy schedules to discuss ideas and read and comment on portions of the manuscript, as well as to be there for me when I seemed to be dragging. I am indeed grateful to: Judy Bluebond Seelig, Carol Fuchs, Mary Frankel, Augie Hermann, Drew Humphries, Robert Kastenbaum, Suzanne Langner, Coral Lansbury, Bryan Lask, Phyllis Magaziner, Dale Perkel, Lynne Quittell, David Rosen, Tory Rosen, Daniel Schidlow, Enid Schildkraut, John Stewart, Liesa Stamm, and Toby Zinman.

This book has also benefited from the careful reading and thoughtful comments of Jill Korbin and Patricia Marshall, reviewers for the Press. I wish that I had been able to incorporate more of their suggestions. I shrink in horror at the thought of what this book would have looked like without the careful attention to detail given by "my copyeditor," Bob Brown. As many at the Press know, only Bob would do. Bob has taught me the true meaning of the blue pencil. I also appreciate the efforts of Gail Ullman, who acquired the book for the Press, and Mary Murrell, who shepherded it through the reviewing and approval process.

I would also like to thank the Department of Anthropology of Case Western Reserve University and the Childhood and Society Seminar, Institute of Education, University of London for inviting me to try out some of my ideas on my colleagues in anthropology here and abroad. I hope that some of the questions that I could not answer then are answered here.

Similarly, I would also like to thank the Cystic Fibrosis Foundation; Institute of Child Health; Department of Psychological Medicine, Great Ormond Street Hospital for Children; and the Departments of Pediatric Pulmonary Medicine at the Royal Brompton Hospital, London; the Departments of Hematology and Oncology, Royal Victoria Infirmary, Newcastle upon Tyne,

England; and the Department of Pediatrics, Portiuncula Hospital, Ballinasloe, Ireland, for inviting me to speak about my work to those directly involved in care and treatment of children with cystic fibrosis and other chronic, life-threatening and fatal illnesses. Their probing questions and incisive comments increased my desire to write a book that would be of clinical value. If this work proves useful in clinical practice it is in no small way due to the efforts of these dedicated clinicians.

For the opportunity to present my work to parents of children with cystic fibrosis I would like to thank the Cystic Fibrosis Centers at St. Christopher's Hospital for Children, Philadelphia; St. Vincent's Hospital, Dublin, Ireland; and Children's Hospitals of Akron, Ohio, and Winnipeg, Manitoba. The comments that I received from parents have informed not only the content, but also the structure and format of this book.

Most professors have a list of graduate students to thank for their assistance on a project. I have a long list of hard-working undergraduates at the Camden campus of Rutgers University, who must be recognized for their most able assistance: William Fugee, Lynn Gault, Reed Gladey, Alicia Moschini, and Christina Wileczek for assembling the bibliography and abstracting articles; Johanna Green, for observations in the waiting room; Ursula Marrolli for coding transcripts; Xenia Tuton for the selection and organization of pseudonyms.

Analysis of the data was greatly facilitated by a computerized database and indexing program designed by Howard Lubert and George Lesser. This program made it possible for me to locate and code, in a variety of ways, every recorded utterance and observation made over the nineteen months I spent in the field. My mother, Claire Bluebond, and cousin, Rene Schwartz, did all of the data entry. My father, Mahlon Bluebond, tirelessly photocopied pages and pages of transcripts and field journal entries that computerized searches indicated were relevant for examination of particular points.

Verbatim transcripts were flawlessly prepared by Donna Douglass and Robert Arendt. Thea Dugan prepared the charts for copyediting on less-than-state-of-the-art equipment. Jessica Bluebond-Langner helped with corrections in the final stages of copyediting. Laura Mansnerus was invaluable in dealing with the page proofs.

Funding for this project was provided by grants and fellowships from the National Science Foundation, Howard Foundation, American Council of Learned Societies, and Rutgers University Research Council and Faculty Study Leave Program. Without their financial support neither this book nor related research projects and publications (see works cited) would have been completed.

This study would not have even been possible, however, without the cooperation of the staff of the Cystic Fibrosis Center and families at St. Christopher's Hospital for Children who, owing to agreements with the human-subjects-review committees at both St. Christopher's Hospital and Rutgers University, must remain nameless. The staff could not have been more helpful, graciously introducing me to families, patiently answering my many questions, and providing me with a space to work when I was at the center. The families opened their homes to me and gave unstintingly of their time and of themselves. I am indeed privileged to have known them. This book is dedicated to the families.

Part One

INTRODUCTION

CHAPTER 1

The Impact of Cystic Fibrosis on Well Siblings

THIS CHAPTER introduces the reader to some of the previous work on well siblings and to the present study. In the first section I review the literature on well siblings with cystic fibrosis (CF) and other chronic, life-threatening illnesses, and I suggest that the real shortcoming lies not in its lack of consistent conclusions, but in its underlying approach.[1] In section 2 I describe the population and collection and coding of data for the present study. In section 3 I acquaint the reader with two basic concepts that emerge in the analysis—the strategies that parents use to contain the intrusion of the illness into their lives and the natural history of the illness.

1. APPROACHES TO THE STUDY OF WELL SIBLINGS

Much of the research on well siblings to date has been from what Drotar and Crawford (1985: 360) call "a deficit or disease perspective." In these studies

---

[1] This review of the literature includes studies of the well siblings of children not only with cystic fibrosis but also with other chronic, life-threatening, physical illnesses (e.g., cancer, diabetes, hemophilia, kidney disease). Further, the review does not include literature on well siblings of children with physical or mental handicaps or psychiatric disorders, except those who are part of studies of well siblings of children with chronic, life-threatening physical illnesses. In the main, physical disabilities (e.g., cerebral palsy, deafness, blindness) or mental handicaps (e.g., developmental delay, mental retardation) are not life threatening. The prognosis is, as we will see, a significant feature of cystic fibrosis (CF) and the diseases listed above with it. CF should therefore be distinguished from those illnesses which are not life threatening. Findings from such studies may be of benefit for work in CF or other similarly categorized illness, and similarly some of the work in CF and other chronic, life-threatening illnesses may be of use in the study of other physical disabilities and mental handicaps.

This review also does not cover literature on the impact of the death of a sibling. It is worth pointing out, however, that that literature is plagued with the same sorts of problems as the literature on well siblings of children with chronic and life-threatening illness.

I do not include a full review of this literature since the death experience was a very small part of this study. Not enough children in the study experienced the death of a sibling at the time of the study to do a meaningful study of the experience. Also, in the case of CF and other chronic, life-threatening illnesses death is increasingly less of a part of the well siblings' experience. They are often grown or have left home by the time the death occurs. With advances in medical science children are living longer with these catastrophic illnesses and the chronic character of the illness is a more prominent feature of the well siblings' everyday experience than the dying.

investigators "have searched for evidence of psychopathology or major dysfunction as the primary impact of catastrophic disease on individuals and families" (Carpenter and Sahler 1991: 194). To accomplish this they often turned to standardized instruments thought to measure social and emotional adjustment in children. These measures, "for the most part, were normed in psychiatric populations" (Carpenter and Sahler 1991: 194). They then analyzed the results in terms of variables that had proven meaningful in other studies of social and emotional adjustment in clinical populations (Delisi 1986).

The types of studies these investigators conducted reflected their motivation, background, and training. These researchers were interested in improving the lives of well siblings. They wanted their work to be of some use in clinical practice (a value I share). Some were in clinical practice and all had some clinical background or training. Given their orientation and background, their approach to the question is not surprising. In clinical work one prefers to rely on controlled studies with large samples, with clearly defined and delimited predictors of outcomes, and to make recommendations based on those findings.

This literature, however, is marked by contradictory findings and divergent interpretations of those findings. A substantial portion of the literature evaluates negative effects on the well siblings. Researchers report a panoply of problems: psychosomatic disorders,[2] somatic disorders,[3] accident proneness,[4] behavior disorders,[5] behavior problems,[6] hyperactivity,[7] irritability,[8] bedwetting and soiling,[9] regression,[10] stealing,[11] fire starting,[12] aggressiveness,[13] generalized hostility and rebelliousness,[14] poor social adjustment,[15] laziness,[16] withdrawal,[17] poor school performance,[18] learning disabilities and learning problems,[19] low

[2] Burton 1975: 190; Lindsay and MacCarthy 1974: 193; Allan, Townley, and Phelan 1974: 193.

[3] Tropauer, Franz, and Dilgard 1970: 430; Sourkes 1980: 63.

[4] Burton 1975: 200; Sourkes 1980: 63.

[5] Rosenstein 1970: 29.

[6] Cimini 1986: 2153.

[7] Meyerowitz and Kaplan 1973: 52.

[8] Lavigne and Ryan 1979: 624.

[9] Burton 1975: 200; Allan, Townley, and Phelan 1974: 139.

[10] Lindsay and MacCarthy 1974: 193.

[11] Allan, Townley, and Phelan 1974: 139.

[12] Ibid.

[13] Burton 1974: 190.

[14] Burton 1975: 198.

[15] McKey 1973: 93.

[16] Burton 1975: 200.

[17] Lavigne and Ryan 1979: 623.

[18] Meyerowitz and Kaplan 1973: 52.

[19] McKey 1973: 93.

self-esteem[20] and feelings of being socially stigmatized,[21] social isolation,[22] rejection,[23] anxiety,[24] depression,[25] anger,[26] resentment,[27] jealousy,[28] guilt,[29] shame,[30] fear for their own health,[31] and negative body image.[32]

At the other end of the spectrum are those who find that chronic, life-threatening illnesses do not necessarily have negative effects on well siblings and may actually have positive ones. For example, in a study of the well siblings of children with cancer, Kramer (1984: 49) found that "the effects of the leukemic illness on the well siblings were not all negative. The same experiences that engendered the negative feelings of isolation, frustration, anxiety and resentment also brought about positive and adaptive responses in the healthy siblings and their families." In a similar vein, Harder and Bowditch (1982: 118) in their study of the well siblings of children with CF noted that the "occurrence of cystic fibrosis apparently has helped some siblings to be less self centered; . . . having the disease in the family improved their ability to empathize and communicate with the ill and to cope with difficult circumstances." Some investigators have even gone so far as to characterize the presence of a seriously ill child in the family as an opportunity for the well sibling. Gayton, Friedman, Tavormina, and Tucker (1977: 893) called attention to researchers like Pless and Pinkerton, who suggested that "handicapping illnesses do not invariably result in maladjustment and that on the contrary in some instances may provide opportunities for the growth of personality." Iles (1979) found the well siblings of children with cancer became "more compassionate, tolerant, empathetic, and appreciative of their own health" (Kupst 1986: 176). In her survey of the literature on the well siblings of children with cancer, Walker (1990: 358) cited studies with evidence for such positive effects as: "increased ability for empathy and sensitivity, enhanced personal maturation and self concept, an increase in family cohesion, and a perceived ability to cope with negative changes."

There is also a midrange of studies which reject both positive and negative labeling (Gayton, Friedman, Tavormina, and Tucker 1977: 888; Drotar and

[20] Carr-Gregg and White 1987: 64.
[21] McKey 1973: 93.
[22] Cairns, Clark, Smith, and Lansky 1979: 486; Chesler, Allswede, Barbarin 1991: 21.
[23] Burton 1975: 11; Lindsay and MacCarthy 1974: 192.
[24] Lindsay and MacCarthy 1974: 193; Cairns, Clark, Smith, and Lansky 1979: 486.
[25] Myerowitz and Kaplan 1973: 52; Farkas and Schnell 1973: 208; Rosenstein 1970: 29.
[26] Burton 1974: 190; Lindsay and MacCarthy 1974: 192; Kramer 1981: 160.
[27] Burton 1974: 190; Burton 1975: 193; Rosenstein 1970: 29.
[28] Burton 1974: 197; Burton 1975: 17; Kramer 1981: 160.
[29] Dooley 1973: 72; Burton 1975: 195; Lindsay and MacCarthy 1974: 192; Kramer 1981: 160; Sourkes 1980: 58–59.
[30] Sourkes 1980: 58–59.
[31] Cairns, Clark, Smith, and Lansky 1979: 486.
[32] Ibid.

Crawford 1985: 355; Tritt and Esses 1988: 218). Some would like to have investigators "define competencies rather than deficits" (Carpenter and Sahler 1991: 194). Some of these researchers and clinicians find the well siblings to be "within the normal range of social competence" (O'Brien 1987: 5075-B), "not any less well adjusted than controls" (Binks 1982: 43), and not deviant or disturbed in the way that many of the studies would suggest (Switzer 1984: 1926-B; Gayton, Friedman, Tavormina, and Tucker 1977: 888). Kupst (1986: 84) and others find that "while the experience of serious illness in a brother or sister may present several upsetting and uncomfortable situations for a child, most of them appear to be able to cope with it, especially over time." Others, like Carpenter and Sahler (1990: 202), take the position that "these children do not appear to be at risk for major psychological disturbance. On the other hand, by clinical experience, minor dysfunction as an indicator of distress occurs frequently."

Several of these researchers urge their colleagues to examine particular domains of psychological function and social adjustment before concluding that chronic illness has a negative impact on well siblings. For example, Drotar, Crawford, and Bush (1984: 109) argue that "the general mental health of siblings is not necessarily impaired, but their social adaptation may be vulnerable." Breslau and her colleagues put a finer point on this. They found that "siblings of disabled children [study included children with cystic fibrosis, cerebral palsy, myelodysplasia, and multiple handicaps] did not manifest higher rates of severe psychologic impairment or greater overall symptomatology when compared to control subjects. [However] on two scales measuring interpersonal aggression with peers and within the school, siblings of disabled children scored significantly higher indicating greater pathology in these behavioral domains" (Breslau, Weitzman, and Messenger 1981: 350). Similarly, Cadman, Boyle, and Offord (1988: 119) found "little increased risk for psychiatric disorders or social maladjustment. The two exceptions appear to be increased risk for emotional internalizing disorder, including depression, anxiety or obsessive-compulsive thoughts and actions as well as difficulty getting along with peers."

Evaluating the results of studies of well siblings is no easy task. Most often one is not comparing equivalent pieces of work. There is a tremendous range of variation in: theoretical perspectives or orientations (e.g., family systems, coping, crisis, and stress),[33] study populations (e.g., disease[s], severity), period in the illness (e.g., time of diagnosis, physical deterioration, quiescence or terminal phase), type of study (e.g., research, clinical, quantitative, quali-

---

[33] These categories are used by Brett (1988) in her review of the literature as a way of dividing the literature on "the well siblings' response to chronic childhood disorders." Whether one accepts these particular categories or not, the point that theoretical perspective plays a significant role in one's studies is well taken.

tative), sample size and criteria (e.g., age, sex, socioeconomic background), informants (e.g., well siblings, parents, teachers), assessment approaches and instruments (e.g., observational accounts, psychological scales, behavioral checklists), terminology, and reported findings. And this is just to name but a few of the differences. It is not surprising that the studies often appear to contradict one another.

Even within the same disease population researchers' findings vary. Consider these three examples from studies of the well siblings of children with CF. Allan, Townley, and Phelan (1974) found numerous problems in the well siblings. Gayton, Friedman, Tavormina, and Tucker (1977) did not. Allan and his colleagues worked in what Brett would define as a crisis-and-stress paradigm, whereas Gayton and his colleagues worked in what Brett would call a coping paradigm. Is the difference in their findings a function of the paradigm and the methods of research, analysis, and interpretation that follow from them? As Brett (1988: 44) comments, "The investigators' choice of perspective (whether overt or covert) has major implications for the resultant research questions, data collection and analysis methods and most importantly for the interpretation of findings."

Looking at a specific finding like generalized hostility and rebelliousness, Burton (1975: 198) found it and Rosenstein (1970: 29) did not. Burton's findings derive from a study of the parents, Rosenstein's from a study conducted as part of clinical practice. Is this difference because of the differences in their approach, methods, or sample?

Lindsay and MacCarthy (1974: 193) reported regression in well siblings of children with CF, but did not mention bedwetting and soiling, as did Burton (1975: 200) and Allan, Townley, and Phelan (1974: 139). Does the omission of bedwetting and soiling from the list of problems mean that bedwetting and soiling were not problems for the well siblings that Lindsay and MacCarthy studied? Or is it that since bedwetting and soiling are hallmarks of regression, and regression is reported, there is no need to mention these problems specifically? Is the problem one of terminology or of substance?

After presenting their research design and findings, the authors invariably give an account of what they see as the possible or probable explanations for their findings. These vary as much as the designs and the findings themselves. The problems (or lack thereof) of well siblings of chronically ill children have been variously attributed to: the patterns of communication between parents and well siblings;[34] the degree of parental involvement with the ill child;[35] the patterns of communication between parents and well sib-

---

[34] Burhmann 1970: 587; Tropauer, Franz, and Dilgard 1970: 430; Denning and Gluckson 1984: 470; Kramer 1981: 159; Chesler, Allswede, and Barbarin 1991: 21.

[35] Myerowitz and Kaplan 1973: 50; Lindsay and MacCarthy 1974: 191; Dooley 1973: 72; Chesler, Allswede, and Barbarin 1991: 21; Binks 1982: 62.

lings as well as the degree of parental involvement with the ill child;[36] family functioning (including family patterns of communication, cohesion, and adaptability; problem-solving ability or skills and how the family manages relationships among physically and healthy children);[37] family environmental influences;[38] and "the degree to which the family has accepted, understood, and incorporated the illness into their daily lives."[39] Consideration has also been given to the impact on the well siblings of the changes that occur in: emotional alignments within the family;[40] family patterns or rhythms[41] and image;[42] members' roles, responsibilities, and expectations of one another;[43] and parents' (especially mothers') mental and physical health.[44]

Seeking to explain the responses (positive, negative, and neutral) that they find in well siblings, researchers also have looked variously at: age;[45] birth order;[46] gender;[47] socioeconomic status of the family;[48] parents' marital situation;[49] problems in the family prior to the onset of the illness;[50] number of ill or deceased children in the family;[51] nature or character of the illness (e.g., genetic or nongenetic, visible or invisible handicaps, changing or stable course, imminently fatal or of long-term duration);[52] severity of the illness;[53] when in the illness the problems occurred[54] as well as the nature of the ill child himself;[55] well sibling's relationship to the ill child;[56] well siblings'

---

[36] Burton 1975: 190, 201.

[37] Drotar and Crawford 1985: 358; Delisi 1986: 67–68.

[38] Gallo, Breitmayer, Knafl, and Zoeller 1992: 26.

[39] Denning and Gluckson 1984: 470.

[40] Kramer 1981: 159.

[41] Crocker 1983: 140; Kramer 1981: 159; Chesler, Allswede, and Barbarin 1991: 21.

[42] Crocker 1983: 140.

[43] Ibid., 141.

[44] Breslau, Weitzman, and Messenger 1981: 352; Leonard 1983: 3360-B; Cohen 1985 in Walker 1990: 351; Treiber, Mabe, and Wilson 1987: 87; Delisi 1986: 20, 67–68; Gallo, Breitmayer, Knafl, and Zoeller 1992: 18.

[45] Lindsay and MacCarthy 1974: 191.

[46] Myerowitz and Kaplan 1973: 36; Lavigne and Ryan 1979: 624; Drotar and Crawford 1985: 356.

[47] Breslau et al. 1981: 350.

[48] Burton 1975: 10; Cairns, Clark, Smith, and Lansky 1979: 484; Cohen 1985 in Walker 1990: 357.

[49] Cairns, Clark, Smith, and Lansky 1979: 484; Leonard 1983: 3360-B; Ferrari 1984: 473.

[50] Burton: 1975: 10.

[51] Burton 1975: 191; Myerowitz and Kaplan 1967: 260; Buhrmann 1970: 587.

[52] Lavigne and Ryan 1979: 617; Drotar and Crawford 1985: 360; Breslau, Weitzman, and Messenger 1981: 351; Lobato et al. 1988: 407, 402; Magrab 1978: 3; Sourkes 1980: 56.

[53] Binks 1982: 55; Magrab 1978: 3.

[54] Sourkes 1981: 54; Lobato et al. 1988: 400; Carr-Gregg and White 1987: 64; Spinetta 1981: 135; Cohen 1985 in Walker 1990: 357; Kupst 1986: 173.

[55] Burton 1975: 191; Myerowitz and Kaplan 1967: 257; Breslau et al. 1981: 352.

[56] Drotar and Crawford 1985: 358; Delisi 1986: 20.

knowledge of the illness;[57] perception of the impact of the illness on the family, particularly parents;[58] well siblings' understanding of their parents' emotional responses;[59] and competition for parental attention.[60]

One looks at these lists and wonders how to proceed with research. There is clearly a need to consider a multiplicity of factors as well as questions about how they interact with one another (Lobato, Faust, and Spirito 1988: 399; Drotar and Crawford 1985: 358; Brett 1988: 47–48, 53; Carpenter and Sahler 1991: 194). But how does one select which factors to consider? There are, for example, those who argue that, on the basis of their findings, the severity of the disease is not an issue and hence need not be considered in constructing the sample; and other researchers who find the severity of the illness an important factor deserving consideration in sample selection and analysis (Binks 1982: 55; Magrab 1973: 3).

We leave this review of the literature confused. Still before us is the issue of whether or not well siblings experience social or psychological adjustment problems. The precise causes, nature, incidence, duration and severity of the problems, or lack thereof, remain unknown.

In our understanding of the well siblings we are still, many studies later, in the words of Anselm Strauss (1984: 110), "in the realm of terra incognita." We have neither a clear answer to the question of how chronic illness affects well siblings, nor an idea how to obtain one (Chesler, Allswede, and Barbarin 1991: 33–34). As one investigator described his study of the well siblings of children with CF, "These results are consistent with the inconsistency of previous findings" (Delisi 1986: 67).

I argue that the absence of satisfactory answers lies in the way researchers approached their investigations. Implicit in their approaches is the notion of the disease or illness as an entity that has x, y, or z effects. Looking at any chronic illness or handicap in this way is inappropriate. Response to chronic illness is a complex process. "This process . . . defies simple causal reduction to some . . . fixed set of determining events. Although it is possible to detect, *post hoc*, certain regularities in the process, this is not to say that its end-states are wholly contained in its beginnings" (Davis 1963: 10). The task of the researcher is to discover the patterns of response to a chronic, life-threatening illness.

I see ethnographic research as essential for the task at hand. Ethnography, with its emphasis on immersion in the world of those we study and analysis of what we observe in the context of the world view, values, and social groups in which these people participate can provide us with insights that are otherwise unavailable. Arthur Kleinman, in his seminal work on

---

[57] Crocker 1983: 141; Kramer 1981: 159.
[58] Carpenter and Sahler 1991: 196.
[59] Crocker 1983: 141.
[60] Crocker 1983: 140; Chesler, Allswede, and Barbarin 1991: 20.

chronically ill adults, *The Illness Narratives: Suffering, Healing and the Human Condition*, argues for the use of ethnography in the study, as well as in the care and treatment, of the chronically ill and their families. He objects to the quantitative research that dominates the literature. He finds that it not only fails to capture the experience of chronic illness, it also distorts it, and in so doing offers the clinician no assistance in caring for the ill and their families.

> Symptom scales and survey questionnaires and behavior checklists quantify functional impairment and disability, rendering quality of life fungible. Yet about suffering they are silent. The thinned-out image of patients and families that perforce must emerge from such research is scientifically replicable [although in the case of well sibling research we do not even find that to be the case] but ontologically invalid; it has statistical, not epistemological significance; it is a dangerous distortion (Kleinman 1988: 28).

Chronic illness is woven into the fabric that is the life of the ill and their families. As such, any approach to studying chronic illness or its impact must include an understanding of peoples' everyday lives, their lived experience with the illness, as well as how they view the illness and the meanings that it has for them, over the course of the illness. The work that follows, ethnographic and nonquantitative, embodies such an approach.

2. AN ETHNOGRAPHIC APPROACH

With funding from the National Science Foundation and a study leave from Rutgers University, I was able to do nineteen months of uninterrupted fieldwork from February 13, 1985, through to September 18, 1986. The families who participated in this study came from the patient rolls of the Cystic Fibrosis Center of St. Christopher's Hospital for Children in Philadelphia, one of the largest and most respected centers in North America. During the first five months I spent the major part of my time meeting and talking informally with 175 of the 320 families followed at the center. I was introduced to the families by the physicians either in the context of an outpatient visit or on rounds in the hospital. I saw and spoke with members of single-parent families, families with one ill child and one or more well siblings, and families with more than one affected child and one or more well siblings. The conditions or status of the ill children ranged from newly diagnosed to dying. At this point in the study I interviewed physicians about CF and the families, reviewed charts and attended "outpatient" and "inpatient" rounds and conferences. Observations, notes from review of charts and from interactions with family members and staff, as well as personal reflections and ideas of a more analytical nature, were handwritten in 5-by-8-inch spiral-bound notebooks I always carried with me.

In the remaining fourteen months in the field I focused on 40 of the original 175 families. These families were representative of the original 175, in terms of structure and ill children's physical condition. I observed and spoke with the well children, their ill siblings, and parents whenever they came to clinic or to the hospital as well as in their homes at various times throughout the project.

The data I collected were in two different forms. There are field notes which I took while in clinic, on hospital floors and in rooms, and during home visits. In addition there are verbatim transcripts of audio-taped conversations and interviews. Some of these conversations I participated in; others are simply free-flowing ones recorded in the clinic, hospital, or family members' homes. For the interviews with family members I wrote a series of open-ended questions and a specifically related list of probes to remind me of what I needed to cover in order to insure that the same issues were covered in all of the interviews.

While in the field I realized that before I could address any issues of concern to me I would need to develop a means of systematically identifying, locating, and retrieving relevant information from the thousands of pages of typescript I had collected in the course of fieldwork. By the time I left the field my field journals (typed versions of material in spiral notebooks) filled twelve three-inch binders, and an additional fourteen binders held the verbatim transcripts of all of the audio-recorded interactions and interviews. I also had two binders of notes taken from hospital charts indicating when, where, and for what reasons children had been hospitalized.

I desired a system that would be flexible enough so that as I proceeded in my work I could explore issues I had not thought of when I started, as well as changes in my conceptualizations of particular issues without doing endless recoding or retyping of the field journals or transcripts. Also, struck by how much variation there could be in an individual's views on a given issue, not to mention the variety of views in any household, I wanted to be able to capture all of the different views that an individual gave on the same issue at the same or different points in the illness trajectory. Then, upon retrieving bits of text for analysis, I wanted to be able to identify the specific speaker or observer, as well as when in the course of the illness the particular statement, action, or interaction occurred or was observed.

Transcripts of all of my field notes and all conversations and interviews were coded. Passages were marked off on the basis of content. They were then coded for the speaker, the topic, who or what was being spoken about, the period in the illness when the interaction took place, and the period in the illness to which the content of a passage refers. I had a database management program designed so that I could search using any or all of the relevant factors as keywords singly or in combination. The field journals and transcripts were thus completely and compatibly referenced. Computerized database searches delivered every instance of a note or remark about, for example, a particular topic or made by a particular person at a given period in the illness.[61]

3. A FRAMEWORK FOR ANALYSIS

The Intrusion and the Strategies

In 1985 when I began my fieldwork, I expected to find children who were different from children who had no ill siblings. From reading the literature I did not know what the differences would be—better adjusted, less well adjusted; more mature, less mature—but I did expect differences of that order of magnitude. My initial round of interviews and conversations with parents, clinicians, the ill children, and the well siblings themselves did not reveal such dramatic differences, nor did observations of them in their homes, the clinic, or hospital.

I was puzzled. How could these children appear appreciably no different from other children? A chronic, life-threatening illness like CF is a frontal assault on the family. Chronic illness sets the family and its members apart from others. Plans, roles, duties, obligations, and priorities change as family life is interrupted by the burdens of care and treatment. The disease becomes a constant companion. Each new illness experience serves as a reminder of the disease's unrelenting course and eventual outcome. At risk is the integrity and continuity of the family.[62]

I came to realize that the answer was in the fabric of family life. By looking at the well sibling as a member of a family unit dealing with a chronically ill child with a limited life expectancy, I would be better able to understand the impact of chronic, life-threatening illness on well siblings.[63]

I found that the considerable force brought to bear on these families is met

[61] For a more detailed discussion of the methods of research design data collection and analysis see Bluebond-Langner 1995.

[62] Recently other researchers have come to the same conclusion (Carpenter and Sahler 1991: 202). While they recognize the need to look at the well child in the context of the family and call for "family-centered framework," the ways in which they apply this principle in their work vary tremendously. For example, from this perspective Carpenter and Sahler (1991: 193–94) studied "the relation between siblings' [of children with cancer] perception of family crisis [as measured by results of a mailed questionnaire designed by the investigators] and its impact on the family subsystem and parental perception [as measured by results of questionnaire designed by the investigators] of the [well] siblings' post diagnosis psychosocial adaptation." Gallo, Breitmayer, Knafl, and Zoeller (1992: 27) looked at variations in well-sibling adaptation in relation to the mothers' perception of the illness experience and family life. As the reader will find, what I do from a "family-centered perspective" differs from what these and other investigators (e.g., Delisi 1986) have done from the same perspective.

[63] Lavigne and Ryan (1979: 616) note that in an early study of families of "handicapped children" Jordan (1962) describes illness as "an entity attacking the fundamental social unit, the family."

with an equal and opposite reaction. From the time of diagnosis through to the terminal phases, family members attempt to contain the illness's intrusion into their lives. They endeavor to preserve what they can of their normal way of life for as long as possible. The strategies that family members adopt allow family life to proceed for long periods with some modicum of normalcy, some sense of control.[64] Further, the strategies that parents adopt to contain the intrusion have important consequences for well siblings. The strategies discussed in Chapter 11 are: (1) routinization of CF treatment-related tasks; (2) compartmentalization of information about CF and the child's condition; (3) avoidance of reminders of CF and its consequences; (4) redefinition of normal; (5) reassessment of priorities; and (6) reconceptualization of the future. They set the stage for the views and responses we observe in well siblings, described in Chapters 12 and 13.

This is not to say that parents' actions determine the well siblings' views and responses. To the contrary, well siblings' views and responses are part of a process that involves not only the parents' responses, but also the ill child's condition and experiences. Well siblings interpret their parents' responses as well as the ill child's condition and experiences and forge a line of action based on those interpretations (cf. Bluebond-Langner 1978: 3–12).

Natural History of the Illness

Although many researchers have suggested that parental and well siblings' behavior may be related to the stage of the child's illness, few have taken this factor into account (Spinetta 1981: 135; McCollum and Gibson 1970: 265; Kupst 1986: 173; Lask 1992: 18). I found that changes in parents' and siblings' responses were intimately linked to pivotal experiences or events in the illness trajectory. Family members viewed these experiences or events as what others and I refer to as turning points in the "natural history of the illness" (Charmaz 1991: 210; Davis 1963: 9; Kleinman 1980: 107).

The natural history of the illness, as I use the concept, is a series of events from diagnosis to death, which mark critical changes in the social and emotional life of the family as well as in the clinical status of the child. The natural history of the illness closely parallels, but is not identical to, the clinical course.[65]

Chronically ill persons and family members often use events in their ill-

---

[64] This is not to say these families did not have problems (a point addressed in the Afterword), but to see these families as rife with problems as a result of having a child with CF would be in error (Fosson, D'Angelo, Wilson, and Kanga 1991: 309; Binks 1982: 43). Similarly, it would be a mistake to see these families as necessarily more cohesive because they have a child with CF. The illness is one factor among many in how families function (Delisi 1986: 12).

[65] It is important to note that in the case of the families that I studied clinicians agreed with family members on the significant turning points in the illness.

ness experience to locate events in their everyday life experience. For example, a description of a well sibling's performance in a school play would be prefaced with a remark about when the play came in relation to the ill child's first hospitalization, not the season or month of the year. The periods in the natural history of the illness became the blocks of time bounded by the events that parents, well siblings, and children with CF used to frame their retelling of everyday life events as well as CF-related experiences.

The natural history of the illness can be broken down into six periods, each defined by significant events and experiences. The six periods in the natural history were: (I) time of diagnosis through to the first annual examination; (II) months and years following the first annual examination, when the child is relatively healthy, through to the first major exacerbation requiring hospitalization; (III) recovery from that exacerbation, when the CF is relatively stable, through to the time when hospitalizations begin to increase and lose their predictability; (IV) development and increase in complications (e.g., Pseudomonas cepacia [now known as Burkholderia cepacia], diabetes, shortness of breath, intermittent use of oxygen during hospitalizations) through to the discussion with the physician that the disease has advanced; (V) increased deterioration (e.g. regular use of oxygen, activity restricted by the disease, permanent central lines) through to the conference where the physician tells the parents that the child's condition is terminal; (VI) terminal phase through to death.[66]

———————

Having concluded that the well siblings' views and responses must be understood in the context of family life over the course of the illness, I was faced with how to present this context to the reader. How could I convey a sense of the siblings' thoughts and concerns as they themselves and others see and express them, in the context in which they emerge?

I decided to write a series of accounts of family life at different points in the natural history of the illness. In Part II, family members speak in their own voices, revealing how they integrate the tasks of care with the thoughts and the feelings that accompany the rhythm that is everyday life with a child who has CF. We learn how family members perceive one another and the role of these perceptions in their relationships. Only after the presentation of these detailed accounts, where the reader can learn of the various forces that are shaping individual reactions, does the analysis begin.

[66] A brief overview of the cause, course, and treatment of CF is included in the Preface. At the end of the book is a glossary of terms used by family members and clinicians when they talk about the illness.

Part Two

PORTRAITS IN WAITING:
NINE FAMILIES

Introduction

In Part II I present the ethnography through a series of portraits of families. Each of the chapters introduces the reader to life with cystic fibrosis (CF) at a different point in the natural history of the illness. For example, Chapter 2, "The Daleys," provides insight into what life is like for families of newly diagnosed children, while Chapter 8 ("The Fosters") shows what it is like when complications of the disease increase and the child's condition begins to deteriorate (see Table 1). Each portrait consists of material from a single family. Neither the individuals nor the families are composites. The names of all individuals who were in any way connected to the study, including staff, have been changed.

Like the population of families of children with CF, the families depicted in Part II vary in terms of the number of affected children in the family, ages of parents and children, household structure and composition, religious beliefs and practices, and socioeconomic status. Each portrait generally consists of three parts. The first and last parts are scenes taken from my field journals which occurred in the hospital waiting room. In the middle are conversations and comments by family members including those not present in the waiting-room scenes. Statements on a given topic are grouped together. When the comments of a speaker were not made in the presence of the person who preceded him or her, I show this by changing the mood or tense of the verb used when the speaker begins. This allows the reader to see the variety of family members' views on a topic as well as what each will or will not reveal in the presence of another—a point that must be kept sight of in working with seriously ill children and their families.

The statements ascribed to speakers are taken from field journals and transcripts (see Chapter 1). Except for deleted words or phrases (e.g., "uh," "you know," "I mean") that interrupt the flow, their statements are unaltered. At times I fill in nonverbal or background information that may be needed to follow a family member's account. I also alert the reader to changes in time, place, and speaker.

All of the waiting-room scenes in the nine portraits are written as if they take place on the same day. In fact, they did not. I have written the section in this way so that the processual character of the experience, moving from diagnosis to death, may emerge.

TABLE 1.
Locating Family Accounts in the Natural History of the Illness

Periods in the Natural History of the Illness

Families	I		II		III		IV		V		VI	
	Diagnosis	*First Annual Examination*	*Years Post Annual*	*First Exacerbation*	*Recovery From First Exacerbation*	*Increased Hospitalizations*	*Development, Increase in Complications*	*Conference With Dr./Team*	*Increased Deterioration*	*Conference With Dr./Team*	*Terminal Phase*	*Death*
Chapter 2 Daleys	│											
Chapter 3 Shermans			│									
Chapter 4 Farringtons					│							
Chapter 5 Campbells						│						
Chapter 6 Reynoldses						│						
Chapter 7 Chases						│						
Chapter 8 Woodwards							│					
Chapter 9 Fosters									│			
Chapter 10 Baileys									│			

Note: │ indicates where family members are in the Natural History of the Illness at the opening of the chapter. While the chapter focuses on family members' thoughts and experiences at that point in the natural history, the chapter is not limited to their thoughts and experiences at that point. For example, in the case of Baileys, the account moves beyond, to just after the child's death.

CHAPTER 2

The Daleys

(Individuals mentioned by name, in order of appearance)

ALICE DALEY: Infant with cystic fibrosis
MRS. AUDREY DALEY: Mother of Alice Daley
MR. COLLIN DALEY: Father of Alice Daley
DARRELL DALEY: Three-year-old well brother of Alice Daley
MRS. RHONDA SNYDER: Mother of child with cystic fibrosis
MRS. MADGE DALTON: Mother of children with cystic fibrosis
ERIKA DALEY: Two-year-old well sister of Alice Daley
THEA WRIGHT: Outpatient clinical nurse specialist

"When will it be our turn?" the three-year-old inquired, just short of whining.

"Soon! Soon!" his mother replied, tightly and a bit distractedly. "Sooner, later," she mumbled, "what difference does it make?"

Five months ago Alice, the baby, was diagnosed with cystic fibrosis (CF). The doctor had said, "Alice has cystic fibrosis." And for Mrs. Daley, "Nothing has been the same since."

"You see," Mrs. Daley began to explain, "we never had any hard times except for when Alice was diagnosed. Everything was so happy and we never experienced death in our families."

"It was just the biggest disappointment," Mr. Daley put in, "It was just disappointing. At first I just sorta saw everything go up in smoke."

Mr. Daley paused and Mrs. Daley began again, "Darrell was in the hospital, two months old, with meningitis and that was like our worst thing."

Mr. Daley laughed sarcastically.

"That was our worst," Mrs. Daley repeated.

"And that was so easy."

"'Oh my God,' I said, 'Meningitis? Oh my God, he's never going to walk or play sports.' I had him crippled, like a vegetable. He was in the hospital five days."

"And came out," said Mr. Daley, finishing his wife's sentence.

"And I can just picture it now."

"Yeah," agreed Mr. Daley.

"When they came in—meningitis—I didn't know what the hell meningitis was. And we were crying and crying, crying." Mrs. Daley paused. "Then when Alice was diagnosed, I said, 'Oh, it won't be like Darrell, where we come home happy.'"

There was a brief silence, before Mrs. Daley continued. "You know, I'll never forget when she was first diagnosed. I kept thinking I didn't want to get close to her. I wanted her to die then. It's a horrible feeling. And I sat up that whole night in the hospital, talking to Rhonda down the hall. Her son was diagnosed a week before. We sat up the whole night talking about it. And by the end of the night, at like four in the morning, we were really going crazy, saying we'll fix them up together 'cause he'll be sterile and Alice won't care 'cause she. . ." Mrs. Daley didn't finish that thought. She simply reiterated, "We got really crazy at the end. But, we shared our feelings. I kept saying, 'I really don't want to get close to her.' I was just afraid of her.

"But now that's changed. I want to give her everything I can. I want to take her to Disney World. Now is that a normal life?" Mrs. Daley laughed. "I just want to take her everywhere, let her see the world. Just let her live a life in a shorter time, if that's what's gonna happen. Live a good life. That's our main goal."

Mr. Daley weighed his thoughts. "I guess sometimes the way I feel sometimes about it is that unfortunately, she was born with cystic fibrosis, and it's not that there's nothing you can do because, I mean, you have to do treatments, and medicines and so forth. I think that we'll try to give her the best care in the world. But there are a lot of other diseases out there, like cerebral palsy, and I think that you have to put CF in perspective. Let's face it. It's a fatal disease, but there's other things that could be worse. I mean there's things that could be worse."

"Definitely," Mrs. Daley affirmed.

"You know there are children born retarded. And I guess maybe that's my inner security blanket."

"They just lay there. They're like vegetables. I thank God I have what I have. That she can walk and talk and be normal like everybody else, that it's inside and not showing. I would take that any day. I just thank God she has everything else."

"There's a lot of bad. You see it at the hospital. It's sad. But, boy, sometimes you just thank God that you have two healthy children and . . ."

As Mr. Daley paused, Mrs. Daley began, "I always think to the future myself, and how she'll be. Everybody that you meet when you go to the doctors'; I sit there and look at them and think, 'Doesn't look like it bothers them much.'"

Mr. Daley added, "I'm sure there's bad, good times and bad times. But when they're healthy, there's a world of difference. 'Cause you really don't think about it; other than doing the treatments. You don't tend to dwell on it too much." Mr. Daley paused. "I used to think about it a lot. I used to think about it going to work, coming home. Normally when you're by yourself. I used to think about it a lot. But, anymore I don't. I don't think about it. I don't tend to dwell on it as much as I used to.

"Yeah, I don't sit there and get upset," added Mrs. Daley reflecting on her own thought patterns.

"I don't get upset over it anymore. That's for sure," Mr. Daley emphasized.

"I think we got upset when we were first told," Mrs. Daley explained.

"I keep it to myself more. I used to think about it a lot. I thought about it a lot. A lot of different things go through your mind. But I don't get upset anymore. No. Not really."

"I guess when you're told, it's a big shock and you get emotional, and you cry and you think, 'Why me?' But then when you have her home and she's normal really, besides the treatments; you look to somebody else's troubles and think, 'I have it pretty good.' That's the way I look at it.

"And I think my outing is talking to other people that have it, other parents. I seem to do that all the time. If I'm down, I call up Mrs. Dalton, or I call Rhonda. And we don't sit there and talk about it. We'll laugh. But, we have something in common—where nobody else does."

Mrs. Daley paused and as if clarifying an earlier statement continued, "When I do think of CF I just think of when that day is when Alice's going to get sick. And I think of the kids. When I think of Darrell and Erika having to face death, I get upset." Mrs. Daley's voice trailed off and her husband continued.

"That's pretty much how I feel. And I know it's not going to be easy but I pray to God that it's going to be as easy as possible. Hopefully, she lives a relatively normal long life. But then of course, you have to think of the other thing; where if she's going to be very sick, well you know, she may not, you know." Mr. Daley had difficulty. He stumbled. "She may not live all that long. You know, you never know." He paused and recovered his professional actuarial voice. "The statistics are varied. There's a big variation. You just can't think cut and dry."

Mrs. Daley seconded her husband's remarks. "Yeah. I never hear of any younger kids. You never see how many people die of it, young. I mean they tell you twenty-four. Well then, I think when she's twenty-four she's going to die on me."

"It's deceiving."

"It's like she's going to twenty-four years, and I think, 'Oh, that's great, twenty-four years.' But, really, she can go any time. I shouldn't say that like that, but she could get really sick."

As in a game of hot potato, the prognosis was passed back and forth. In Mr. Daley's hands, "It's deceiving what they say. I guess they told us what the average age is. I think they said the word 'average' was twenty-three. Now, average to me means, there's a big difference in average, and what's the other one?"

"Median."

"Median, yeah, median. Also you hear different things too. I've heard that girls can have it worse than males. I don't know whether that's true or not."

"Where did you read that?" Mrs. Daley asked.

"I might have read that in that book, in *Alex* come to think of it.[1]

"That's why I had to put that book down."

As Mr. Daley tried to recall where in fact he had read this bit of information, Alice started to whimper. Mrs. Daley reached for the bottle, but unlike with her two other children, Mrs. Daley just couldn't put the bottle in Alice's mouth. There were the enzymes that had to be given each time Alice ate.

Darrell and Erika often re-created the feeding scene with their dolls. They would break the capsule and try to catch the beads that got away. Like their parents they would be frustrated when the doll refused the enzyme-laced applesauce or when the formula dribbled down the baby doll's chin. Sometimes Darrell would find an enzyme capsule or some beads around the house, in the car or on the street and bring them in to his mother. Mrs. Daley noted, "That's when I knew he knew what they were. Darrell also knows that Alice needs treatments.

"And he wants to come to clinic, too. I think to make sure that they don't put Alice in the hospital. But I bring them down so that they can be a part of what it's like for Alice, to see where her doctors are and to get used to where Alice goes all the time. I think that will be good if they understand."

Mr. Daley agreed. "All in all for being young, I think they've handled it pretty well. There's no outward jealousy, that's for sure. I haven't seen it. No. I haven't recognized it at all. Really."

"Like with therapy," noted Mrs. Daley, "Darrell is usually watching television, his cartoons; and Erika will usually go and get her doll or something. She'll wander off. She knows that's the time for me to be with Alice. In the morning when I do it they're not up yet. Well no, Erika is usually up, come to think of it."

"Occasionally Erika will come over and she'll want to play with you, but then you just say, 'I have to do this.' And she'll leave. There's no outward sign of dissatisfaction or anything. They kinda take it in stride pretty much."

"I think that if it's just the normal thing like growing up they will take it in stride. But taking enzymes all the time and getting sick, getting this treatment done and their sister getting clapped, getting PT [chest physical therapy]. I think that should be hard to see."

"I think both of them are going to have to make an adjustment. I mean they're going to be in a different situation from most kids, knowing they have a sister with a chronic illness."

[1] *Alex: Life of a Child*, is Frank Deford's account of his daughter's struggle with cystic fibrosis and death at the age of eight. It was later made into a telemovie and aired in the course of this study. Both the book and the telemovie were the subjects of discussion among parents.

"Yeah," agreed Mrs. Daley. "Sticking up for their sister if anybody ever teases her or something."

"Well I guess that's the way. I mean, once they begin to understand she has a serious illness. I guess there's got to be a social adjustment there."

"And I guess Erika in a way is beginning to work it through. She does it with her dolls. She goes over and gets her baby dolls and gives them the treatments [chest physical therapy]. And then the other day I found enzymes all over her Cabbage Patch doll. I left them in a little cup with the applesauce 'cause Alice didn't eat right away. They were all over. So obviously Erika is seeing everything."

Mr. Daley agreed and then went on. "I think Erika might be able to handle it easier than Darrell."

"Easier than Darrell, definitely," said Mrs. Daley, nodding. "Maybe boys hold it back. But I'll be anxious to see what it's like." Mrs. Daley paused for a moment. There was more to say about Darrell. "Darrell's very emotional. Like the first time when we left Alice in the hospital, he didn't understand. But the second time, when we didn't come home with her, he cried, and that just struck me. I didn't think he really understood what was going on, but I guess he did. And he really cried.

"You can tell there is emotion there. He gets very upset. I often wonder what they think of when I'm doing the treatments. Darrell has never asked us. We've tried to explain to him as we do it."

"We talk about St. Christopher's like it's part of our family. We talk about how we're taking Alice and the medicines and everything." Mrs. Daley looked to her husband as if to say, "It's your turn."

Mr. Daley responded. "I think Darrell realizes Alice's different. He said something to me once about lungs. So he knows that. . ."

"Alice has bad lungs," Mrs. Daley finished her husband's sentence.

"Bad lungs," echoed Mr. Daley. "I think he associates her colds with her lungs. But Erika, Erika doesn't really seem to know, to have an understanding."

"She's too little."

"To have an understanding."

"Give her about two years. In two years she'll probably be so close to Alice that it'll be terrible for her."

"I think it's going to be hard on both of them."

But the problems for Darrell came sooner than the Daleys had expected. Seven months after Alice was diagnosed, Darrell began stuttering. Mrs. Daley explained, "Not long after seeing *Alex*, Darrell started stuttering."[2]

"I wanted to watch and Darrell wouldn't go to sleep," Mr. Daley interjected.

---

[2] Referring to telemovie Darrell saw.

"Darrell was in the living room on the landing," Mrs. Daley continued.

"On the sofa," Mr. Daley corrected.

"Anyway," Mrs. Daley went on, "we thought he wasn't watching, but he took in quite a bit. Because on Monday when Erika scratched Alice in the face for taking a toy, and her face started bleeding, Darrell started to scream. 'She's spitting up blood like Alex.'[3]

"We told him that it wasn't the same. Alice wasn't spitting up blood. I called the pediatrician twice and he tells us Darrell will grow out of it. But I'm worried. In the car Darrell said, 'Alex had CF. I hope Alice doesn't spit up blood.'"

Mr. Daley shook his head. "I feel so bad for letting him see it. But I just didn't think he'd watch. I wanted to see it and I didn't want to go up then and lay with him."

"Bed time is a bit of a problem," Mrs. Daley interjected. " I lay down in the bed with one of them, 'til they go to sleep. I'm too tired to listen to them screaming up there. I don't have the patience by then.

"My days are long. I start maybe six, six-thirty, and we come down and we do our enzymes and give Alice a bottle. And then when I'm giving her the bottle, I go in and I have my coffee. And then usually after that, Darrell and Erika wake up. It seems I wait until they get up and then I do her treatment, about an hour after she eats. And we give her her treatment and then I run around the house and I get all the beds made and all my chores done. And then by afternoon it's time for the treatment again and the enzymes. I feel like I feed her a lot, because she really doesn't eat cereals and that, that much. I get her a little bit now. But it seems like I'm constantly feeding her enzymes and giving her a bottle and trying to get those enzymes in her mouth. Chasing beads down her chin, those little things. There's more under her neck than there are in her mouth. It's real nerve-wracking.

"Then two days a week my grandmother comes. If it wasn't for her, I think it would be a lot harder. If I had one to worry about, if I had just Alice, it might be different. I'd probably give her a lot more attention and care, you know. But being that they're so close, some days are really hectic, because Erika's screaming for attention. She's a baby herself. So, some days are really bad. But, I think of those two days, if my grandmother didn't come, I don't know how else to say it, my days would be terrible.

"Oh, I get out. Like when my grandmother comes and I bring Erika and Darrell out. If we go to the store, that's an outing for them and it's time for them too, some time with them. And then usually in the afternoon there's some time. Darrell goes to school two days a week, on Tuesdays and Thursdays in the afternoon. So that's like a little break because if Alice's in bed, then I have Erika to play with and give my time to her.

---

[3] Alex died shortly after episodes of vomiting blood.

"I feel bad because I have Erika. Erika's the in-between one and she doesn't get as much attention as she should. Sometimes I kick myself for not planning it better. They're so close in age." Mrs. Daley sighed, "And then at night when he comes in I say, 'Here they are, Collin. *Here they are.*'"

"Yeah, it's tough."

"And I feel bad because I don't really, I don't think Darrell gets any attention now. He doesn't."

Mr. Daley shook his head and repeated his last statement, "It's, just tough. I think it's tough. It gets tough with Alice being an infant. And on top of that, you have the treatments and you have the medication."

Mrs. Daley agreed. "You're always worried about the medication and . . ."

"You're always doing something," Mr. Daley added.

"It's always on your mind, because you're doing it three times a day, the medication part. The enzymes, every time she eats. And she eats pretty much." Mrs. Daley smiled. "And if you go out it's packing everything up, remembering the enzymes, remembering her bottles and like other just normal baby things."

Mr. Daley shook his head in agreement.

"You just can't grab a bottle and go out, 'cause then when you get to where you're going and say, 'Oh, I forgot the enzymes.' It's the most important thing. You have to run home and get them. So your mind's always going."

"I think it's going to be easier once Alice's able to walk and swallow and that kind of thing. Hopefully, it's gonna be a little bit easier." Mr. Daley paused for a moment and added, "On everybody." He drew a deep breath and sighed. "But, right now, it's work.

It's work," he repeated. "Three kids are just work, I guess."

––––––––––

"OK, Mrs. Daley, you can bring Alice in now." Mrs. Daley rose in response to Thea's command. Darrell and Erika followed close behind.

CHAPTER 3

The Shermans

(Individuals mentioned by name, in order of appearance)

KATRINA/TRINA SHERMAN: Eleven-year-old girl with cystic fibrosis (CF)
MRS. EUNICE SHERMAN: Mother of Katrina Sherman
THEA WRIGHT: Outpatient clinical nurse specialist
LIAM SHERMAN: Thirteen-year-old well brother of Katrina Sherman
MISS COLEY: Teacher of Liam Sherman
MR. HARLE SHERMAN: Father of Katrina Sherman
LORETTA HAMILTON: Social worker
OLIVER MATHERS: Cousin of Katrina Sherman with CF

BOOKS opened on their laps, Katrina and her mother looked around the waiting room. Katrina's smile is broad, almost as big as her eyes that look out through thick glasses. Her mother's smile is no less bright, but more controlled, polite.

"I didn't know we were scheduled for an annual," said Mrs. Sherman.

"I'm afraid you are," Thea, the outpatient clinical nurse specialist, smiled back. She handed Katrina a specimen cup.

Katrina took the cup and shrugged, an "OK, if that's the way it is," kind of shrug, and walked over to the lavatory.

"I didn't realize we were up to an annual again," Mrs. Sherman began. "As it is we have all these visits regularly scheduled and I'm never sure how good an idea that is. It just brings it up when we don't really need to be dealing with it. I suppose it's good for her to just check up on it. I could be happy with fewer visits, so that it's not so much of a thing, built into her life, so that she can forget about it."

Katrina returned and took up her place beside her mother. They had already been to X-ray. Now they would wait to be called for the pulmonary function test. With that test completed, they would wait some more before seeing the doctor.

Katrina's brother knew some of what happened at a clinic visit and at an annual, but not a great deal. As he said, "Maybe I should ask more, but I don't. We don't talk about it much. We forget about it most of the time. I don't know whether my parents are constantly thinking about it, but I'm not. It doesn't affect us a whole lot. I really don't think about it at all much. I just don't think much of it at all.

"Maybe I should think about it more, considering that my sister has it. Maybe I should think about it and read about it more, but why should I think about it considering she's not, I mean she's not any different really. I don't think she thinks . . ." Liam paused for a moment. "Well, she probably does think about it a lot, but I don't. I don't see why I should; besides I just don't think about it a whole lot."

Liam remembered. "But I did a report on it, in fifth grade, on cystic fibrosis. I think Miss. Coley, my teacher, kept it. I wrote it from the pamphlets and stuff we had in files and stuff. From time to time when we get stuff we put it in files. It's useful information.

"I don't think I have it [the report], but I do remember some things. First it's sort of an inherited disease. I did the whole diagram on this. If a mother is a carrier but doesn't have it, and the father is a carrier but doesn't have it, it's a hundred percent sure to have one child . . . Hold up a minute. With four children, if one of them is a carrier and one isn't, you're a hundred percent sure to have one a carrier. It's real complicated. I can't remember everything about it. Well, anyway, it's an inherited disease. You can't catch it or anything.

"I forget most of how they test whether you have it. They can do a sweat test and if you're more alkaline, I mean more, well, if you have more, if you're more sweaty, if you have more salt in your sweat; they can measure whether you have it or not.

"And they don't know whether I'm a carrier or not. Unless, like, I marry somebody and one of our children has it then, then I have it. But they don't know whether I have it until one of my children has it or something.

"It [CF] has to do with mucus. Her mucus is thicker and stuff. The aerosol is used to bring up the mucus or at least thin it because it clogs. And it's good for her to have a lot of breathing exercises so it doesn't get quite as thick and stuff, and it gets brought up a lot. Like thumping is to bring it up. And trampolines and swimming now are good.

"I've tried giving therapy. Well, I've messed around but I've never done it a whole session. I don't know all the different positions. They say that when you get older you can do it. But I've never done anything. I just know to cup the hands and do it wherever she tells me to, but I don't know it that well."

Liam paused and reached back into his memory for more information from his report. He thought out loud. "I'm not sure about the lungs. They get like contracted or dilated or something? I'm not sure how the passages get. I'm not sure exactly what happens. It's harder to breathe, anyway. It's tougher to breathe or something, because the mucus gets clogged and you have to deal with that.

"It's [CF is] a lot to do with digestion too, the pancreas. It's a lot to do with the pancreas. She takes Cotazymes. She has to take a lot, not a whole lot of them, actually. Our cousin in Australia, he has it. I'm not sure whether he takes more of them or less of them than would be normal. She takes about four. Like she might take eight of those pills every day and then some of the others. There's a whole bunch on the kitchen table, in a basket. There's water-soluble vitamin E and stuff there too.

"They change the pills and other stuff too sometimes. They kind of messed up,'cause first they were telling us not to have much fat at all and then they say that's nothing, that it should be the opposite—make her have more fat. So we stopped getting skim milk and started giving a lot of whole milk and ice cream and stuff. We completely changed what we used to be doing. It's weird 'cause it was completely opposite. Before they were saying no, not much at all. And now they're saying more than normal. We started out one way and now she doesn't have any restrictions."

Liam stopped again. He appeared to be going back into his memory bank for more information. He concluded, "I'm not an expert obviously on cystic fibrosis. I obviously don't know a lot about it. I think I should know more.

"For my report I read that thing that comes out sometimes, the magazine, I can't remember. It's called *Cystic Fibrosis and You*, or something. I don't read that a whole lot actually. I just read it occasionally. But I know a bit about it, but not a whole lot.

"I guess Katrina knows more. I'm not sure. I'm not sure how much she knows, but they probably told her a lot more about it than I know.

"We don't talk much about it, Katrina and me. No. Not much, actually. Most of the time I forget she has it because the things become quite routine. So, we're having therapy in the morning. It's like, I don't even think about it anymore. It's just sort of normal. I don't look at her as having it at all. I just forget about it. I don't think about it a whole lot.

"I used to notice it more when I was little, but not now. I never used to really think about it a whole lot. I just took it in, I don't know," Liam shrugged, "I don't think about it a whole lot.

"Having a sister with CF is just normal. I think I just act about normally, like anybody that has a sister who's a brat. But that's the way it is with all sisters. I made sure. I talked with my friends. They all have brat sisters. She's OK. She's fine. I don't look at her any differently. I don't think anybody does. No. Not at all. Except for that hour she has to have therapy and stuff and aerosol. It's nothing more than that and taking pills."

According to Mrs. Sherman, "Liam likes to be cool about it. He doesn't want you to tell him things about it. He doesn't want to know. Most of the time he really doesn't need to know anything bad about it, but he might after her future."

Mr. Sherman agreed. "He's quite quiet about it. I think he'd probably just as soon have it all go away. I don't mean just for jealousy, but because it is a painful thing for him. So I think, judging from the way he deals with some other things, he's working out of a, 'if you don't talk about it, it'll go away,' kind of concept. I had to work my way out of that myself. Just keep abreast of it as best you can with information. You know, a more adult pattern.

"I think pretty soon he's going to have just about the same sort of relationship to it I have; that we have. Eunice and I have sort of a suspended reaction to it. That gets you through pretty well.

"It's a very worrisome disease, because it doesn't have any clear-cut thing. All you know is your child has it. But you don't know how much, or when, and everything else is up in the air. And it seems to stay up in the air. You always know after the fact."

"It's always there in the backs of our minds. There's the uncertainty of it all. You've got to act as though there is no uncertainty, as though everything is fine and she's doing splendidly at the same time thinking somewhere in the future there's something else down there and you have to prepare for that too.

"There will be periods now where I don't think about it, whereas when she was little there weren't many periods when I didn't think about it. Now she is in sort of this good stretch, so I'm really interested in what other things she wants to do, not to feel that nothing's worth doing.

"I just wish they would hurry up and find a cure for it. I think that more now than I used to. It was very interesting at the beginning and didn't seem, I mean, it was very threatening then too. But now it's less. I mean, I worry about her specifically less, but I really want them . . ."

Mrs. Sherman did not finish her sentence. She shifted in her chair and began again. "I see her at ten or eleven, eleven now, she just had her birthday. It's more important to me now that they find some cure for it, because she's just getting into her teenage years, doing nicely, and I would want them to come up with something. I hope they can come up with something that will control it at least. I'm sort of interested in all the research and stuff. I don't know whether it's going to be soon or if they'll find something or what."

Mr. Sherman picked up on his wife's thoughts. "In addition to being a background worry like that, it's also a race, because you can see the National Institutes of Health working on it, and the hospitals. And you can—I don't think it's entirely just imagination—imagine that something good can come of this, fairly soon. And so you say, well, it's just a question of how soon can they get there; before lung involvement takes place with my child. And so it's that as well. And it makes you really aware of that whole side of things, the research end of it.

"And then, also, it makes you aware of the fact that a lot of work is being done, but an awful lot is not understood. And doctors can mention a whole lot of different ways of that. So I'm just saying we don't know this, we don't know that. Some of them say it in a much more elegant way, but it's the same message. And at times you feel you know almost as much as the doctors know about it."

Mr. Sherman hesitated and then burst forth excitedly. "But by God, there should be some way of solving this thing. When you think of all the fronts they're working on: genetic, pulmonary, and just medications; amazing things, brilliant things. In fact, therapy itself is pretty brilliant considering it's free and it does have a lot of effect in many patients." Mr. Sherman settled. He became quiet, reflective again.

"There's that kind of thread of optimism. It works through, I guess, all parents. If that's the word for it. Optimism or hope, I guess is all that it really is. But that, the fact that CF for many patients like Trina lurks rather than manifesting itself, makes it a very strange thing to live with."

Mr. Sherman paused and added, "I used to think, well, of course, death is lurking as well. So it's not as though they won't lose a life, no shadows at all, but it's a medically discernible problem and it is threatening. I think it's sort of hanging over our heads and all.

"Sometimes I think just pretty simple things like, 'How long is my daughter going to live?' Oh, all sorts of gruesome items. I even dream about it as well. It gets into your dreams. I imagine her choking to death, coughing to death."

Without a breath, Mr. Sherman continued. "I don't know very much about the digestion end of this thing, but it just doesn't seem so threatening. But it is bad. And Trina suffers much more there now than she does with her lungs. Often she gets tummy aches and I think some of that might be from not getting the balance of the pancrease, Cotazyme, and the fat content and so forth.

"It's just an ongoing problem that she's had. I think the stomachaches she's had, other kids would be screaming their heads off with. She's just used to it. And she's used to that kind of misery, fairly often. Every week she's bound to have a stomachache. And I think every day, she has a little bit of one; for a while, in the morning. So there's that bit of misery."

As Mr. Sherman shifted topics his voice changed. No longer quiet and reflective, it became louder and more determined. "I have to learn more about the human body. I don't know anything about the body. And I find I know all these special things about cystic fibrosis, but I don't know what the pancreas hooks up to. So, although I talk to the doctors and I get this feeling that I'm just about abreast of their information, I'm not really at all, because they know the body in a much more intelligent way.

"So I guess one thing CF's done is it's made me interested in going back to my biology books. And I think that would be somewhat more satisfying to me anyway. At least it'll make some sense, get some sort of a rational basis for understanding what's happening. I can't bear complete mystery. I don't like this mystery. At least you want to know some sort of cause and effect. You want to get some sort of grasp of the things."

Mrs. Sherman shared her husband's drive to understand and to learn as much as possible. "My way of coping in the beginning was sort of finding out everything and writing about it, or going to conferences. That sort of thing was helpful to me. When Katrina was first born [Katrina was diagnosed at birth] I did a CF parents' newsletter. The foundation ran it off for me and sent it out to all the parents.

"We also started a parents' group around the time she was born. I think we were the first group that had parents from all the three clinics. Some of the doctors were sort of worried about it, that we might be comparing notes or something. But actually it was quite good. And we met out at somebody's church in the Northeast and we, we used to have speakers or we'd just talk about things among ourselves.

"I remember this one guy we knew in the group, the one whose daughter has just died, in fact, he just died too. Well, this guy didn't believe in talking to his daughter about what she had at all. He had had two other kids that had died of CF. And he didn't take her to the clinic and he wasn't doing therapy. He had his own methods of dealing with it. I used to talk to him quite a bit on the phone, and a lot of what he said made sense, as Trina got older. Because his daughter was older. Because what he was basically saying was, 'I want to get her to get on with her regular life and I don't want to spend all her time thinking of CF.' But I think he wasn't very good about it. He didn't take her to clinic. He didn't have the regular checkups. But what he was basically trying to do was deal with it himself, try and protect her in his own way.

"I don't know what Trina's way of coping with it will be. I have a feeling she'll grow up to be a bit like me. She'll want to find out more about it and read and write and stuff. I'm not sure exactly how she'll cope with it. But she's so healthy. And here she is ten, eleven; I think she needs to be thinking about other things really.

"Anyway, the group went quite a while, a good while, until our kids were at the stage where we were less interested in talking about CF, and they were ready to go on. We wanted to just be doing normal things."

Mr. Sherman agreed. "We didn't need the group anymore. We decided we didn't need it anymore. But I think that sort of thing may spring up again, from time to time in our lives—parents' groups."

Mrs. Sherman continued, "I think we must've sent a letter out to all the parents asking for anyone who was interested. And anyone who was interested showed up. And we got down, we got to a group of about ten to fifteen who would regularly show up. And we met. I can't even think of how often we met now, but it was fairly frequently for a few years.

"I was doing the newsletter during that time. I did that for about five years altogether. I did that about four or five times a year or something. That was very helpful to me because I was very sort of concerned about CF at that time. More than I am now, really. I was sort of thinking about it all the time, so things that I wanted to ask, I would ask a doctor and then he'd write the answer in the newsletter. And when people wanted to write something, they did. So, that was quite helpful to me.

"And I got very involved in CF stuff, too. I went to some conferences, like I attended that conference at the university. That was all in that stage where I was very sort of obsessed about it [CF].

"And I was involved in something that was being put together in Washington. It was sort of a state-of-the-art meeting. It was a bunch of working groups and I was in one of those working groups. I can't even think which group it was, but it was the one that had social workers and psychologists. We had a couple of parents and a dietitian. It was sort of social services to CF patients, I guess.

"I think it was funded maybe by the National Institutes of Health or whatever that is. I can't remember. And it put out some huge reports at the end of it all. I have a copy of it all stashed away somewhere. It was sort of medical groups that were looking at the state of CF research. There were five, four or five different groups.

"It was sort of fun because I got to go to Washington and spend a couple of days there. And I was involved with that, so it was all kind of interesting.

"But, as Katrina got older, I got less interested in that and more interested in just dealing with her usual, the normal school problems. I just didn't want to focus on CF. I think it was probably because she was doing well and I started to realize I couldn't go on being this involved forever. It wasn't going to be doing her any good. Before she was five, it was alright because she wasn't aware of what I was doing anyway. But I started to get more interested in how she was going to cope with regular school stuff."

Mr. Sherman explained, "Now she's pretty much like any other kid. It's pretty difficult to perceive any difference between her and Liam or anyone else."

Mrs. Sherman laughed, "That's certainly the way Liam sees it. Like when she has a clinic visit and isn't going to school he'll get a bit irritated and say, 'Well there's nothing wrong with her. Why does she need to do that?' He used to be annoyed about the attention she got from therapy. But he doesn't seem to care about that now."

Mr. Sherman continued, "A few years ago he used to sort of hang around during therapy; as though he had nothing else to do in the morning. I don't know. It would be very hard to translate this as jealousy. I suppose there could have been some jealously there. I know that sounds funny, that there should be jealousy there. But I suppose there could've been some. It did cross my mind. But he's got better things to do now. He's pretty good about her therapy and her condition generally."

"I'm not sure how he is going to feel in the future. He is very close to her, so I don't know how he'll cope."

Liam did not talk about being close to Katrina, but he did acknowledge talking and playing with her. And while Katrina talked about the time they spent playing together she also said, "I'm just an embarrassment to him. I do anything and he gets embarrassed."

According to Mrs. Sherman, "They're just sort of very normal, arguing and all that stuff. They get along a lot better than a lot of brothers and sisters. At least that's how they feel. Trina says when she goes to other people's houses she notices how they [the other people] fight more. So I really do think they get along well.

"They do argue and box each other and there is a fair amount of bickering that goes on, but generally they are pretty attached to each other. And they still do play with each other quite a lot. They're just sort of very normal.

"They get the Playmobiles out, or they like to play with the trains. Since they're stuck together, they figure something out to do that will suit them both.

"I don't want CF to be something big between them. Because he doesn't need to be worrying about her or feeling sorry for her. He has to be what he would be anyway for her. So if Liam doesn't want to know that much about it [CF] that's probably good as far as the relationship goes.

"I've talked to him, but I don't know how much of it he really took in, or how much he remembers, because that was back a ways; that he actually had to read stuff and write about it. He always says he's not interested, and he doesn't need to know, and what's the big deal. There's nothing wrong with her as far as he can see." Mrs. Sherman chuckled. "I think he sort of knows that there's something wrong with her. He does know, because I've told him. I mean I've told him what the problem with CF is, that people, children do die of it.

"Katrina knows too, I think. She knows that children die of CF sometimes, but that you can't really tell how you're going to do unless she's doing very well and blah blah blah. She knows that it does cause a shortening of your life, probably. I think that's what she knows. I think Liam knows that too, but he never, never says much or asks much about it.

"Katrina doesn't ask much about it now either. She has in the past. She's had spells when she's really concerned about CF. I remember it struck her, I think when she was about eight or nine that maybe this was more serious than she had thought. It hadn't occurred to her before that. And then she started asking questions. It sort of struck her that this could actually be life-threatening. She managed to gather that information.

"So we set up with the social worker at St. Chris, Loretta, who she really liked. Katrina talked to her a couple of times. I think it was a bit traumatic for her, because she learned some things she didn't know before, about how long most people live through CF.

"I think maybe it was just sort of time for her to start learning a bit more about it. And I think partly it was she didn't have enough to do in school. This was right at the end of Essex [school name]. She had done very similar work the year before. She was really under-occupied at school, and wasn't challenged enough. So she had time to think about herself and worry about herself. And also, because of her age, she was getting very interested in it. So that was rather a difficult time.

"She missed a lot of school that fall. And looking back I can't quite remember why, but she was sort of sick on and off a lot. She didn't want to go to school and seemed to have a lot of difficulty staying, being there every day, without feeling or saying she was sick. But she seemed to get through that, and she had quite a good second half of the year.

"Then this last year she's had a good year, except the work has been quite hard. But I think that's been good for her, hard work. The teachers have been telling her she's got to be more organized and so she's had to think about that stuff more. But I think she does think about it [CF] and she does talk about it sometimes. Late at night she still talks about her worries about CF.

"She talks to me and I think she probably talks to her dad, too. But, I've been trying to get her not to make too big a deal out of it [CF], especially at school. Because I think she has used it in the past as a sort of way of getting attention. And I don't think kids always appreciate that. So I've been trying to get her to take it in stride and say, 'Well, I have to take these pills.'

"But I know the gym teacher said, 'Is there anyone who has any illness, who shouldn't do this sport?' And she immediately went up and told him she had CF. And I said to her afterwards that having CF didn't mean she could get out of doing sports. Although he needed to know about it, it wasn't anything he needed to know.

"So I'm trying to persuade her just to sort of take it, try and take it in stride a bit more. Just cope with it as she goes along, without her always thinking of herself as this person who is sick or has a handicap or something.

"But I know that she's always aware of it. She's concerned about it. It's always there in the back of her mind. She worries about dying young and I guess that's sort of basically her worry. She's heard now from Loretta that the oldest person who had CF is about fifty or something and she didn't realize that before. And although fifty's a long way off, she's sort of aware that there are children who die of it younger. So although she knows she's healthy, she's pretty healthy, she's aware of it, hanging over her. So the only thing I can think of to do is to try and get her interested in other things. I mean she's not gonna be unaware of it, but to try and get her to want to do other things to see those as very important.

"And sometimes she says peculiar things. When I said, 'I hope they'll find a cure for CF one day,' we were talking about research and stuff, she said, 'I don't want to lose my CF.' I guess because she sees it as very much a part of her. She's always had it and it's very important to her. She could accept the idea of their controlling it, but she couldn't accept the idea of there being an actual cure; getting rid of it altogether.

"She had a lot of worries about me dying, which I'm sure is very understandable. She was sort of worrying about me dying, but I think she was really worrying about her dying. And so she thought if she stayed nice and close, then nothing's going to happen to me; if she could keep an eye on me. And maybe nothing would happen to her as well.

"So, it seems to me there is more going on between us than say, between me and Liam. In terms of worrying and concern, I think she's getting better about being willing to do stuff away from me. Or maybe I'm getting better and letting her. I don't know. I can't tell.

"Liam's always been willing to go away from the house. He's always been quite adventurous. I don't know whether the difference is in the fact that she has CF, or he's the oldest or what. But it's been harder for her and she was babyish longer than some of the kids her age.

"We are all very sort of emotionally close, Katrina and I. Liam and I are too, but in a different sort of way. She can't see quite, she can't get hold of the idea that she might not live here one of these days. She might be living somewhere else, in her own setting. She says, 'Oh, I'm always going to live here. This is going to be my house.' She doesn't see herself as very separate, but she has gotten better. Like this is the first year she's ever agreed to really, to willingly go off just camping this summer.

"She had this two weeks of swim camp and she enjoyed it a lot and had a good time and said she'd like to go next year. And I'd never heard her say that before. We've always sort of pushed her into going for a short time, for a week or for a morning session sometime; just so we could just sort of get her into the idea of doing it really. Because otherwise, if she was given a choice, she'd always be here." Mrs. Sherman smiles and continues.

"And I think school has been good for her as far as that goes. Her new school has been good for because it has taken her mind off—off her worries. And when she worries, I worry. That's when I get depressed. If I get depressed about it, it's when she's depressed about it, and I have to deal with her worrying about it. That really worries me, because I'm not sure quite how to deal with it and what to say to her, what the next stage is. I don't know what to do. So that's hard work. I don't spend much time specifically worrying about it, except when it affects her."

Katrina, however, did not portray herself as concerned or worried about her CF. "I don't like to call it a disease, 'cause it's not. It's not that big. And I have a mild case of it so I really don't need to call it a big disease and all that or a handicap or whatever. I feel like any normal kid would, except I'm rather hoarse sometimes.

"I just kinda say, 'I have [CF] and it's . . .' I usually have to explain that it's kind of like asthma, and my mucus is thicker than yours. And I used to have to ask them, 'Do you know what mucus is?' And I say, 'My mucus is a little thicker than yours and so I have to take my pills and . . .' Well actually, when people ask me, 'What are you taking those pills for?' I just say, 'It makes my stomach not hurt.' And so I don't have to go through the whole thing with them.

"And I say that I take my pills because if, now I get this all mixed up, I don't take my pills, I can't go to the bathroom and if I take too many, it goes, it's runny. And so, I have to take these pills. I have to take my vitamin Es, my aquasoles, and my multivitamins and my cortisones.

"And then I have to do therapy in the morning. I usually show them how. I say, 'You clap your hands.' And they usually do a couple pounds on me. And then they usually say, 'Is it deadly or something? Is it?'

"And I usually tell them I'm not contaminating either, cause once when I told somebody what I had to do they shrieked. And I said, 'No, I'm not contaminating.' And that's just about all I would tell somebody. I don't know much more, but I know a bit more."

Chatting as she looked for the file in her mind, "I can't think of things. I can usually do things and not think of things. Liam usually thinks of things to play. But I do them with him."

The file retrieved, Katrina continued. "I know how I got it. Mom had her genes [for CF] and Dad had a gene [for CF], and all my relatives, I guess, have genes [for CF] and stuff. We don't know if Liam has one, though. And so when the genes do whatever, when they have me or Liam, it doesn't matter which, they pick at random. They say, 'Okay, I'm gonna do Katrina this time, not Liam.' And so when they put their genes together they get one child with cystic fibrosis. But if only one parent has it—this gets all confusing—if one parent has a gene and the other doesn't, then you might have a child with just a gene. You'll at least have one child, I think, with the gene. And if you have two parents with the gene, then you're bound to have a child with this, with the disease.

"And there's other stuff. One in every two thousand people have it. That's not much, considering how many people there are in the world.

"My cousin has it. His name is Oliver. And I remember he came here once and he was really quiet, and he wouldn't say much; not just about CF, but about anything. He just wouldn't say much. He was real quiet. He was ten or something, about my age. He has to take a lot of pills a day. He has to take double what I have to take, thirty-two or something? He has to take a lot of pills a day. He has to take five at lunch and I only have to take three at lunch. It's a worse case than I have, but not that bad.

"And one of my friends has asthma. I know a lot of people with asthma. CF is less frequent than asthma. I only know one person with CF, and it's my cousin with CF. And I know a lot of people with asthma. I know about five people with asthma.

"When I went to Great Adventure, I met a couple of people [with CF], but I didn't know a lot of them. It was a trip for people with CF. I don't know anybody, really, that has CF except me.

"When I want to know things Mom and Dad tell me. Well, I also kind of feel I have a right to know about it because I do have it. And so they tell me everything about it and stuff.

"And, they didn't tell me that the stork brought me or anything like that, or that they found me under a mulberry bush or anything like that. They told me the truth. They said I got the sweat test when I was little. And now they have this new one. They put it on your wrist and it turns green if you have it. It's really neat. It turns green if you have CF or if you have more sweat or something. It's just one of the tests. They did another kind [of sweat test] on me.

"They put me and Liam in this really sweaty incubator or something. So we're sitting there, sweating our minds out and I guess they were seeing, testing the sweat or something. They put us in this place and it made us sweat a lot. And I guess they were just seeing what the sweat was like, if it had more salt in Liam's or something. Liam's didn't have as much salt as mine. But I have it [CF] and he doesn't.

"They know he doesn't have it, but I think he does have the genes. Pretty likely, because Mom and Dad both have it [the genes]. My relatives have the gene."

Katrina moved on from the diagnosis. "Mom says that if they lined up three kids with me I would be the same. They'd just have to take X-rays and everything to see what it would be like. Because now I know I don't have much wrong with me. Mom said, 'Someday they'll find a cure.' And I say, 'But I don't want a cure, it doesn't bother me.'

"It did once though, when I went and talked to Loretta and she told me. I got really scared when Loretta told me. I was real young. Well, not real young, but I thought I was gonna die real soon. That was a couple of years ago. I heard someone with CF died. And I got really scared, and I thought I was gonna die at ten or something. There was a woman, the oldest living woman [with CF] so far was fifty-two. And then mom told me that that was just the one who had died [the one who was fifty-two]. That means there was still growing up.

"And we Shermans live a while. My great grandfather just died a couple weeks ago, and he died when he was ninety-seven or something. He was pretty old. And my great grandmother, my other great grandmother, my mom's grandmother, she died when she was ninety-two. And my other great grandfather, my mom's grandfather, died when he was in the war. I think he got some stuff in his lungs or something. And her grandmother, my great grandmother, died when she was ninety-two. And my great grandma and my dad's grandmother is still living and she's ninety-five now. And my dad's grandfather died when he was ninety-seven. It gets more confusing."

After a recitation of the survival rates in her family, Katrina returned to her own condition. "There are things I like about my CF. It's fun taking pills, because I've never taken pills. And I get my shots and stuff, and Liam says, 'Oh, I hate shots.' And I say, 'But I like them, they're fun sometimes.' It depends how you're getting them. And then when I'm doing therapy, I can just sit there and get pounded. So that's pretty fun. I like therapy. It's fun. When Dad tells me stories and Mom tells me about Morris Mucus and you see it's fun. I mean," Katrina clarified, "I don't exactly, I don't really want it. It's just, I was born like that, so why not accept it?"

"For Katrina," Mrs. Sherman would explain, "CF is part of who she is. I'm not sure she would want to give it up."

"It's there," added Mr. Sherman. "But I don't believe it has, at this time, much of a strong effect at all on our life. There are other things that come up that have as much of an effect as that. When we talk about other problems that might make our children or Trina separate from others, like religion perhaps or different philosophies in life, I don't think it [CF] really has taken its place here as a major factor. I mean, it's not really something that's so much taboo to talk about. We talk freely about it. But it just doesn't loom very large."

––––––––

"OK Katrina," Thea called from the receptionist's desk, where she was looking over the morning schedule. Katrina and her mother got up and walked toward the open examining room. Thea followed them in and closed the door behind them.

CHAPTER 4

The Farringtons

(Individuals mentioned by name, in order of appearance)

CODY FARRINGTON: Seven-year-old child with cystic fibrosis (CF)
MRS. VERA FARRINGTON: Mother of Cody Farrington
HOLLY FARRINGTON: Thirteen-year-old well sister of Cody Farrington
HEATHER FARRINGTON: Ten-year-old well sister of Cody Farrington
THEA WRIGHT: Outpatient clinical nurse specialist
MR. MAURICE FARRINGTON: Father of Cody Farrington
MRS. JENKINS: Kindergarten teacher of Cody Farrington

CODY sat on the chair next to his grandmother. Every so often she would rest her hand on his thigh as if to stop his legs from swinging. He would stop momentarily and she would return her hands to her lap. Next to her sat her daughter, Cody's mother, who just stared straight ahead. Next to Mrs. Farrington sat Holly, her elder daughter and Cody's sister. Holly's feet almost touched the floor as she bent forward in her chair, her arms resting on the armrests and hands clasped together. Heather, the middle child, was not in the clinic that day. She did not enjoy coming to the clinic as much as Holly did and had made plans to spend time with her friends.

Thea Wright, the outpatient clinical nurse specialist, walked over to Mrs. Farrington and knelt down to her eye-level. "Have you thought any more about the prednisone study?"

"Yeah, but I'm still not sure."

"Do you want to think about it some more?"

Mrs. Farrington nodded.

"Perhaps we can talk about it if you'd like?"

"OK."

"Excuse me," said the resident as she smiled at Mrs. Farrington and turned to Thea.

Thea rose and looked to the resident.

"I need you for a moment," the resident said.

"Would you excuse me?"

Mrs. Farrington nodded. Thea followed the resident into one of the examining rooms.

"I don't know," Mrs. Farrington sighed. "We decided to do it, but I don't know. With that kind of stuff you don't know what to do. It can have these side effects. You think, 'Well I have enough problems. We don't need all this to go with it.' That's the part that gets to me. When you stop and think about it, that's just going to add to everything else. But I don't know.

"Then they said that a lot of drugs that he takes now can give side effects too, which I never really thought about. Because I don't think I've ever asked the question about them. And they said that if anything would happen they would stop it right away. If he had a reaction to it or anything they would just stop it. And then they said that if you don't do it you may be sorry that you didn't do it." Mrs. Farrington paused.

"No! No! My Jesus!" exclaimed Mrs. Farrington, just as she did on the phone when the nurse called. "See they called me because I hadn't answered the letter they sent.

"I'm on the phone. I'm thinking, 'Oh geez, how am I going to get out of this one?'" Mrs. Farrington let a giggle escape. "Because I didn't like the idea of the side effects. But then, when I was talking to Thea on the phone, she said, 'You know if you don't, you might wish you had. You might feel sorry in four years.' Because that's how long it's [the study] for, four years. So then you don't know what to do, when they say stuff like that.

"I don't know what to do. It's one of those things, you don't know what to do. So I just asked my husband. And he said, 'Well yes.' He trusts them down there. He really does. Anything they want to do, he goes along with it. Because, like I said, he really trusts them. He has faith in them. And so he said, 'Go ahead and do it.'

"But I don't know. Once you do it, then you start thinking about it, the bad parts and all. I don't like to think about it. No. It's funny. When he was first diagnosed I used to just sit and think that it'll go away. That's all I kept thinking—it'll go. And someday I'll go down there and they'll say, 'He doesn't have this.' That's just because that's what I wanted, when it first happened. That's why I said, 'I don't like to think about the bad part so much.' I don't know if that's good or bad. But I don't like to do it.

"Of course when you first find out, when they sit there and tell you your son could die. Whoa!" Mrs. Farrington laughed nervously. "That's kind of hard to handle. And then they say the average life span is about twenty-one, depending on how severe and how this and that. The thing that scares you is they say they can't tell you anything. They can't judge anything. Like they can't tell you how he's going to do next year, or the year after. They said they can't tell you anything like that. 'It's out of their hands.' That part's scary. Because he does so good, and I sit here and think, 'Well, gee, I can't believe that it's possible that next year he could be, well say, twice as bad as this. How can that be?' But they say it can happen, but they can't tell you if . . ." Mrs. Farrington didn't finish her sentence. She began anew.

"Each one progresses different. I don't know. I guess it's better not to know, rather than have them come out and say, 'Well, this is going to happen, and that's going to happen.' Maybe it's better not to know that. And then again, maybe it is!

"But when he gets sick, then I start worrying. Like when he was in the hospital last time, or if you hear it on TV or something. It's like you're thinking about him being sick, but you're not thinking about what's going to happen. I mean, it's in my head all the time that he has it. It's just I don't think about what's going to happen or what could happen. I don't like to think about that. But it makes you kind of, probably overprotective of him. Like, when he was younger you'd be afraid to let him out of the house, be around other kids and stuff. And they used to tell me, down the hospital, 'You can't do that. You have to let this kid be normal.' It's just your first reaction is to do that, to hide him or something; so he doesn't get a cold, or whatever. And once you get over that it's easier.

"And then I kept him out of school a year too because of that. Because all I could think of was, he's going to come home every day and he's going to be sick. Or every week he's going to get a cold. So we kept him out a year. He should have gone to first grade, and we just put him into kindergarten. We just figured, 'Well, we can't keep him out again. We have to send him.' He'll be behind, but Holly is too. She had to be put back and repeat kindergarten.

"But it was scary because all I could think of is, 'Geez! He'll come home with everything! He'll get sick, and we're going to have problems.' And it wasn't that bad. I was surprised. It wasn't as bad as what we thought it was going to be. I mean, he got colds and all, but he didn't get so bad that he had to be hospitalized for pneumonia or anything. And that's probably what we were afraid of. Even my husband was afraid to put him in school. Because that's all we could think of—'He'll be sick *all* the time.' But it wasn't like that.

"I just kept him out a year because that's what we were thinking about, him getting sick and being ready to deal with all that. After having him do so good, for six years, and then go putting him in school and having to deal with him getting sick and going in the hospital. We didn't want to deal with that. Then we put him in this year and he did good. Yeah. He didn't do bad; not as bad as we thought. Of course, he did get more colds than if he wasn't in school. But it wasn't as bad as we thought it would be.

"When he did go in the hospital it was mostly his weight, his lungs weren't in trouble. He wasn't that sick. They just wanted to get some more weight on him, because he started losing weight. And so they put him in mainly for that, and to clean out his lungs completely with IVs and all. And it wasn't too bad. Like I said, he wasn't really sick, it was mostly his weight. So I knew that his lungs weren't in trouble.

"I took the girls to see him and all. Just to watch what he goes through and all. That was new to them, to see all that, with the IVs and all that stuff. They were real good with him. They'd go down there and sit there and play with him, and keep him occupied. They weren't . . . they didn't get scared or anything like that. But that was the first time they've seen him in the hospital like that, and seen what happens when he's in there and all.

"It was the first time he's been in the hospital since he was diagnosed and that's been six years. It's been a long time. Some kids go in there more often. I hear people down there saying that some kids go in there more often than that. I can't imagine that, living with that all the time. It must be hard on the family.

"My husband felt that I should be there all the time, around the clock. He couldn't be there, because he would work. And he'd get mad if I came home early or something. And I mean, how long can anyone stay down there? There's nothing to do down there. And he'd get mad and say, 'How come you came home so early?'

"I want to be down there too, every day, but I don't want to be down there twenty-four hours every day." Mrs. Farrington laughed. "I've got other things here. I've got two kids home and that part of it bothers me, because he thinks that I should be down there all the time. And when he [Cody] was in, he wasn't that sick either. And he [my husband] couldn't go down because he works. But he just expects me to stay down there with him. I always found that strange.

"I know it bothers him [my husband] a lot, but he doesn't talk about it. No. We don't talk about it. He just keeps it in I think, because when Cody gets sick, he gets upset. More so than I do because I take care of Cody and I kind of know. I can try and judge how sick he is. I can tell pretty much.

"And he just doesn't want to think about it at all. Like when Cody gets sick he'll say, 'You better call the doctor.' But he doesn't know what Cody gets in the way of medicine and stuff like that. He doesn't have any idea. I find that hard, kind of strange, because if something should happen to me, he should know all this stuff. He should learn to do the therapy and all, but he doesn't. Holly knows more than he does.

"Holly pretty much knows what I know. The younger one, Heather, she doesn't ask that many questions. They know he has to have enzymes every time he eats, about his vitamins and this and that. But they don't ask, come out and ask me questions. They understand that when he gets a cold that it can get real bad and he will have to go in the hospital. I don't think I've actually come out and said that he could die from it. I don't think I've done that. I don't think I can do that. Maybe when they get older. I don't know.

"They think we spoil him; which we do. That was easy to do. They say we let him get away with a lot of stuff. And we do. And when my mother lived with us, she spoiled him too. We had three of us there to do it." Mrs. Farrington laughed.

"I guess we do because of the CF. When I go down the hospital and I see some of those kids in the clinic, they really look sick. That scares me. I don't like to see that. 'Cause, I don't know, I just . . ." Mrs. Farrington's voice trailed off.

"Some of them are so thin, and they cough, cough continuously. And that scares me. I don't like to see that. See, Cody, he's not like that. He doesn't cough. And if he gets sick, he'll lose weight; and I'll notice it. But, he's not real thin, not like a friend of my sister's. Her daughter was real, real thin, and she was real sick.

"But the girls, they don't say that we spoil Cody because of the CF. They say it's because he's the youngest. That's what they say. I don't know. Maybe the older one might think that it's because of the CF. I don't think the younger one thinks that. She's still young yet.

"Holly just thinks we let him get away with too much. She'll say, 'You can't just let him get away with everything because he's sick.' And then I'll say, 'Well that's easy for you to say.' And she says she understands, 'but you can't have the kid turn into a monster.'" Mrs. Farrington laughed.

"I tell her something could happen to him," explained Mrs. Farrington, her voice becoming increasingly somber. "And she knows that." Mrs. Farrington nodded. "And then I just say something could happen to him and we would feel bad or something.

"The youngest one doesn't ever say anything like the older one. It's just the older one that says, 'Well, you can't let him get away with everything because he's sick.' I just ignore her. It doesn't make me not do it anymore. I still do it.

"Holly says those things when she gets mad. See, if we tell him 'No,' not to do something, and if he goes ahead, if he keeps doing it, we don't just stand there and yell at him, and say, 'Don't, don't, don't!' And she doesn't like that. But I think that even in a normal family, the youngest one is likely to be spoiled. But with Cody it's just even tougher.

"Holly knows now that you can die from CF. I told her just in the past year, after he was in the hospital and she was on me about spoiling him. She's older now, and I can tell her, and she understands. She's thirteen. She's old enough to understand what that means. But I didn't tell the other one because I don't think she would [understand] yet. She'd probably ask me a million questions, like I ask down at the hospital." Mrs. Farrington smiled and chuckled.

Before Cody's first hospitalization, months before her mom spoke to her about the fact that one could die from CF, Holly thought that CF was "something you're born with. And if you get a real bad cold then you get congested in your throat and in your lungs. So when you get a real bad cold, then it gets pretty bad. When you cough, when it has like this tickle in there, then it stays there a long time. You have to take all this medicine and treatments to clear your lungs and stuff. And then when you get a cold you get this stuff in your lungs. They get clogged up and you cough. And if you get running around and stuff, you wheeze. Sometimes if it's real hard to breathe.

"We have a stethoscope and we play with that, hearing him breathing. When he has a cold and stuff you can hear the stuff rattle inside.

"Cody gets colds sometimes, real bad, and he has to take medicine. Otherwise he's an active kid. If he doesn't have a cold or anything, it's really like he really doesn't have it. But if he gets a cold, it's pretty bad. He coughs a lot.

"Now he has a cold, but I don't think it's real bad. It's just a small cold.

"Mostly it's like he's a normal kid. If he doesn't have a cold or anything, then it's like it's not there. But then if I have friends over and if he has to take his treatment or his enzymes before we eat, like lunch or something, they ask us what they're for. And I tell them he has cystic fibrosis, and it's a lung thing, and when he gets a cough or cold it clogs his lungs. And he takes his machine thing, mask; where the steam comes out the holes, whenever he has a cold, and once in a while if he doesn't.

"He takes enzymes too. We always have to remember to give them to him. Sometimes he forgets. Sometimes my mom says, 'Holly, get him the enzymes.' Or other times he says, 'I need my ennies.' He calls them that.

"If he doesn't take them, he can't digest his food and then he has to go to the bathroom a lot.

"Sometimes I wonder how it is going to be when he gets older. Like the other day I asked my mom and grandmom if as he gets older, how many enzymes will he take. Before, he only had to take one enzyme. Now he has to take two, and when he gets older I said, 'How many does he have to take; a whole bottle of enzymes when he gets older?'

"He has to take vitamins too. And if he has a cold he has to take his treatment. And my mom has to pat him on the back and stuff. And he has medicine if he has colds, pink medicine.

"They don't usually give him the treatments unless he really needs it. Sometimes we give them once in a while.

"My mom pats him on the back sometimes, but mostly we give him this little blue thing and he puts the mask on, and my mom puts the medicine in, or tells me what to put in. And me and my sister have to keep him busy while he keeps it on. We play cards or something while it's on.

"He doesn't do it every day. If he has a cold he'll have to do it every day, because he coughs a lot. Other times he just gets it once in a while."

For Heather, the middle child, "CF's a harm to Cody. It was born with him. He had it when he was born and he had it all his life. And it stays all your life." Heather said that she did not know what happens from having CF, but that she did know what you had to do to take care of it. "Like he has to take his enzymes before he eats, but not before he drinks, just so he can eat. He can't eat without them or he'll have to go to the bathroom all day.

"And he has to go on this machine. When he takes his machine you have to put medicine inside it so it can take all that stuff out of his nose and stuff, so his colds can go away. The medicine goes around in the mask and in his nose and when there's no more medicine in the thing then it's done. And it takes about twenty minutes or so.

"After he does the machine Mom gives him a treatment. When he was four she just went like that," explained Heather, cupping her hands and pounding them against an imaginary surface in the air. "She had to have her arm like that," Heather added, holding up a bent and angled elbow, level with her shoulders. "And she'd pat him on the back."

Heather did several more demonstrations in the air before concluding her description of the chest physical therapy treatments. "Now she only does all that when he coughs really bad. Usually he just does the machine. She doesn't clap him as much.

"Now with the cold he has, he gets on this machine three times a day. Sometimes he yells and screams. He says, 'I don't want to take it.' He doesn't like the machine because he doesn't have anything to do. But now me and my sister play with him when he's on the machine. We play cards with him.

"We just go there and play with him. We made that up so that Cody won't scream and holler. He would scream and holler. He just doesn't like it [the machine with the mask]. He was bored when he had it on. He was just sitting there watching TV so we started playing with him, like when he has colds and has to be on the machine.

"When you have CF you get colds and stuff all the time. Me and my sister feel sorry for my brother because he has to take medicine and everything. We talk about it, me and my sister. When my brother gets silly and everything we talk about it because we don't understand why he's silly. And we say he's a pain some days.

"Like the other night he was being really bad. When my mom yelled at him he wouldn't listen. My mom had to give him a spanking because he was being hyperactive, and going in front of the TV so we couldn't see it. And when my mom spanked him he didn't cry or nothing. He kept on laughing and everything, jumping on the couch. So then, a few minutes later when he had to go upstairs to get ready for bed, we all had to get ready for bed, he realized what he did. He probably realized when he was on my mom's bed. And he felt sorry for himself. He realized that it's bad enough to do that because you know you're going to be sorry. He started crying and my mom came up.

"When I get mad at him and I say, 'You're a pain,' and all; I feel sorry for him. And I say I shouldn't do that because it's mean to do that to your brother and your sister, especially a brother with cystic fibrosis.

"When he gets sick I don't yell at him. I don't get mad at him. If he does something I get mad, but I don't say anything to him. I say not to do that because he's sick. I'm not the same with Holly when she gets sick. It's only when Cody gets sick. He has cystic fibrosis and I understand how he gets sick.

"Holly is like any of us. We get sick from the cold. If it's winter and we get a stuffy nose it's not from CF. It's just from the cold; that it's really cold outside from the winter. It's different because we don't get colds from cystic fibrosis, only Cody does. And we don't have to take a machine or we don't have to take that kind of medicine that Cody does. We take just aspirins and stuff if we get sick. We take different aspirins if we get sick.

"My mom treats us the same, but if we have colds at the same time she treats Cody better, because he has cystic fibrosis and his cold might get badder. Mine and Holly's doesn't.

"I feel sorry for him when he gets colds and everything. He once went to the hospital for a hernia, not his CF. My mom and dad stayed with him because they wanted to see what they would do, because they didn't know what they would do. So my mom and dad slept over and when my brother got home my dad and my grandmom got him a present. We got him a present when he came home from the hospital.

"If he gets a cold I think he'll go to the hospital and I get worried, because if he has to get something done to him that I don't know of. I get mad because I don't know what's going on."

The wait in the waiting room was getting longer and Cody was growing increasingly restless. His dangling legs no longer waved gently. They seemed to be moving faster and faster with each passing moment. "I'm hungry," he called to his mother.

"I don't have anything with me, Cody."

"At school I have snack."

"I know."

"How 'bout if I get something?" his grandmother suggested.

"Well," his mother began.

"Mom?"

"Did you bring his enzymes?" Holly asked.

Several days earlier when a friend was visiting and Holly was telling her about Cody's enzymes, Cody volunteered, "At school I have a whole bottle [of enzymes]. I take the bottle into the nurse and she gives it to me when I eat. Like when we have lunch they just give them to me. Sometimes when the nurse goes to another school she just gives Mrs. Jenkins them. She'll put them on her desk 'til snack time and she gives them to me. She's leaving. She's not going to be the kindergarten teacher."

Suddenly Cody stopped his long discourse and asked his mother, "Will I have to take them . . .?"

No one seemed to be able to understand the rest of the sentence, but before anyone managed to ask him to repeat what he had said Cody had another question, "Will I die or something?"

"What?" asked Mrs. Farrington.

"When I grow up?"

"What?" Mrs. Farrington repeated.

"Will I still have to take them when I grow up?"

"Have what?"

"Enzymes."

"Yes."

"Even when I die?" he pursued.

Mrs. Farrington laughed.

"When I'm big like you, do I still have to take them?"

"Yes," his mother answered.

"Until I die, too?

"I guess. Forever"

"I'm not taking those things forever," Cody countered. "I hate them."

"How can you hate them after seven years?" Mrs. Farrington laughed, but Cody remained quite serious. "You should be used to them by now."

"I hate them. I hate . . ."

———————

With the negotiations for the snack still incomplete the nurse returned. "Cody, Mrs. Farrington, do you want to come with me?"

Cody and Mrs. Farrington followed the nurse to the examining room. Holly waited in silence with her grandmother.

CHAPTER 5

The Campbells

(Individuals mentioned by name, in order of appearance)

JEREMY CAMPBELL: Ten-year-old well brother of Zoe Campbell
ADAM CAMPBELL: Ten-year-old well brother of Zoe Campbell
MRS. MERYL CAMPBELL: Mother of Zoe Campbell
ZOE CAMPBELL: Ten-year-old child with cystic fibrosis (CF)
TAD CAMPBELL: Sixteen-year-old well brother of Zoe Campbell
ADAM ELIAS: Grandfather of Zoe Campbell
JEREMIAH ISAIAH: Grandfather of Zoe Campbell
ARIEL CAMPBELL: Sister of Zoe Campbell who died of CF
MR. LLOYD CAMPBELL: Father of Zoe Campbell
DR. EVERETT REESE: Pediatric pulmonologist
DR. LENORE HASTING: Pediatric pulmonologist
DR. MYRON GROSSMAN: Pediatric pulmonologist

"I'm hungry," Jeremy announced.

"Me too," echoed Adam.

"Can we get something to eat? Please?" pleaded Jeremy.

"Not right now," their mother replied.

"When then?" the boys asked in chorus.

"When Zoe's finished."

"When will that be?"

"When she's been examined."

"But that's a long time."

"It won't be long, she's in getting weighed."

"Please can we go?" Adam begged.

"No. We'll wait 'til Zoe's been examined."

"Can we go by ourselves?" Jeremy offered.

"We'll come right back," Adam assured.

"No!"

"If Zoe wanted something to eat you'd get it for her right away."

"Yeah. You'd let her eat."

Mrs. Campbell did not respond. She continued to look straight ahead, her expression unchanged, while the boys pouted in their chairs and waited for Zoe to return.

"They're triplets," Tad, their sixteen-year-old older brother, explained. "And they're all pretty much the same. Zoe's the girl, and it has nothing to do with CF. They're all just normal. They're all the same. They have different personalities and everything, but they don't say anything about her, like about CF. They never . . . you know, it's never brought up. She goes to the St. Christopher's Hospital and that's just another checkup. She's just a normal girl.

"It doesn't show, the disease, so it's nothing really. It's not a part of her. We wouldn't think of it. I don't think of it when I think of her. She's really normal.

"She is the girl of the family, and she's in the third grade, and the boys are in the fourth. The first year she was in school she was falling back and she had to be put in a special class. She had bad classmates or something. She wasn't accepted and she didn't like school. She didn't have the interest either. So she went to a special learning class. Then she took first grade again the next year. But they [Jeremy and Adam] don't treat her like, 'Oh, she's a third grader.' Because they're all equal.

"Right now she's learning really to be responsible. The boys are terrible with their rooms, all messy. And she has a really nice, clean room and everything. She's getting to know responsibility and a mature side of things.

"She's bigger than the other two, and if any of them try to beat her up, she can beat them."

Jeremy would agree. "She hits back a lot. When I want to do something she hits me in the back. She does. I'm not kidding. She's good in sports. She hates my friends."

According to Tad, "Jeremy is stubborn. He gets on my nerves. He doesn't want to do wrong. We're trying to get through to him about that. He has a temper and if he doesn't do something right he'll just try to hit something or make up. But anyways, he's a good kid. He has a good outlook. But I used to get mad at him because he would act the wrong way. And they're all trying to help him. But otherwise he's fine. Any other time he's not bad. But he's stubborn. I like him a lot.

"Adam is the opposite of Jeremy. He's generous, giving. Jeremy's the bad sport, and Adam's the good sport. And Adam is, you know, he's really good, but I guess he saw Jeremy and said, 'Well this isn't really right.' He took the good side of him. He's just really a good kid. And when I think of him, I think of what his grandfather might be because he has the name Adam Elias and Jeremy has the name Jeremiah Isaiah. Isaiah is my grandfather who is just like Jeremy. He's stubborn and all that stuff. And from what I've heard about my other grandfather [the one Adam is named for], he died, so I've only heard things about him, but he was supposed to be very generous. That's what I think of them both as.

"My parents had another kid who died of it [cystic fibrosis]. I was three when it died, when she died. I don't remember anything. We just have pictures." Tad paused for a moment. "I know what my parents went through and all that stuff, because around three years ago I went to Toledo by myself, my first plane ride by myself. And I went and stayed with my grandmother and she told me all about it. And stuff that I didn't know. That's where I found out just what they went through, what they did, what Ariel was like, what I did.

"We went to Walt Disney World afterward [after Ariel's death]. We left the house to get away. We went to Walt Disney World. Then I heard that I had a thing about her [Ariel], because we came back to the house and everything was out of her room and I was like, 'What's wrong? Where is she?' and my parents are like, 'Oh my gosh!' And I heard there was some funny thing. I would always ask them where she went. And they said to heaven. And I would be thinking about that.

"I just was constantly wondering where she was. I don't remember. And then there was some instance where I finally realized that she was gone.

"My grandmother always said she went to heaven and I'm glad my grandmother finally told me. I knew she died and everything, but I didn't get it. I didn't realize it because I was too young.

"My grandmother told me what I asked her and everything. We were just talking. We talk a lot, but we were just talking and it came up and then I asked more and more about it. And we spent most of the day talking about it.

"My brothers and sister know about Ariel, but I don't really know if they know it was from CF. I think we're afraid to talk about CF and Ariel to Zoe, and I don't think they want to bring it up. At least I haven't heard my parents talk about it."

Mr. Campbell would concur with his son's assessment. "I guess we just sort of avoid the subject. And I don't know if we should set them down and say, 'You guys want to ask about it,' or we should set them down individually and see if they have any concerns. If they ask us point blank we try to explain it I think: in a positive way. Again we'd try to avoid the down side of the discussions, down-side risk type things. Because we want things to be positive and I think Zoe's mental outlook on life is important to her well being. So we just try to emphasize the positive."

"Further reasons for holding it back," Mrs. Campbell added, "is so she will feel good about herself. I feel like at each stage we've kind of maybe decided she could handle a little bit more. But you're afraid to talk too much because knowing that her sister died of it, it's been something we kind of hold back. I don't even know if she realizes it now. I've always kind of squashed the conversation whenever it's come up."

"I think we bullshit in a lot of ways. We've been through it. We've seen what can happen, the worst possible thing. And we've always tried to raise her just like the other two; the same kind of treatment and not show favoritism or anything else. And, fortunately, she's remained fairly healthy so it's a lot easier to do that."

"We've been fortunate."

"If she was real sick, then I think it'd be another problem with what we would do. But we don't openly discuss the down-side risk of the whole situation with her or with any of the kids. I think with Tad we probably talk a little bit more about it with him. In fact, last summer or two summers ago, when he went home and he had a discussion with my mother about it, he said he figured that Zoe was going to die soon. We knew we hadn't talked to him about it. My mother told me, so we sat down and talked to Tad about it. We tried to explain to him. His remembrance of what happened [to Ariel] is probably what he's applying after her [Zoe]."

"He doesn't remember Ariel. I think he was just too young. He was four when she died. Or almost four. Of course, the pictures we have, but maybe he doesn't really remember her. So that's whatever we share with him."

"Remember," Mr. Campbell interrupted, "the night at the dinner table when they asked about how, why she died or something like that."

"We always said she was very sick," Mrs. Campbell picked up. "We kind of kept it very vague. We just didn't feel like or just didn't think she could handle it."

"I guess when they get a little older it'll be different."

"Well then we can reason with them. We can tell them it was misdiagnosed and it was something where if they'd known what it was she'd be with us today."

"See, we never really cared for Ariel in the CF sense. By the time we found out that she had it, it was over."

"It was too late."

"We don't see any purpose in discussing Ariel in terms of why she died. Someday, yes. Right now, I don't think they're mature enough to deal with it in the proper framework. So we just don't talk about it."

"And they can bring it up on their own, you know, like Tad, he asked what he needed to know. He brought it up."

"Tad's different. I mean, he's older."

"We once did sit down and talk to them, come to think of it. I think it was right, shortly after we moved in, when they found out she [Zoe] had CF. Our neighbor's a nurse. She must have discussed something in front of the kids about Zoe's gonna die. They went through this really open, right to the point, of what it probably used to be. So of course he [the neighbor's child] shared with Zoe. And it just threw them. The kids were just floored because they never heard a thing like that. Oh, that of course we had to explain. It used to be that children did die young, but you're in such good shape and you've done very well. It just won't happen to you.

"And I guess the other time is, there's been little time slots on TV. And of course they put the worst possible example they could put in there, because sadly enough that's how they get more money. So there again we had to explain that this is what happens to some of the children, that you're not necessarily in that category and don't worry about it. It's not you. So there's been those times that's kind of like shocking. Cutting to the core. Scared."

"They know she has CF," Mr. Campbell explained. "Basically she's got to take her pills with her meals and everything."

"That's something she is always going to have to deal with," added Mrs. Campbell.

"I don't think we've ever talked about the potential seriousness of it or anything like that."

"We've told her what it involves in the body. And she's been very open about it. She told other kids about it and she tries to exploit it to her friends.[1] And she doesn't seem to hide what she has, which I think is a healthy attitude."

"Like when she was in the hospital a couple of years ago, that kind of struck home a bit."

"That's what you call a crash course. Everything you wanted to know and more," Mrs. Campbell laughed. Mr. Campbell joined in. "She had two girls in the room who were veterans," Mrs. Campbell continued. "One was from Palmyra, New Jersey. A teenager, probably what? Fourteen? Fifteen?"

"Yeah."

"And the other girl next to her sounded like she spent a couple of long times in the hospital. She weighed about the same as Zoe, maybe a pound heavier, and she was at that point, she was, what, three years older than Zoe."

"Three or four years."

"Yeah."

"She's from Harrisburg, I think."

"She was from a . . . wasn't she from a divorced family?"

"Yeah."

"Yeah?"

"No. I can't remember if they were divorced."

"But they kind of took Zoe into their room. She had problems with her IV's hookup sometimes, and they would help her get, not help her get hooked up again, but they knew how to flush it and all this business. They had been through it a couple of times. In a way they were a help to her. Maybe that probably opened her eyes, too, to what all this could involve. Although she knew that she's I think in a lot better shape than they are."

"As for the boys, well, we haven't said you have a potential of being a carrier or anything like that yet. I guess we just . . ."

---

[1] Mrs. Campbell said exploit, but I think she meant to say explain.

"No, we haven't told the boys," Mrs. Campbell confirmed.

While Mr. and Mrs. Campbell have not talked to the boys about carrier status, Tad seemed to be aware of the genetic component of the disease. As he explained it, "CF's in the genes. My parents know a lot about it because they had a kid die of it. So they learned a bunch about it before they had the triplets. They wanted to know the chances. And just Zoe got it of all of the three. So we were relieved too, when we felt like we had a second chance too.

"It's a lung disease," Tad continued. "And it affects the pancreas. But I don't really see that much of it, because Zoe's not really affected all that much.

"You have to take pills and you have to take a lot of vitamins because your body doesn't take all the nutrients the food gives. And your bowel movements," Tad giggles, "are affected. And PDs. You have PDs, postural drainage. We have the table downstairs.

"She also watches what she eats. She doesn't eat much greasy stuff. Like if we go to McDonald's or Burger King, she'll skip the fries and have something else. If she watches. She's very thin. She's not too thin. She's fine. I used to think she ate a lot," Tad smiled. "I used to always say, 'You eat more than I do. Why are you doing this?'

"I just think of it," the smile fading from Tad's face, "as a condition that sometimes gets too out of hand and it drains the body. Because one of the people I knew in Alabama[2] was very thin and that's only because not much of the food got to the body itself. I know that some people have lived until thirty-five. They're really healthy. And, I don't really think about Zoe dying early. But she says, 'I'm going to be this when I grow up.' And I always think about it. Just for an instant, though. I don't give it. I thought about when she would die. I don't want to think about it. It's not what I plan to do either.

"I think about maybe pancrease[3] and that the kids can grow up—some can, some can't—and that my sister has it. There. That's about what flashes through my mind.

"But I don't like to think about it very long. Maybe because it goes through the death thing. But it's also, I don't think I talk about it as much because it really doesn't affect anyone. That's usually why people don't get into all this stuff or don't give to Cancer Societies and that stuff. Because they're not affected. But, I am, sort of, but not really, because Zoe is normal, as I said many times."

Adam's and Jeremy's knowledge and views of CF are somewhat different from Tad's. For Adam, "CF's like a living thing. You're born it. And it's like a disease or something. And Zoe takes pancrease, that's her pills, and she

---

[2] Where the family lived when Zoe was diagnosed.

[3] The speaker is referring to a pancreatic enzyme taken by children with CF, often, but not always, a brand named Pancrease (see Glossary).

comes here [to the clinic] every once in awhile when she gets sick or some-thing. And she takes some pills too, but I don't remember what they're called. I don't read the labels or anything. She just takes them. She takes six pills at a time. I can only take one. The pancrease is to help digest the food.

"When she was littler, she got Ps [chest physical therapy]. That's what we called it. And she'd lie down on this thing. My mom would go push, push, push. And then she would go on the other side and go push, push, push. But she doesn't do that anymore. I'm not sure I know why. I would watch and like wow and see if—ask her if it was any fun, 'cause it was weird to see—bong, bong, bong. But she stopped, I think it was when she was eight or nine.

"One time she was sick. She had something wrong with her—I forget what it's called, but she had to come to the hospital for about a couple of weeks. It was frightening, but she came out, so—I was glad. That she doesn't get hurt a lot or anything. Like she might get like sicker and die or something because." Adam stopped for a moment, the word "because" holding his place.

"We were like, 'Where's Zoe?' 'She's at the hospital.' And then my mom and dad went there in the morning. I went to see her one time when she was in the hospital. And it was weird because she wasn't here [home]. When she got back everyone was happy and everything."

Jeremy also recalled Zoe's one hospitalization. "She was in the hospital for pneumonia. She had pneumonia. I gave it to her. I knew it because I had it before she did and she just got it. Sometimes I think it's my fault and it bothers me." Jeremy drew a deep breath and looked down for a moment. Looking up, he added, "Zoe told me she might be cured."

Zoe did not remember telling Jeremy about being cured or anything else for that matter. "They don't ask me [about CF]. When they were little they always asked Mom. I used to too, when I was small, but not now." However, Zoe has thought about the issue. "I think about it every day sometimes, almost every day—a way to cure it. People say that they are trying to cure CF, but it's hard though. I wonder if they could discover how they could get rid of cystic fibrosis and discover a new way. Now I have to take pills.

"At clinic I get more pills. I have to get more pills today—pancrease and sweat pills and Vitamin E. I need my pills to help digest my food. My CF has a hard time digesting my food. It just goes right through, and so my pills help stop and digest the food so I get energy and help keep up my work.

"The nebulizer helps me when I cough and my mom does PDs [chest physical therapy] on me. I have a PD board for PDs. I use it when I have a cough. Well, if my cough gets real bad, my mom starts doing PDs. And once when I was at the hospital, stayed there, I felt very sick and I threw up so I couldn't have the PDs. But I don't like the PDs. We have everything if I have a cough, but I don't cough anymore.

"You're born with it, the CF. Somebody can't catch it from me though. Nobody could catch it from me.

"I could get pneumonia and I'd have to go the hospital like I did for twelve days when I was out in first grade and my brothers' class and my class gave me flowers.

"If I get pneumonia I have to stay at the hospital. When I had pneumonia I had to stay in the hospital. I had pneumonia and I didn't like it. I had these shots, they killed," said Zoe pointing to her wrist. "It killed when they put it in. When I first got my shot it was all puffed up so I had to get another one and one fell out at night. And I had like nine of them. I got a lot of blood tests. Right when I got up I got one. I didn't even know.

"I had a roommate. Her name was Ariel. I don't know her second name though. My sister's name was Ariel. I used to have a sister who's dead. She died. She was very sick. I hadn't seen her before, only in a picture.

"When I have pneumonia I really get scared. I'm not sure if I'll get better. I hope it gets better. I know that when I have pneumonia I have to go to the hospital, but when people usually have pneumonia they stay at home, but I have CF pneumonia. But otherwise I'm the same. I play soccer and take gymnastics. Sometimes people have a lot of CF, but I don't."

Mr. Campbell's assessment of Zoe's condition was similar to her own. "It doesn't seem like she has a lot of lung involvement. She had the episode of viral pneumonia when she was real small, around when she was diagnosed, and then this last episode that was pretty bad, real bad and landed her in the hospital. But we just came to the conclusion that she's sick or she isn't sick. If she isn't sick, she doesn't cough up a lot of stuff and doesn't appear to be having a problem, so then we don't have to do the PDs and the nebulizer."

"The doctor recommended that we do," Mrs. Campbell interjected, "But I felt like why put her through this? It doesn't seem to be making any difference. I talked to Dr. Reese about it. I talked to Dr. Hasting about it. And there haven't been any studies made, from what they were saying, to show that it makes any difference."

"They just sort of say, well if it seems to be working for you, well just continue with the same thing. It is not something I want to do anyway. It takes a lot of time, effort. If we had to, we would. I'm not being lazy."

"It doesn't seem to make a difference. She rarely coughs anything up."

"I think when we got her out of the hospital the last time we were doing it twice a day for a while."

"Yeah, we kept up with it. I know at one point they had her on a 'bronchial dilator' and I put the dosage in they told me to use and she started to have the racing heart and it scared me half to death. So I called to be sure that I had put the right dosage in and I had. So from then on I didn't use it anymore. I used the other, with the white box, 'phener' or whatever it is. But I said, 'Why should she have this reaction at home?' And they said, well maybe the difference in equipment, what they use in the hospital and what we use here. I don't know if they gave the answer I was satisfied with, but I said I'm not using it anymore then. And at that point I think it was just kind of that she really didn't need it anymore. She wasn't wheezing anymore. Mainly we were just kind of gradually working her off it."

"The doctor in Alabama."

"Dr. Grossman," Mrs. Campbell filled in.

"Dr. Grossman I think it was. I think Dr. Reese's the same way he is. He's sort of 'Whatever works for you' kind of thing. Dr. Hasting, she was kind of the old strict . . ."

". . . Treat them all the same," Mrs. Campbell finished her husband's sentence. "But she was really not for nursery school for Zoe."

"Don't expose them."

"Yeah, don't expose them. Well, if you don't expose them, you're gonna expose them when they start kindergarten. What's the difference?"

"So I guess we tried to apply a little common sense; what we think is common sense. It may not be, but it's what we think it is. With the doctor's recommendations we kind of go from there."

"And work it into our lives. What works there."

"Of course I hope she continues to do well, and I think it's going to be tough, because she has been so active; if she does start having problems, it may be a little difficult for her to understand why she can't play soccer anymore, which I don't know if she'll want to continue to play soccer when she gets older."

"It may be field hockey."

"I hope she can stay active on her own. I know we've read some studies where they had CFers running and doing a certain amount of that kind of exercise and it seemed to help."

"It's very good for the lungs. That's done her as much good as postural drainage. I know there were times where she would run, be running the field, and she would bring a little bit [of mucus] up. Remember that?"

Mr. Campbell nodded in agreement.

"So it was like jarring it loose, running."

"You do her PDs on her when she's not sick and you just don't get anything out of her."

Mrs. Campbell laughed, "It's like you're beating on an empty drum."

"You can't seem to generate anything. So we didn't think it is necessary. When she is sick she coughs it up. When she starts having a cold or gets bronchitis or something we start her on the nebulizer."

"And the postural drainage," added Mrs. Campbell.

"Yes, the PDs. But she hasn't been sick for a while. So we haven't done it. She just takes her vitamins and her enzymes and that's about it."

"She's an active child. Soccer is a lot of running."

"We try to keep her involved in sports, the running, that type of thing and the soccer. She hasn't had any problems with it. Well, she had one problem with it."

"The first game, wasn't it?"

"Yeah, I think it was."

"It was 95-degree weather! Anyone could've. Her brother was pulled off too. It was just a lousy day. And the coach said, 'I probably shouldn't keep her in the whole game.' Because last year I guess we had to, I finally explained to him that she had cystic fibrosis. She probably could stand a breather in there, but he's evidently forgotten that, because she's one of the best players, so he's kept her in and she hasn't had any more episodes. So I think it was just the type of day it was.

"Zoe's got a good attitude about her CF. I mean she doesn't seem to be embarrassed about it. She's almost proud of it in some ways."

"Probably because she doesn't understand about it."

"Yeah, but she doesn't hesitate to tell kids about it."

"I don't think it has affected any of her friendships or anything like that, that I'm aware of. You never know what the parents are thinking about."

"Yeah. Well, we've done the postural drainage and she's had friends in that have watched her being beat up on."[4]

"Yeah. We've never tried to hide that."

"No."

"That's just the way it is. That's Zoe, and she's got cystic fibrosis."

"Yeah."

"And that's it. You're born with it and you got it and you're gonna have it, and so we're not gonna tell her friends not to come in because she's getting her PDs or anything like that."

"No. I think having a child like Zoe makes other children, your children, other children in the house, a little more aware of, accepting of, everybody, of children and adults that are different, physically or mentally different."

"Yeah, I agree with that too. It changes the way you look at other people. You accept the people for who they are."

"Some children never had the experience of being exposed to a different person or a different child, and they don't know how to handle themselves around them. They just don't. They don't know how to. They're really no different than they are, but," Mrs. Campbell's voice trails off. And then in full firm voice, "I'm glad we've got a cystic in the house!" With that exclamation she laughs.

"That's a big rationalization, that's for sure."

"Yeah," Mrs. Campbell smiled. Her expression once again serious, "When I

---

[4] Referring to the technique of cheast physical therapy, where all the lobes of the chest are pounded with cupped hands.

had polio I felt, 'kids are cruel.' They don't know how to treat you at the same level. I guess I was always self-conscious of being different and I didn't want Zoe to have to go through that. And I guess that's why I'm proud of the way that she's handling it, that she's so open and accepting."

"Yeah. I think we probably push the kids a little bit in the way that they treat other people."

"Kids are naturally curious, and I think it's important to explain to them, maybe after you're out of sight of that someone, to explain about what might have happened to that person."

"I think it may have affected a little bit the way that we treat the kids too, in terms of if they want something. Some things of course we say no, but if there is something special we usually say OK. Not to the point of spoiling them, but when they all make up their minds that they want a bike for Christmas, we usually come across with a bike."

Mr. and Mrs. Campbell laughed together.

"We don't give them any real big major disappointments, I don't think, without going overboard. Wouldn't you say?"

Mrs. Campbell nodded, "Yeah."

"Of course, maybe we would be that anyway, who knows?"

Mrs. Campbell raised her shoulders.

"But I think Zoe's made a difference in our life. I think it's for me a little more of the 'live now' kind of attitude. Sure we'll put money away and everything, but on the other hand sometimes you just say, 'We're gonna do it.' And we probably won't do as much as we could, but on the other hand I think we try to. I think it just makes us feel like we should live now rather than be very conservative in our lifestyle and plan for the future. I think it's one way that's gonna change my outlook on life."

"I think it kinda makes you appreciate life more when you have a special child."

———

Zoe came out of the room where they weighed the patients before the examination by the doctor. She walked right over to her mom. "I gained two pounds and grew an inch."

"You always do," Mrs. Campbell replied, withdrawing a pen and notebook from her purse. She jotted down the gains. "You're taller than your brothers."

"They said we could go in there now." Mrs. Campbell looked over to Zoe's brothers, who were sitting in the chairs, their eyes roaming about; she got up and went with Zoe into one of the examining rooms.

CHAPTER 6

The Reynoldses

(Individuals mentioned by name, in order of appearance)

Mrs. Deana Reynolds: Mother of Carl Reynolds
Mr. Craig Reynolds: Father of Carl Reynolds
Carl Reynolds: Five-year-old child with cystic fibrosis (CF)
Stuart Reynolds: Seven-year-old well brother of Carl Reynolds
Beverly: Playmate of Carl Reynolds
Thea Wright: Outpatient clinical nurse specialist

Mrs. Reynolds sat two seats away from her husband, she with an unopened book on her lap, he with the newspaper. The seats could have been filled by Carl and Stuart, but they were kneeling by the kindergarten- or coffee-table-size table (depending on your perspective) littered with very old magazines and toys of about the same condition.

"Carl, look there's your picture on the bulletin board," Mrs. Reynolds called, pointing to a newspaper clipping about Carl on the bulletin board across the room and behind him. Carl looked neither up nor back. He continued to fondle the plane he had taken from the pile of worn and broken toys in the center of the table. Her exclamation did not rouse Stuart either. Without looking at the screen, he fiddled with the dials on the old Etch-a-Sketch he had retrieved from the table.

A little girl, tall, but not more then three or four, walked into the waiting room with her parents. She came right over to the table. "What's your name?"

Neither of the boys answered.

She grabbed the plane Carl held. Now Carl was mobilized into action. He immediately got up and went over to his mother. "She took my plane," he whined.

Mrs. Reynolds responded with about the same degree of animation that Carl had displayed when she had called his attention to the bulletin board. "Go play with something else."

Carl went back to the table. Instead of taking another toy from the center of the table he tried to wrest the Etch-a-Sketch from Stuart. Stuart now firmly and rapidly twirled the knobs clockwise and counterclockwise, whipping them like window wipers on a car. Carl whined, "I want that." Stuart spread his body over the Etch-a-Sketch, but didn't lie on it. He continued to twirl the dials.

"I want it. Please can I have it?"

Stuart didn't answer. He didn't even look up.

"It's not fair. Please can I have it?"

Stuart still did not answer, his gaze fixed on the toy.

Carl now addressed his pleas to his mother, "I want that. Please. Can I have it? Why can't I have it?" He didn't wait between whines for a response. His mother continued to ignore his plaints.

"Carl, would you come with me to get weighed?" the nurse inquired as she approached the children's table.

Carl got up and followed the nurse in to be weighed. His mother was right behind him.

After Carl was weighed, mother and son returned to their positions. Carl knelt back down next to his brother and resumed whining about the Etch-a-Sketch. Mrs. Reynolds sat back down two seats away from her husband. She shook her head at him, "Carl has not gained any weight."

Carl finally gave up and went for a drink from the water fountain. When he returned to the table, Stuart handed him the Etch-a-Sketch.

Just as Carl started to fiddle with its dials, the little girl put down the plane and reached for the Etch-a-Sketch. As she reached out, her father swooped down and carried her off to change her diaper.

Carl fiddled with the Etch-a-Sketch no more intently than Stuart had before it had become an object of desire. He soon lost interest and put it back on the table as absentmindedly as his brother had first acquired it. Both he and his brother sat in silence.

The little girl bounded out of the room where she had been changed and quickly took the Etch-a-Sketch. Stuart's interest renewed, he tried to get it back from her. She mightily held it aloft and out of his reach. Once again her dad swooped down. While he spanked her, her mother took the toy from her daughter's hand and put it back on the table.

"Mom, Mom," Carl called to his mother repeatedly.

"Yes."

"Can you go to the car and get me a toy to play with?"

"Not right now Carl. We have to wait to see the doctor."

Carl looked down and pouted.

"OK." Mrs. Reynolds turned to her husband, "Honey could you go get Carl a toy?" Mr. Reynolds got up from his chair. Stuart followed him.

"Most of the time, especially in the summertime when they can play outside, they [Carl and Stuart] don't get along too badly. But in . . ."

"They have more good days than bad," Mr. Reynolds interjected.

"When they're cooped up they get at each other," explained Mrs. Reynolds.

"When Stuart's with Carl, with me, or with her by ourselves, he's fine; you couldn't want for a better kid. He'll do anything you ask him to. But when they're together, then it's a different Stuart. It's just like a Jekyll and Hyde."

Mr. and Mrs. Reynolds laughed.

"Stuart's basically a good kid," Mr. Reynolds continued, "But he just does some things to get attention. I don't know what else to say. He's a good kid, but he wants that attention."

"I'm trying to think of a sentence that would describe Stuart."

"Because he does. If you ask him to do something, he does it. He may not do it the way you want to do it, but he does it."

"Stuart wants to be in control of lots of situations. So, if you can learn to trick him into thinking he's in control of that situation and still doing what you want him to do, only having it his way, then . . ."

"It saves trouble."

"He's fine."

"He's Stuart."

"Stuart is Stuart. Stuart and I are the same, and Carl and Craig are the same. So I'm drawn to Carl like I am to you, dear." Mrs. Reynolds playfully smiled at her husband.

Mr. Reynolds smiled back. "Stuart is too much like her."

"I think there would be a difference between the way Stuart and I are and the way Carl and I are even if he didn't have the disease, just because." Mrs. Reynolds quietly searched. "Carl's easygoing," she found.

"Well, yeah. He's . . ."

"He's pretty mild-tempered until he's pushed too far, and then, he fights back."

"But he likes attention too. He'll do things to get Stuart in trouble; just to hear us holler, 'Stuart!' He's sneaky, a little. Isn't he?"

"But he does it in a cute way."

"Yeah, but he still does it."

"Which makes it . . . well, yeah. Yeah, he does it. But he can do the same thing that Stuart does and not get in trouble with it because of the attitude. The tone of voice is different."

"If that was Carl's drink there and he didn't want it, that'd be fine. But if Stuart wanted it, as soon as Stuart grabbed it, Carl would want it back."

"Oh, yeah. But I think that's normal."

"It's a rivalry I guess. But he's slick at it. It's hard to get mad at him."

"He just does it in such a cute way. He grins, and his eyes sparkle. When Stuart does things the horns show; instead of smiling and being cute." Mrs. Reynolds paused. "Well Stuart goes through spells where he seems to be more jealous than others. I guess, though, that Carl never acts like he's jealous about Stuart." Mrs. Reynolds turned to her husband, "What do you think?"

"Can't think of anything. But they have their days where nothing neither one of them does suits the other one. But, I'd say it's four to one. They have four good days to one bad day. At least four to one. But they have always played outside. We have a big sandbox and they'll play in there. Well, they used to. Now they have bikes and stuff to ride. But they used to play in there for three or four hours at a time. And then other days, they couldn't play in there for five minutes."

"Can't even look at each other," Mrs. Reynolds added. "Like the day Carl came to the hospital. That was a day. Nothing suited either one of them. And I was on edge. And when I'm on edge things tend to be even worse. Or maybe I just react.

"And sometimes it's hard for me too when Carl's doing real well. I just sit there and look at him and think, 'Your insides are not right. The insides of you are not working right.'" Mrs. Reynolds shook her head as if shaking off the thought.

"Often times I think," she continued, "that it [CF] does add extra stress. Sometimes when I hear other parents talk about their kids, it really doesn't sound like Stuart's problems are added to by Carl's disease, but . . ."

"I don't think the problem is, but some of the attention is."

"I still have to think it does."

"A result of it."

"Because times when Carl's sick, all the phone calls are, 'How's Carl?' Everybody who sees Stuart, 'How's your brother doing?' And all the presents. Carl gets all the presents. It has to have some kind of effect on him [Stuart]. Like the last time Carl was in the hospital, my mother-in-law dropped off a box of toys, presents to bring down to Carl. And she didn't stay. She just came in and she didn't ask how Carl was making out. She didn't ask me if I was tired, nothing about me, how I was feeling. Nothing about Craig, how he was making out. Nothing to do with coping with any of the things. No concern about how Stuart was handling any of it.

"She gave Stuart a present and we were invited to go over to one of the sisters' houses for cake and ice cream for her birthday. And I said I didn't think we were going to come because Stuart wanted to go to the movies and for a present, for him. And I felt that he and I needed to do something, just the two of us. But I would give him the option. If he wanted to go to the party, then that's what we would do.

"Well, he wanted to go to the mall, to the movies. And I don't think they really even understood that, because when I told her I said, 'Well, Stuart is a little put out because of all the presents so we are going shopping to get him something and to just do a little something special for him.' And she goes, 'Well, OK.' And it was like no compassion."

"So we do try to keep our minds on Stuart a little bit," Mr. Reynolds added, "so we don't shut him out completely. But every now and then you forget."

"And even though you want to do maybe what you truly would want to do, there's things you can't."

"Yeah."

"Although when Carl was in the hospital when Stuart was in kindergarten, and the teacher asked each child to tell what they were thankful for at Thanksgiving; Stuart said that he was thankful for his brother coming home from the hospital.

"Oh, I can feel it coming now," a smile came to Mrs. Reynolds's lips, "there's hope yet for Stuart." Mr. and Mrs. Reynolds both laughed.

"Seriously," Mrs. Reynolds continued, "I think it must be tough for Stuart. I can't imagine if my sister had a disease like that. I mean it's bad enough that Carl has it, but this is a mother-and-son type thing; but for siblings and to be close in age. But in the same respect, Stuart's pretty protective of him. Different people have said that when they're out some place that he's protective as far as, 'Did you take your enzymes Carl?' And when Carl coughs, Stuart sometimes kind of guards him and doesn't fuss over him and doesn't make any kind of explanation, but he's there.

"And sometimes Carl will have to leave the table and go to the bathroom because if he's eating, he'll throw up. And I don't go with him right away. I wait 'til he's done and then I go in because I have to see what's there. But we try not to, 'Oh Carl!' He hates that. He really does. He tries to suppress it."

"And it doesn't bother Stuart. He doesn't say, 'Well there he goes again.'"

"And Stuart was so proud to be trick or treating for cystic fibrosis. He said, 'Because that's what my brother has.'"

"It goes in stages too."

"Yeah, it does," Mrs. Reynolds agreed. "Sometimes I know Stuart resents that Carl gets to stay up later if we've missed his therapy in the daytime; we do it at night. Sometimes we do give in and let Stuart stay up too until Carl's finished, just because it is hard to put Stuart to bed."

"Well it's usually only for ten minutes. We go upstairs and get ready for bed and we forget his mist. So Stuart goes to bed and Carl goes back down, does his mist, and it's only for ten minutes. And Stuart's asleep before we get back upstairs. But he's still had to go to bed."

"And he'll say, 'Well, Carl's going to watch TV.' Or even if Carl's asleep, he'll still say, 'Well, Carl's downstairs.' 'Well yes, Stuart, he's asleep.' It doesn't matter. That doesn't matter. Just the fact that Carl's not going to bed.

"And when Stuart is sick, when he has a cold, maybe he needs to do the mist, maybe he needs the vaporizer. He stresses for some attention when he just has a little cold. So I try to make a bigger thing out of a little cold for him. I maybe let him stay home an extra day, if he acts like he has a cold.

"Sometimes he likes to create sickness and hurts—'Oh my leg hurts'— because he gets attention for that. He's already walked with crutches. People would say, 'Oh Stuart, what happened to you?' Or he'd wrap his leg with an

Ace bandage because then people would say, 'What happened to your leg?' And that was real important to him.

"Stuart does react to things, not so much now, but when he was smaller. I think he reacted the way he did to certain stimulus because he got attention. And he didn't get the same kind of attention Carl did."

"Carl sits on her lap for two hours a day while we pound him. And Stuart's on the floor or something. He's watching TV. He doesn't sit there and stare at us and bawl or anything, but it has to affect him. Carl's being held and he's not."

"Plus," Mrs. Reynolds added, "Carl's more lovable as far as he wants you to hug him and kiss him and he likes you to sit holding him. Stuart doesn't. He's not into hugging. As a matter of fact, I have to wrestle with him to hug him. And I think he fights me because the more he fights me the more I am going to hug."

"Well I think some of that is from . . ."

"That, attention," Mrs. Reynolds finished the sentence.

"We've always held Carl, and Stuart kinda got slid aside."

"Yeah, 'cause when Carl . . ."

"We didn't put it, 'Now you go away while I do this.' But to him it had to look that way. He was only two, he wasn't quite two."

"He was two years and three months old," Mrs. Reynolds clarified, "when we started doing Carl's therapy."

"Yeah, so . . ."

"So from the very beginning when we were doing Carl's therapy, we tried to explain as much as, give him some kind of explanation. But, I refused to stop to get him his drink or do anything like that. If Stuart got demanding while Carl was getting his therapy I just said, 'Whoa, you can't do this. You'll have your time when we're done.' If it would have been maybe a once-a-week type therapy situation, I maybe wouldn't have been like that, but it wasn't. So now he doesn't even question. He doesn't."

"But now the tides have turned a little bit, 'cause when it's time to do Carl's therapy, Stuart goes outside to play and Carl has to stay in."

"Yeah. When Carl was little, like eighteen months, two years old, we made Stuart come in too. Then we made the other kids that were there playing come in the house until Carl was done with his therapy. Well now, Carl's gotten kind of, 'Well, I'm not doing my therapy if they won't come in.' But yet, he'll waste more time arguing about it than doing it.

"And when he does come in, then it's kind of a hassle to get him to do it. And I think, 'Well now he's old enough to know that if he cooperates and gets it done, the kids will wait for him. But if he's going to fart around, there's no sense in making the kids wait.' So then I let the kids go back out to play and then he has a fit. But I let him. I figure that's one thing . . ."

"A learning process," Mr. Reynolds put in.

"He's got to learn."

"Carl's stubborn. He's going to have it his way."

"Who knows? Maybe he's figured, even though he's basically, as I said, an 'easy-going' personality, when it comes to something like that, I think he probably figures—well, I've already lost, the kids are already outside, now I'll make Mom or Dad be miserable." Mrs. Reynolds laughed.

"It seems that way," Mr. Reynolds smiled.

"Certainly, because he doesn't gain anything from it because he knows we're going to do it. We don't give in. He knows he's going to get pounded, one way or the other. One end or the other," she smiled.

"Carl's stubborn."

To Stuart, "Carl's neat. He's funny. He makes pig oink oink noises and stuff like that. I play with Carl the most of anybody. He's fun to play with. We play basketball. I'm a good basketball player. And we play soccer and stuff like that. In the summertime mostly we have our fan on and we play in our room. Sometimes we have Matchboxes [matchbox-size vehicles] and we make roads with blankets. Then we get the Matchboxes and play. Sometimes Mom takes us to the mall with our money and we get to buy Transformers.

"But now I'm trying to save up my money for our horses. Carl and I haven't used our money yet. We're trying to save it for our horses. That's what I'm saving it for. Gram pays us 'cause I drive the 1086 [tractor]. They put a bucket on it. The men came over and they picked the pumpkins. We disk the pumpkins off the plants so it's easy to pick them up without pulling them off [the plant]. And then I drive the tractor down the rows, a couple of rows. Then we get it up and dump it in a big trailer. I can't do that. Mom has to do it. I got hit in the head once. I fell off the bucket. I fell off the tractor and came down and hit my head.

"My mom's fun too. We get in the swimming pool. We swim laps. My dad gets in with us and swims laps with us too. Carl even swam a couple of laps with us once. Carl and I get in with Dad after work and we get in there and we swim laps. Carl's not that good. I teach him how to dive and stuff.

"Sometimes I get to pound Carl. I help my mom pound Carl. My mom usually does it in the morning and when he gets really sick sometimes in the evening. But he usually gets them in the morning. I just usually sit and watch. Sometimes I do the mist too. My mom teaches me how to do stuff."

"Stuart's learned just from us talking about it," Mrs. Reynolds would explain. "In the very beginning, even when he was only two, when Carl was diagnosed, we told Stuart, because he needed to know. Well, all I could do was cry. I would say for the first two weeks that's all I did. And Stuart kept telling me, 'I'm sorry Mommy.'

"He didn't know why I was crying. So, I was trying to explain from the very beginning. Stuart would probably never be able to remember learning about CF. It's going to be like riding a bike."

"Or walking."

"Stuart will never be able to remember not pounding Carl. Because, he was little enough and that way, I'm glad they're close in age. We've always pounded Carl and that's all he's grown up to know.

"So, we just kinda told him as it goes on. And certain circumstances require explanations or whatever, then you tell him.

"I think Stuart knows that it's serious. I don't think he can absorb that statistics-wise, Carl's only got a 50 percent chance of being twenty. I don't think he can understand that, but I think he knows that we have to take care of him. That he has to take care of himself—learn, if it's cold out, you wear a coat. I think he understands that much of it. He knows that he has to eat good and he'll . . ."

"He knows his [Carl's] enzymes too," Mr. Reynolds interjected.

"Yeah, he knows and he understands that if he [Carl] doesn't take the enzymes, that he's going to have diarrhea, which means that food just went right through him. He understands that. They understand what the enzymes are. When I say 'they,' I've told Carl, but I'm not sure if he can actually understand. But I have explained that this is what is in your system, only Carl doesn't have that. He has to have this pill. So, if he doesn't take it, his food is not going to do him a bit of good. I'm hoping that way it's going to be a very natural thing to remember the enzymes, and not remember every four hours I have to take a pill. Sometimes, you forget that. But, if you understand that this enzyme is doing the job that my body doesn't have.

"I really think Stuart remembers that 'cause he's told different people when Carl was at their house, 'Don't forget Carl's enzymes.' He's kind of protective in that way. He'll tell them.

"And he understands that Carl has to cough. And of course, he's seen the mucus. And I've explained when we butcher our turkeys. I've been able to pull the whole lung out and say, 'This is your lung.'

"Stuart took it to school with him. He put it in water. If you look really close, you can see the little air sacs. Well these air sacs get plugged up with all that junk in Carl's lungs and that's what makes him sick.

"And I showed Stuart the mucus and the thick junk that's in it. He'll go 'Oh yuck! Is that in his [Carl's] lungs?' And I tried to explain where it is and why we pound him. Or he'll look at it and he'll say, 'Euww, that's what the color is?'

"And the color of bowel movements have always been a real topic of conversation in our house. So even for Stuart now, that's a big thing. Even his own, he has to tell me what color it is. He'll say, 'I think I might have diarrhea, it was yellow.' The kid's never had diarrhea in his life," Mrs. Reynolds chuckled.

"So I think because we're so aware and in tune with what Carl's things are like," Mrs. Reynolds continued, "Stuart feels, 'Nobody cares what my poop looks like.' Or these other important things."

"He never talks about it, but the way he acts, you can tell it bothers him. You can tell something eats at him. But, he doesn't say anymore, 'Well, Carl did this and . . .'"

"Speaking of pooping," Mrs. Reynolds interrupted, "Remember when Carl told us he wished he could be Stuart? 'Then I wouldn't have to do PT [chest physical therapy].' And Stuart said, 'You wouldn't want my problem.'"

"Oh yeah. That's right," Mr. Reynolds recalled. "Stuart does call pooping in his pants his problem."

Later, Stuart himself would say, "I was born with it."

"Stuart understands a lot. But I don't think that he understands that you can die from CF."

"No," Mrs. Reynolds agreed.

"Stuart treats it [CF] like it's no big deal. He just takes the pills and he's going to be better."

"Carl too."

"Well, both of them."

"Yeah."

"As long as he takes his enzymes there's no problem. Once in a while he may catch a cold and get sick, come to the hospital, but . . ."

"One time Stuart asked me if Carl was going to die. One time, I'm trying to remember if it was when he was in the hospital one time or, I just don't remember. And I told him, 'Yeah, someday.' And I said, 'So are you someday.' So, we didn't discuss it. We didn't drum on it anymore because we don't dwell on that. You know it's reality, but we don't talk about it. So for Stuart it's just Carl has a disease that he takes enzymes for, and sometimes he gets sick, and sometimes he has to be in the hospital, but that's as far as it goes."

"He has gunk in his lungs, that needs pounding out."

"Yeah."

"That's about it, I think."

"Yeah, I think that's probably it. And I think at his age that's probably all he can understand."

"Yeah."

"But," Mrs. Reynolds rejoined, "since the movie [*Alex*], Stuart has asked me if Carl is going to die. And from kids at school, I think some kids at school had watched the movie and then asked him. I don't know what he told them. He didn't tell me, and I only found out from the teacher because the teacher asked me if he watched it. I sent a note to her the day after the movie to say, 'He didn't watch it. Please don't talk about it.' And so she didn't, but she asked me then because she knew these other kids were talking about it.

"I told him that people do die from having CF, but that Carl has been really healthy so far and that with all the new research and all the new medicines and everything that we just didn't think about that. But that yes, it is a possibility, and that's why sometimes he doesn't understand why I say, 'No, Carl can't go out to play in the mud puddles because it's raining.' And different things like that; because of catching colds and that sort of thing.

"I try to use those times to explain to him why I make the choices that I make sometimes. And he seemed to accept that answer and he's never brought it up again.

"But Stuart did ask me not too long ago if they could watch the movie, 'cause the tapes are right there. I let them put in the cartoon tapes and that sort of stuff themselves. I don't know where Craig has since put the tape of *Alex*.

"When he asked me if they could watch it, I told him that it was a story about a little girl that had CF, that died, and that it's a real sad story. And her disease was a lot worse than Carl's. And that I just didn't think any of us were ready to watch it.

"A neighbor called me that night after the movie, just to see how I was. And Craig and I did not handle the end of that movie well at all. I'm glad that we didn't have anybody else in the house to share that with, 'cause we just needed to cry and not . . ." Mrs. Reynolds didn't finish the sentence. "I mean, I guess we and everybody else that I know saw Carl in that movie; anybody that knew Carl, that is.

"And so this girlfriend called to see how I was, and I needed that. And other people called or other people asked me then and my answer was always that it was such an impact because now I felt like I had a different aspect of the disease to deal with. And I know that's a possibility, but I don't want to learn to deal with that. I don't. When the time comes, if Carl gets sick and that's the answer, then I'll deal with it." Mrs. Reynolds laughed anxiously. "There's too many other things that you have to deal with 'til you get to that point. And as long as the child is being really pretty healthy, you don't need to think about that part of it.

"The book was sad, but watching it on TV and knowing that that was a real story, and knowing that the movie followed, so many movies don't follow a book or the real story line, but that movie did. I had the book in my hands while the movie was on and during commercials I would check up on things. And it did work, almost word-for-word. It really did match as far as that goes. But I've wondered if it had the impact on other families that it had on us?"

According to Stuart, "My mom taped *Alex* and I want to see it. I want to see how she died and stuff. But my mom hasn't let us watch it yet." Stuart shook his head in disappointment. With renewed brightness he claimed, "Some people are trying to make a potion that stops cystic fibrosis. I saw it on TV. Carl was born with it. You can't breathe through your nose, 'cause you can only breathe through one side of your nose.[1] Some people die because of it.

"Sometimes I think about that Carl is going to die. Mom had a dream once. There were these people that wanted to adopt Carl and Dad said, 'Oh sure you can adopt him.' I wouldn't like that. I wouldn't feel very happy. I would deck my dad. I really don't want to lose my brother 'cause he's fun."

"And with Carl," Mrs. Reynolds would explain, "he knows the name of it. He knows the same way, looking at the lung [of the turkey]. I say, 'This is a lung. Right here is your lung. And this is . . .' It [turkey lung] really does look very similar and you can see the branches and everything."

"Blood vessels and stuff."

"And, how much of it he [Carl] absorbs, I don't know. Enough that he doesn't ask questions. He knows. He'll even say, 'I can't go down to Beverly's today 'cause she's sick.' So, we don't try to really draw him out a lot, but he needs to try and learn."

"But he knows that if somebody's sick, or somebody's smoking he's supposed to get away from them."

"And we try to too. . ."

"Stuart said that too," Mr. Reynolds pointed out.

"Stress the germs as far as, 'You [Carl] better wash your hands right now because that had germs on it and if those germs get in your lungs, they might make the other germs grow.' And he understands that he needs to grow and to gain weight. Although, it doesn't make him want to eat any more."

Carl would say that, "With CF you start coughing and sometimes you have to get sick sometimes too. You have to kind of throw up too and do all that stuff. And you have to take pills—vitamin pills and purple pills. And there's my therapy. There's a machine that I have to breathe in ten times. And then my mom does PT [chest physical therapy]." Carl paused and compared, "My brother doesn't cough and throw up and all that."

"No, just Carl does," Mrs. Reynolds would corroborate. "Carl goes in spells where he coughs up a lot."

"Three times in a week," Mr. Reynolds noted. "That's about normal too."

"Yeah, but you know, he also goes through spells where he throws up a couple times a day. Remember?"

"Yeah, well . . ."

"Where, geez, he's throwing up every time. It kinda depends. If he's eating and gets a bad coughing spell he'll throw up."

"And then he's done eating."

"And then he won't finish."

"He won't finish," Mr. Reynolds reiterated.

---

[1] A reference to nasal polyps, which many children with CF, including his brother, have.

"But he throws up easy."

"First time, I didn't feel like eating after he was done." Mr. and Mrs. Reynolds both laughed.

"Kinda ruins the . . ."

"But he needs to go back and finish something, and he won't. And he'll get indignant about that."

"Meals get to be a battle ground with him. We even made a video to show him how bad it was."

Stuart also would comment on family mealtimes. "Carl usually doesn't eat everything, but I do. Sometimes, when we have ice cream my mom says, 'You're not going to get any ice cream unless you eat.' He says, 'I don't want any ice cream.' And then at midnight, he wakes up in the middle of the night and goes over and says, 'Mom, I'm hungry.' She says, 'Go to sleep.' Sometimes when Carl stays up in the night he goes down and eats some more supper or a candy bar or something like that."

Carl would just say, "I like to eat a lot."

"You have to try and work the eating with the coughing," Mrs. Reynolds would explain.

"With the treatments, an hour before eating, which we don't always wait. An hour after the therapy. We don't always wait an hour, but we never pound him after he's eaten."

"No, and after he eats a big meal we try to make him be quiet for twenty minutes or so."

"Yeah, go over and play with his cars or something."

"Play quietly instead of racing around, because that sometimes will make him cough."

Stuart knew the rules, "After dinner Carl's supposed to sit down and rest a little. So I sit down with him and rest, and in twenty minutes we're allowed to go play."

"Mealtimes are hard," Mrs. Reynolds would reiterate. "Like sometimes when Carl says the blessing; he'd never say that he'd wish they'd find a cure for CF, but he wished he didn't have it. And it gets you thinking." Mrs. Reynolds looked down in a moment of silence.

Once Stuart had remarked, "I wish Carl wouldn't have CF. It's sad."

Mrs. Reynolds picked up her head. "I guess my first thoughts are that it is fatal. It's always uppermost in my mind."

"It's pretty much the first thing," Mr. Reynolds agreed. "Not when you're talking to somebody, but when I look at him and think, 'Some day he's going to die.'

"Yeah, and I often think, 'Geez I don't want it [death] to be at this age. I don't want it to be at this age.' I try to picture, because even now, Carl's older and he has more friends and I think, 'Oh geez, you know, in another five years he's going to have that many more friends.' And I don't think any parent wants to lose a child before they die."

"Now I could arrange that," Mr. Reynolds quipped, trying to lift the pall. Mrs. Reynolds laughed for a moment too.

"I think that's probably the first thought," she finished.

"Or something will come that will remind me of it," Mr. Reynolds added. "Or he'll do something funny and I'll think, 'Well, how many more years is he going to do something funny?' But I kinda lock things out of my mind. And I just go day to day, don't think too far down the road. Now she's not like that."

"No, I don't. I'm worse when he's [Carl's] worse. When he's sick, when he's starting to catch a cold, then that's it. Then I start thinking, 'Geez how many more colds? What so far has happened to your lungs and to your heart to make the progression worse?'

"I try not to dwell on it. I don't want to or I'll make myself a basket case."

"She'll lay at night and just think of this and that."

"Yeah. My mind just races from one thing to another. I've already pictured him laying in a casket and thinking, 'Oh God! How am I going to handle that?' I guess I do look ahead if I think, 'How am I going to handle that?'"

"Well, I thought of that when Carl was in to have his tonsils out. I went to work that morning and couldn't do anything. I had knots in my stomach, and I said to the boss, 'I'm going to Philly.' And I sat there and I thought, 'His tonsils are out, but God what if he dies or something?'"

"I was glad you came."

"I just got in the car and left."

"He just walked in the room."

"And I told her if he goes [to surgery] at noon to call at my mom's house, and if he doesn't, call home. I was going home early and I'd call her if I didn't hear." Mr. Reynolds looked at his wife. "So I think about it, but I don't dwell on it."

"It," echoed Mrs. Reynolds. "Even at first when we thought about what happens to Carl we considered having more children, just so Stuart wouldn't have to be alone. But then we decided that's really not a good reason to have more children. So we're not."

"Plus the 25 percent."

"Right, the risk is too high. But I think about Stuart. I certainly know; I shouldn't say I know. But I try to imagine how I'd feel if something happened to my sister. And so someday Stuart may have to face that. But then I think, 'Geez, you know, there are a lot worse things.' Being in the hospital makes you realize that. There are a lot of worse things. You pick up the paper and there is always a kid being killed in a crash or whatever.

"I think you always have to think of that and be thankful for what we do have. We've been so thankful he's not been that sick. He's been pretty healthy I think."

"Yeah, he's been good."

"Even though he's been in the hospital five times."

"Yeah."

"He's five years old. So that's once a year. But the times he's been in it's just to be tuned up. It's not been a drastic thing."

"Nothing like these other kids," Mr. Reynolds pointed out.

"And sometimes when I do see the other CF kids that are here, it scares me a little bit 'cause I think, 'Oh gee, I don't want Carl to have to be on oxygen.' Or if I see the older kids and they're not doing well, then that brings me down a little bit. I try to think he's only been in here five times and it's not been real serious each time, but have those five times been enough to start the progression? Have his lungs progressed enough back? Maybe his outlook isn't quite as bright as somebody who has not been in the hospital for those five years. But, you never know. We just take care of him the best that we can. We've only maybe ever, well we've never gone a day without pounding him. We've maybe had a few days where we've only done it once.

"I'd like to know what it's like to have two kids and not have to do that. Sometimes I lay in bed and I pretend, 'Gee, if I didn't have to pound on him today, what all would we do?'"

"Well, just like when we were leaving Carl's room to go down for surgery. I guess that kid in the next bed wanted his candy. So we just gave him his candies. Well now, if somebody did that to Carl, he'd have to have an enzyme. He can't eat anything without an enzyme. So, there's enzymes in all our coats and pockets and glove compartments and just all over. Only twice in the five years we've gone to, well, Grove City is our big town to go to to shop, and only twice we've gone out to supper and forgot enzymes."

"Twice?"

"Yeah."

"I don't remember that."

"It was twice, both in Grove City."

"So, whenever we get ready for a trip the last thing we say, 'Do we have Carl's enzymes?'"

"If we have his enzymes and medicines we can do without everything else."

"And money," Mrs. Reynolds laughed. "Sometimes we add money, but . . ."

"Well we like to take our credit cards," Mr. Reynolds joked back before Mrs. Reynolds could finish her thought.

"Enzymes—always—if we're going. After you've packed and you're kinda going through your mind, 'Do I have this? Do I have that? Do I . . .' As we get in the car, as long as we have the enzymes we kinda . . ."

"And his mist machine [nebulizer]."

"And even that, you can always pound him."

"Yeah."

"So, I don't know what it would be like not to have to do that. But," Mrs. Reynolds paused, "I don't think about the CF while I'm pounding him. I just do it."

"Pound him."

"Unless he's sick; then I think."

"There's been a lot of times I've seen sick kids and I think, 'Boy, Carl's lucky.' Or, 'We're lucky Carl's this good.'"

"But, at the same time I see kids that aren't sick and the parents are 'scuzzy' and they're not taking care of their kids and I just get so bitter."

"Yeah."

"I just look at them and think, 'Ohhh . . .'"

"OK, Carl, it's your turn now," Thea smiled.

Mrs. Reynolds stood up and looked back over her shoulder. Mr. Reynolds and Stuart were just coming back into the waiting room. They followed Mrs. Reynolds and Carl into the examining room.

CHAPTER 7

The Chases

(Individuals mentioned by name, in order of appearance)

JASON CHASE: Nine-year-old child with cystic fibrosis (CF)
MRS. PEGGY CHASE: Mother of Jason Chase
LOUISE CHASE: Twelve-year-old well sister of Jason Chase
REGAN CHASE: Eleven-year-old well sister of Jason Chase
MR. VICTOR CHASE: Father of Jason Chase
YASMINE: Friend of Regan Chase
ADELE: A girl the well sisters met on vacation
TESS: Friend of Louise Chase
YVETTE: Cystic fibrosis poster child
ELYSE: Friend with cystic fibrosis
MARGOT: Friend with cystic fibrosis
NATE: Deceased friend

JASON and his mom walked back to their seats in the waiting room from the Pulmonary Function Lab. Jason couldn't seem to stop coughing. "Everybody hates my coughing."

"Well, I wouldn't put it that way exactly."

"They do."

"Well, look at this way: Maybe you'll have to come in [be hospitalized], and you like that."

"Yeah, no more Louise."

"Jason!"

"Well, she's been a real pain."

"Jason, she's uncomfortable."

"Big deal, she broke her leg."

"It's hard for her to get around with the cast and all."

"Well, Regan hates her too."

"I what?" Regan questioned, catching the end of the conversation, as Jason and their mom sat down.

"You hate Louise."

"Well . . ."

"You fight a lot. You're always . . ."

Before Jason could finish, Mrs. Chase put an end to the discussion. "OK you two. That's enough."

Jason coughed some more. His mother glanced over at him. He looked much thinner than he had last summer, before they all took off on a family camping trip together.

"Every year we go camping for about two weeks," Regan began. "Me, my brother, my sister, all sleep in this brown tent. My mom and dad sleep in the green tent, and the PT [physical therapy] table goes in the green tent. It's a real big tent. It's like an eight-bed, or no—a ten-bed. The PT table goes in the big tent. They have big, big floats. They're like little fluffy floats they sleep on. And the clothes and that stuff goes in the big tent, the sheets and the lamp and all that.

"See, my brother gets kind of sick. He's gotta be out [not in the tent or around the campground], so usually we spend most of the day at the shore. And he gets his machine [nebulizer treatment] more often, like three times a day, when we go camping. Because he has allergies. And sometimes, not all the time, it's just sometimes, after it rains, it gets all like, sick. It's gross.

"It always rains at least once. And whenever it rains, my brother, his allergies start acting up, and he starts wheezing, and then he gets the machine like four times a day. Usually when we go to the shore, he gets it in the morning, the machine, once. Most of all he gets the machine. And when we come back from the shore he'll get his machine. And at night he'll get it.

"Usually this vacation is mostly for my dad, because he loves camping. He used to go all the time. But me and my sister, we just go. It's for two weeks, is all we go. We look forward to it and then we have to leave.

"We usually try to meet a lot of friends. Like this year, oh God, I could have killed my sister. See, there was this girl, Yasmine, that we met two years ago, and this other girl, she didn't look like her, but my sister thought she did—look like this girl we met two years ago. And she goes up—she thought she was this girl—she goes, 'Is your name Adele?' She goes, 'No.' They were up on the slide together. See, there's a lake and then there's a slide. And they go out; it's like a water slide, you get into a lake. And she goes down, she slides down. And so my sister tells me to go and start talking to her. And so she had a lot of friends, she had like all these friends; oh, my God. Since we met her, we had a lot of friends. And this year I think was the best year, and we didn't really want to go. Sometimes we look forward to leaving because it usually is getting kind of boring, but this year we didn't want to go.

"And my sister got her first boyfriend. She had her last boyfriend, too. She met him, but she doesn't have any now. And she met him there. And she was just Tess's friend, that's her name [the one she addressed as Adele]. And then they were going out the last night. It was pretty good, because it was the last night.

"They exchanged things to my sister. A couple days ago she sent her a letter in the mail, wrapped in an M&M package, because she just got done eating M&Ms, and she wrote a letter, and she stuck it in the M&M thing, and she put it in an envelope. She's strange.

"And, well usually when we go, we go to the shore all day, and we come back. It's good, because usually we have little activities every night. Like, every day they have volleyball games, and baseball games, and miniature golf games, because it's like a whole big activity. And they have scavenger hunts every once a week. And they have a Halloween party once; only once, though. We were lucky enough to come on the time they were having a Halloween party. They have movies once a week. No, wait. They have movies every night, usually they're not good movies, but sometimes they are. Like the only movie we really went to see was *Mr. Mom*, but we saw that already, so we left early. They had an ice cream parlor. They have a snack bar, we call it an ice cream parlor because we go in there every night to get ice cream. And they have a store and a lake. And then they also have a place where you go fishing, it's either in the lake or deeper in the forest there's a place to go fishing. And there's bike hikes. It's pretty neat. We used to bring our TV, but we don't anymore, because my dad says we watch it too much. Whenever we're bored, we turn on the TV.

"And besides we have a lot of stuff to go camping. We have the tent that me and my brother and sister sleep in. We have the tent that my mom and dad sleep in. We have, we get a screen tent which we put all our stuff in. We have a bunch of chairs. We have a couple hammocks. We have a lot of stuff for camping, and it's sorta fun.

"Usually we stay up late there. We stay up to 1:00 in the morning, not knowing what time it is, because you don't have a watch. Well, we do have a watch, but usually we don't really look at it, because, my mom, well, one year my mom's watch stopped and we had no idea what time it was and we stayed up late.

"When we go to the shore, we make, we eat lunch there. We spend the whole day at the shore. We drive there. It's only like five miles [from the campground], because we don't like the lake. We used to like the lake, but then Jason's allergies started acting up because it got 'scuzzy.' It used to be clean and then the thing stopped working. It was like a windmill. What are those things called?" Regan paused for a moment.

"Anyway, it was a lake and then at the end there was a barn house, only it's not a barn house. In the middle of the lake, at the very edge where the animals—well, where the frogs are, and there's this thing that used to turn around. I forget what it's called. It carries water. What's it called? I forget."

Regan thought out loud. "It's not a windmill. I forget. It just turns around.

Well, that stopped working. And when that worked, when that spun the water around, it put it, it goes through the house and makes it clean. But that stopped working and now the lake, like ooh.

"So we don't go there anymore. Every once in a while we'll go there and just me and my sister alone, without Jason. But I usually don't because I don't like to get 'scuzzy.' And Louise comes back and she takes a really good shower. The showers are too cold sometimes, and sometimes they're too hot, but you can't control them. Only, there's a bathroom and a shower. Well there's a bathhouse and a showerhouse. If you go in there, there'll be one shower and the shower is good, you can control it. But it's usually taken. And if you go into the other showers it's like a string you pull.

"It's nice though. That's why we like it a lot. The only thing bad is the lake, but we don't go to the lake. We go to the shore. Oh, and we always have people visit us. So we were at home [at the campsite]. We were eating lunch at home, at camp. So anyway the trash people came and Louise saw a bag and she didn't look in it. She thought there was trash in it. And she just said, 'Here! Wait!' And she just threw it in. And it was my brother's pills. And my dad had to go to the trash dump, and he had to find them. And my mom had to get all new prescriptions for all new pills that we needed. And my mom's like, 'Louise, he could have died! Why didn't you bother to check?' And so she got in big trouble.

"And my dad found them. And he also found ten dollars. And he found them, and he came back, and they were still sort of good because it was only an hour, I guess.

"So my mom just gave him them. They were good because they were all in a bottle, but just the bottle got sort of disgusting. But he had to take them until, it was like the next about two days later, we got the other prescriptions [those in the bag and not in bottles] and everything was fine.

"But Louise felt bad. She was like, 'I'm sorry. I didn't know.' She kept on apologizing. And she got in trouble. My mom yelled at her. And the friend who came [the one they were waiting for], well, she started saying how it was her fault, even though it wasn't. She was just trying to cover up.

"See, my mom was real worried because we didn't have the money to pay for it [to replace the medications]. Well, we did sort of. We had a thousand dollars to go on vacation. That's a lot. And it costs a lot just to stay there. She had the money, but we had to cut out stuff. See, that year we would have gotten a little bit crazier than we usually do, like buy more stuff, but we had to cut out on spending. When we went, my mom thought we were going to go shopping a lot. But we wasted practically all the money on the prescription. I don't know how much we had left. All I know, all I remember is my mom stopping to get her check and she says, 'Look at it! A thousand dollars.' Like, oh my God, we're going to spend all that. And then we wasted a lot of the money on the prescription. But it was worth it. I guess.

"It was my brother. I mean, my mom said he could've died. And even if we went home [to get more pills] there was still no pills, because we took a lot of the pills with us. And it was sorta worth it because it [the vacation] lasted longer [than if we had to go home and get the pills].

"See, in the summer I have to stay in a lot and babysit my brother, because we had a babysitter and my mom liked her at first, but then she saw that all she did was watch MTV and let us take care of ourselves; send us down to the Dairy Queen and watch soap operas. So she decided to have me watch Jason because my sister watches my cousin a lot.

"When my brother gets sick, my sister gets to stay home and watch him. When my mom has to work and my dad has to work, that is. She'll miss a day at school, usually only like one a week, whenever he's sick. It's usually only once, because my mom usually gets somebody, my grandmom, but sometimes she doesn't, she can't.

"When Jason gets sick he gets very sick. Like if it would be for me a normal cold, like maybe a 100 temperature, he would be like really wheezy and stuff. And he would have to get his machine [nebulizer treatments] a lot. And every once in a while, if he wheezes, he's not breathing properly. So that usually happens when he gets sick. And like it kind of is a lot worse. It takes longer to get better.

"Usually I think, 'No, he's not going to get hurt, well really sick, like a matter of life and death.' Because I know he's been sick a lot and stuff. I just think, 'Well, he'll get better eventually.' And sometimes I feel kind of sort of sorry for him because he misses a lot in school when he gets sick. Like if I'd be sick two days or something like that; he's usually out a whole week when he gets sick.

"He's been sick a lot this year. He's been sick a lot, really. But I kind of get used to him being sick. And now I just think of it as, 'Well he's gonna be out a whole week; I might as well stop by the teacher and tell him and get his [Jason's] stuff.' So now I kind of don't really worry a lot, because I'm kind of pretty much used to it and stuff.

"It's kind of a shame because he'll be out for a long time, and he'll see that's one of the reasons. He's doing pretty good in school for being out a lot. He's always falling behind.

"And my sister, I just think she's a lot lucky because she gets to stay home and watch my brother. Whenever my mom has work I just think we should take turns because I really want to know what it's like to stay home and watch and take care of my brother for a whole day when he's sick.

"And I know what to do. Every night you [a person with CF] have to get on this machine. And it's because you get all this mucus in your lungs and it's hard to breathe. And when you get sick, you really get sick. And after you get on the machine you have to get clapped. You get that two times a day, in the morning and in the night. And when you're sick you get it three times a day, sometimes four. And he wheezes. Whenever he wheezes that means he really needs his machine [nebulizer treatment]. And you have to kind of take real good care of yourself. You can't really ever smoke or be around smoke or anything, because then your lungs get real clogged up. And, well, you get allergy shots every, I think, month; it might be every two weeks, I'm not sure. And you take a lot of pills. For every meal you have to take some pills. And in the morning you have to take a lot. And sometimes you die at an early age. But I don't think that will happen to Jason, because he's in pretty good shape. That's about it.

"My mom's told me about it and I saw stuff on TV, when they have things for hospitals. I've seen them talk about it. And once they had this special CF program on. And once my mom was on TV because of my brother, and so I saw a couple of them; maybe four or five, around there.

"See, my brother was a poster boy and this other girl named Yvette. She was real cute and she has CF too. So they were both poster boy and girl on the same poster for CF. And I know I saw a lot of people on the TV shows who have it. And one of the twins that my brother knows, that have it, she was on TV. I think it was Elyse. It might have been Margot. One of them was on TV. It was a sponsoring show, and my brother was interviewed by a lot of CF people.

"It's kind of strange," Regan mused, "but I've never really talked to anyone about CF unless they had it. And if they had it they really don't. See, it's kind of strange, because they really don't seem any different from anybody. You don't even know they have it until they mention it. Like with Elyse and Margot, I had no idea they had it. We just had dinner with my dad's friends from work and they invited them too. And I had no idea they had it until they mentioned it. And I was, 'Oh my God, you have that?' It's kind of weird, you don't even notice they have it.

"And then there's this one kid, I don't remember his name, but he was sixteen and I think he died that year [when he was sixteen]. My mom went to his funeral. And this other girl, I forget her name, she had it too. She's still alive. She's fine. I know a girl, she's older, she's a woman. Her name is . . . ? Starts with a W," Regan thought out loud. "Well, she doesn't take real good care of herself. I mean, she would be practically fine; but what she does, she smokes. She never takes her pills. Well, she takes them once in a while. She never goes into the hospital to get her things [to be treated]. So she's not doing too good. Usually she's in her bed a lot because she can't hardly walk or anything and she can't breathe that much.

"Sometimes I think about what would happen to my brother when he gets older. 'What would exactly happen to him? Would he be accepted for some stuff or would he not because he couldn't do? What kinds of things could they do and could they not do? What would actually become of my brother when he grew up because of his thing?'"

Louise, the oldest of the three children, would tell the story of how when their dad was remodeling the attic for a bedroom for her, "Regan and me started arguing. Regan said that it didn't matter because Jason will probably get the room the longest if Daddy and Mommy don't move out. I said, 'So that's four years, Regan.' And my dad said, 'Well, Jason probably will be living at home.' Because me and Regan we're going to move out when we're eighteen. And my dad said, 'Jason won't move out when he's eighteen.' And so I asked him why. And he says, 'Well because he won't be able to find a job because of his cystic fibrosis.' And I felt sorry for him."

"Sometimes," Regan continued, "I think about why he has to get all that stuff. I know it's because it helps him to breathe better and helps him get through, but what is it doing and stuff? Like his machine and getting clapped, I don't really understand that. He takes [uses] the machine and I don't really know what it does. And then right after that he has to get clapped. And you can't eat around it [the therapy session]. I don't really understand what that does.

"And I know he takes pancrease before every meal. He usually takes three before meals and I think one before snacks. Because he'll get a stomachache if he doesn't. And he takes Theodor and Ceclor[1] or something once a day and in the morning, and that helps him get through the day more better. If he doesn't take his medicine he gets like kind of wheezey and he's not as active, I think. But I'm not sure. But I think that's what it is.

"And sometimes it's kind of weird at night. I wonder if someone that didn't have any idea my brother had CF came in, and saw his equipment in our medicine cabinet and lying around the house, he walks in his room and sees this big table, he wonders what it's there for and stuff. And like at night when he gets his machine, they would probably—see I'm kind of used to it now, but if it was somebody that just walked in; I'd think it was pretty strange and all, because there's a lot of weird stuff laying around the house from my brother. We usually get pretty much used to it, and we don't worry about it a lot or anything.

"Like, his bed's here," said Regan, pointing to areas on the table, as if it were the room, as she spoke. "And then his drinking table is here. And if you walked in you'd wonder why that's in there. There's this machine. It's lying on the floor in the corner. If someone saw that they might think that something; that's really strange.

"There's some stuff in the medicine cabinet. They might try to read the labels and they wouldn't even be able to pronounce the names. They would think maybe somebody in this house is on drugs or something. So it's kind of weird.

---

[1] Theodor and Ceclor are brand names for a theophyllin preparation bronchodilator and a cephalosporin antibiotic, respectively.

"Sometimes when my new friends come into my house they would be, 'What's that? And what's that?' And they would go, 'Why is your brother on that thing [nebulizer] right there?' And they would ask me a lot of questions. I try to answer them. But sometimes they're still confused.

"I was only three years old when I found out about Jason. And then all I remember is my mom coming home and saying, 'Jason's got a disease.' And I thought, 'Oh God, I'm going to bed. Wake me, because I don't want to catch it.' That's really all I remember. I don't remember a lot because I was young and I didn't understand what it was. I stayed at my grandmother's until he got home.

"And then he really wasn't very different. It really isn't much different, having a brother with CF. He doesn't really change our lives a whole lot, just a little bit. It causes us to want to eat a lot more because when he eats a lot, it's not fair. My mom has to go out and buy a lot more. Not a lot more, but some more. I don't think it really changed us a lot, a whole lot, maybe just a little bit. Maybe my mom and dad, because they have to spend more time with Jason in the morning and stuff; getting him ready, because he has to get all this medical attention and everything and at night too.

"I don't think it really is hard. I think it's good because it teaches us about a disease most kids don't know, and like we usually know what's happening around with CF. And I think it's pretty good, because he's been in posters, he's been on a couple commercials, he's been interviewed, met a lot of famous people. I think he's kind of lucky, but I'm lucky too. He was born with it.

"I really don't think it really is that hard, except just getting that machine. That [nebulizer treatments] wastes a lot of your time. It wastes about a half an hour in the morning and a half hour at night. My brother gets up. If he wasn't such an early bird, he'd probably should get up at 6:30, just to make it on time. And we get up at 7:00. But really, he gets up at 4:00. Don't ask me why, but he gets up at 4:00. It's kind of hard. See, the one thing hard about this is because when my brother gets his machine, since he gets up so early, he falls asleep at 7:00. He'd be on the machine and then he would just like fall asleep. And he's in the middle of the machine, and we'd always have to wake him up so he could get finished and stuff. He's usually like, 'I don't want to.' You have to really force it to him. Sometime you have to give it to him because he won't even touch it. We have to press this button for him to get it onto him. Sometimes we have to do that. That really wastes a lot of time at night, when you're trying to watch TV. And this thing makes a lot of noise and you're feeding it to him or giving it to him because he's asleep and you can't hear the TV. So it's kind of annoying sometimes.

"And sometimes Jason's a little greedy. Like when I brought these candies home, when he saw them he goes, 'Give me some right now.' He wouldn't ask politely or anything. He's just kind of greedy.

"And sort of a little spoiled. And it's really not my mom's fault or my dad's fault. It's just that when they found out he had CF, they just . . ." Regan didn't finish. She took a different tack.

"He eats a lot more than us, because he has to gain a lot of weight. And at night when he sweats a lot, it's salty and my mom doesn't want him to get under the covers like that. She always sort of treats him a little different. He's kind of, well, kind of like . . ." Regan didn't finish that line either. She began again.

"My mom would usually take his side on some things because he's a little younger. But if she saw the real [what happened] if she really knew it was not my fault, if she was there, or even if she wasn't there, but she couldn't figure out how it would be my fault and she would see that it was my brother's; then she would treat us kind of both the same.

"I really don't mind. I used to mind when I was little, not really little, but like in third grade. My brother would come home and eat all the stuff. I'd say, 'How come he gets to eat more than I do?' Because he gets to eat all this good stuff, like pudding and stuff. And I'd say, 'I want some.' But now I don't. I don't really mind."

Louise would say of her brother's extra eating and special food, "My brother always has to eat more than usual. He can't go without dinner. He has to eat a lot. My mom always buys him these special puddings or something and he has to eat them. He has to gain weight a lot.

"And he has to get PT [chest physical therapy] and get clapped and get the machine. I hate that machine. It makes so much noise. And after he's finished that, my dad claps him, in the morning. He gets up around 5:30. He gets up early. And so that gives him a lot of time to do the thing.

"I clapped him a couple of times when my mom and dad are busy or something. See, my brother wouldn't even let me clap him. He's like, 'Don't touch me.' And I was like, 'Jason, sit still.' We have a table and so I don't like clapping him. I clap him once in a while.

"Oh, and you have to put Intal [for bronchospasm] in that machine. And he has Theodor and Ceclor and Pancrease. Pancrease is like this thing. You have to take it before you eat, because it helps to digest the food. So when you go to the bathroom, it'll all come out right. And you won't digest the food right [if you don't take it].

"And he has to go to clinic to get checkups. If he's doing alright and all that. They take needles. They put needles in him. They take blood and all. And they put one of those things, stethoscopes, up to him to see how he is. And they weigh him and see how tall he is.

"I went once when I was five. My brother usually goes when he has school. But once when I was five I was in there and just waiting. Because that's what I remember when he was getting a needle and he was crying. Because I was out in the lobby.

"It's a disease in the lungs. And your lungs are clogged. And it can be hard breathing. And you're allergic to dust and you can't run. I mean you can't go running five miles. You have to stop. He starts breathing, 'Hhhh hhh hhh.' And you start wheezing a lot.

"I know he's going to wheeze a lot. And then he can't get too excited. Like, once when he was sick I made him laugh a whole lot and he started wheezing and coughing up and I got into trouble, because you can't get him too excited.

"When Jason gets sick, we stay home more. He wheezes a lot. And if I got sick I stayed in for three days. He probably has to stay home for four or five, because he's wheezing a lot. And he's kind of lucky because he always stays home from school because he's wheezing or something like that. But he doesn't stay home all the time. But he stays out more than me.

"And sometimes when he's sick, and that's only because he's sleeping, he's so cute. And then I think about CF. I think about it at the bikeathon [Cystic Fibrosis Foundation fund-raiser] or when he's sick. I think if they're ever going to find a cure for it or not, 'cause we're raising money to find a cure. And a couple of months ago my mom told me they found what causes it or something about it.

"I heard that they don't live to be . . ." Louise didn't finish that sentence. She started anew. "Like if I live to be a hundred, they'll probably live to be seventy or fifty or something like that. They don't live as long as we do. They get not like real sick. Like he's still talking and bossing me around and I'm just thinking he's a pain.

"Well, I don't think he's gonna die right now or soon or something, but in around forty or thirty. By the time he gets older, the medicines will be better, so then he'll live longer.

"I don't know. I don't worry about CF too much. It's not one of my big problems. If Jason were here [in this room] you could never guess in a million years that he has it, because he is always yelling or something or doing something. If he had something else that's more serious, I would worry about that a lot. But he seems pretty healthy to me.

"Once in a while he'll get real sick, because I mean he gets real sick sometimes, real sick. But I don't worry. Not really.

"Once after I read this book, called. . . . I can't remember what it's called. It was about the Capallettis. They lived near here, but they moved away. When this kid Joey [a child] got real sick [with leukemia], he had chicken pox and he was sick all these five months, and he got real sick . . ." Louise didn't finish, she hurried on. "And after I finished reading that book Jason got real sick and I thought, 'Ooh, maybe he could die.' And I said, 'No.' Because I knew he was going to get over it or something like that. He was like over it in a week and back to himself. So I don't worry anymore.

"He's like a regular kid to me. He's like regular. I don't think of him as anything else but a brother. It's normal. And I don't think of him as cystic fibrosis. But I think of him as a brother. I don't know. It's just everyday stuff. Even if he didn't have it, I would think around the same.

"We treat him the same as any other person. But if he was just a regular person, who couldn't run super fast, then we would not let him slide. When we're playing kickball or something like that we know he can't run as fast. He can run fast, but he's not strong. So we let him slide sometimes, because he's cute, smiling."

According to Mrs. Chase, "When Jason heard his sisters were going to be interviewed about having a brother with cystic fibrosis, he said, 'Well why does she want to talk to them and not me?' And I said, 'She wants to see what it's like being a sister or brother with someone with CF.' And he said, 'Well, they don't treat me any different.' He said, 'They just treat me like normal, like I'm normal.' I said [to him], 'Well don't you want to be treated that way?' And he said, 'No.'" Mrs. Chase laughed.

"He feels pretty positive about having CF. He's not ashamed of it. Like Jason will take his ten pills and wop them in his mouth and swallow them with one sip of water, and the kids will be like, 'Wow.' Or up at school he'll come in, and he knows all his medications and he goes to the nurse's office to get them. They don't know what they're doing. He has to show them how to hook up his inhaler and all. He knows what medicines he's on and he'll take them.

"I don't leave him solely responsible, because we sort of check up on each other, all three of us. Because it's hard to remember everything. But he takes pretty good care of himself. He's like an old man sometimes. He's a little worry wart." Mrs. Chase smiled.

"He has to take a lot of medications and he has to always watch it because of his asthma. And that tends to make him a more cautious child. So he's a little worry wart. And he's always worried about this and what this is going to do. And he's a very cautious child. He's not as happy and carefree as an average child.

"I see it because when I was younger I had health problems and so it's real easy for me to identify and see things that probably an average person wouldn't. And then you try to treat him normal, but then you always have to be cautious.

"He's kind of grumpy. You can notice that when he has a long stand where he's real well. He becomes a much happier, more carefree child.

"And there's a lot of stuff he does, like in school the teacher always notices. They were designing T-shirts one day and everybody else was writing this little . . . I forget what. Jason made the bikeathon T-shirt for CF and wrote CF on it. And he thinks about CF a lot. But he likes it at this age."

"I don't know if this comes with cystic fibrosis," Louise would go on, "but he's so bossy sometimes. Once in a while we'll be standing there and say, 'I'm special.' And Jason goes, 'Nah uh. I'm more specialer.' I go, 'Why?' And he goes, 'Because I have . . .' He goes, 'You're not special.' And I go, 'Yes I am.' He goes, 'I'm a special kid.' I go, 'You are not.' He goes, 'Yes I am.' I said, 'Why?' He goes, 'Because I have CF.'

"He thinks it's some kind of . . ." Louise didn't finish. "I don't know. He knows about it and he doesn't take it too seriously. And he thinks he's special.

"Sometimes my parents have to spend more money on him, because I remember something. When I asked for a raise in my allowance or for clothing or something, my mom said once that they would have had a lot more money, if my brother didn't have it [CF]. If my brother didn't have it, we would have a lot more money. But I don't care, because I have a lot of stuff. And they become more involved in the disease and stuff like that.'"

"Whatever the girls may say," Mrs. Chase would remark, "I think they think he gets special things or that he's treated more special. They just think of him as being more special. They'll say things like, 'Oh he's lucky, I wish I had CF.' I'm there, 'Oh no you don't.' But people say things like. . . ." Mrs. Chase didn't finish. She picked up with a specific example. "Louise had this thing last year where she said she wanted to break her arm or leg so that she could stay out of school, and then she would get lots of presents.

"But I think now that they're older they're starting to understand a little better. I think when they were younger I could see more jealousy. They would show more when they were younger. I think when they were younger, I would notice it more; just to maybe think they were doing it in school and maybe I didn't have as much time to give them. See, I think a lot of it may be related back to Victor or me; how much attention, like they're not getting attention from us. Sometimes I think that maybe they get less attention. Well I know when Jason gets sick they do.

"People worry about Jason. Nobody worries about them. They're normal, and if they get a cold you don't worry so much that they get a cold. But you worry whether Jason will get a cold from them. And they know all that.

"And I think they have each other. I think we're probably tougher on them than we are on Jason. That's just the way it's been.

"And in some ways I think it'll be good. Sometimes I think it's good to have something in your life that where everything's not like a rose garden, where everything's not so wonderful. So maybe they learn to be more sensitive, which I hope they do. But I don't know that I see that right now; I think as they get older.

"I wonder sometimes if they worry. I don't know if they do, because they are aware of a lot of the disease, what happens and stuff, because they've known. See, I've become friends with a few people at the hospital. There was a boy a few years back that died. But it doesn't seem to bother them, or they don't associate it with Jason. They don't associate. It's like, 'That's somebody else.'

"Well, if you ask the CF patients at the hospital; they'll see someone die, and this kid is the kid that's pretty healthy and comes in maybe once every year and a half. And they'll go, 'Oh, that's a sin. That poor person.' And they really haven't identified, made the connection that they have the same thing. And I do the same thing. I don't associate it."

Having said that, Mrs. Chase returned to the subject of her daughters. "I really can't say what they know for sure, because even though they've been told things, I don't think they relate back to you. Their vocabulary is much more limited. They just really can't explain things. And I don't really know for sure if this is what they know.

"Well, they know it's a disease of the lungs. They know, I've explained the whole process to them. But I would think they probably think of it more like, 'Cystic fibrosis is where you get colds a lot and you have to take antibiotics and lots of pills and get therapy all the time and you cough up mucus. And you get real sick and your lungs can get all closed up if you don't take care of yourself.' That's what I think they know. But I think I've told them a lot more.

"It would be interesting to know what they know about the genetics. I've told them. They should know, but I don't think they have that much scientific knowledge to know what the genetics is. They know they could be carriers. But I don't think I really have stressed that. I think they'll learn that more when they get older. I don't see any necessity to tell them now.

"Just like I think they know people die from CF. I think they think it can happen to Jason. And I think they know we're worried. And I think that both of them [Louise and Regan] think about the same thing, because they're both the same age. I think they know we worry about it. They probably kind of worry about it.

"They grew up with it. Jason was one when he was diagnosed. So for eight years we've been through the whole business. They just think of it as part of their life. That it's just part of our life. They know that I'm real involved with it. So I don't know what they think about. They probably think I'm crazy." Mrs. Chase laughed.

"I think they've learned everything basically from me. There's always been literature around the house that they could have read. And things they've overheard people saying. Jason, of course, has heard a lot of stuff, because he goes to the clinic and I talk to people [the staff]. I talk to them about it, but it's not like we sit and talk about it all the time.

"And sometimes you wonder, 'I can't believe you didn't know that.' It's like Louise just got her period and two years ago I explained everything to her. And yet it didn't mean anything to her then. So I had to retell her everything. And she didn't. And I think it's like that. I think you can tell them all this information, but it's not going to mean anything. And I think that's why you tend not to talk about it a lot. It's not that I don't want to talk about it, it's just you talk about it when it comes up. We'll talk about it at the dinner table, about something. But it's not something I say, 'You have to understand this.'"

Mrs. Chase stopped and then just announced, "I never told them about it. I didn't tell them about some people that have died. Because I think sometimes you shouldn't stress so much the negative.

"For me, when I think about CF I think it's something that doesn't go away; something that is part of my life. Something that I always wonder about. God, I didn't even know what it was. And I think the big thing you always think about are all the little things—the infections and the pills and this and that. But I think you could cope with all that. But the big thing that you always have in the back of your head is the prognosis. And I think you suppress it a lot. But I don't think there's a day that goes by that you don't think about it. And I think that's how it is for everyone.

"And I think you think about it all the time. And I think if they could control the disease like they can control diabetes or something like that, I think it would definitely change a lot of things.

"When someone is sick at the hospital, really sick, like when someone dies; oh God, then you think about it all the time. No, you think about it. It's not that you don't think about it. I mean it's not like you think about it every day, but it crosses your mind every day.

"You just can't imagine sometimes how you'll ever cope. And you think about it when you think of the future. Like I think when you get married and you have these kids and you have all these goals of what your life's going to be like and then you tend to think of the future and it gets pretty hard." Mrs. Chase began to cry.

"I'm a crybaby," she declared with a smile, wiping away her tears. "But then you have to think that you don't know—that's the thing. It might turn out fine. You have to think of the positive. You have to think of yourself in those statistics that are like the sixty-four-year-old grandmother. There's a sixty-four-year-old grandmother, I think, or something." Mrs. Chase paused. Her memory triggered, she went on.

"An interesting thing happened last year. On Louise's birthday we had a little party with some girls over, and I bought a Ouija board for them. And of course every kid asks, 'How old will I be when I die?' So Jason did it and it turned out that he was going to be ninety-two. So he says, 'Oh God!' He said, 'I thought I was going to be fourteen or fifteen.' And I said, 'Why did you think that?' And he said, 'Because that's what Regan told me a couple of years ago.' And I'm thinking, 'This poor kid. For two years he's been going around thinking,'" Mrs. Chase shook her head, "'no wonder he's so miserable.' He never told me that. And I knew nothing about that, but that was interesting. I think what happened was that was around the time when Nate died. And he was fourteen. And Regan blurts things out. So that's what I think happened.

"But I was thinking, ever since then, 'So he's got this idea of ninety-two, let him believe it. Why not? So he thinks he's going to be ninety-two.'" Mrs. Chase smiled with the thought.

Her face grew earnest. "See, when you hear your child has cystic fibrosis, the first thing you think of is your child might die. At first you think it's going to happen right then and there. You start looking at your child like they're no longer a person. They're this poor thing you feel sorry for. But as you learn more about it; education is a big thing. If I have the knowledge then I'm more in a position to be in control.

"When you meet other people; I've had a lot of negative things with meeting other people. But I've had a lot of positive things, and you learn how to face it. You learn too. I met and learned a lot talking to other parents, people who have older kids, getting involved in the foundation. They have a newspaper that comes around. And just finding out that that isn't all there is to it.

"And then, if I take care of him, I do have control. If you believe that, then I think that's when you stop thinking of it as. . . ." Mrs. Chase didn't continue in that vein. "You see that it's something that you have to work for. You have to do all this stuff if you want him to be OK. And that's what you do. And I really know how to take care of him. And I know just what's going on. And that makes me much more in control.

"But then I don't want to be like this kind of person that drives myself crazy, like, 'I'm going to raise all this money for CF and I'm gonna do all this stuff and my child will not get sick and will not die.' I mean you do have to be that way, but then on the other hand, it might not work. That's the only way it will work, because you can't be setting yourself up for a big disappointment. Because it's true.

"That's another thing that CF has taught me. You're just like anybody else. And sure, it might all work out and you might be lucky. But then again, there's plenty of people in this world that have done everything right and they're not. So you could be in the same position. If something happens and their kid does die, so that could happen. And you have to look at both ways of it.

"But I think I've seen people that are too naive. I don't think it's good to constantly think about it and constantly think you can make this stop happening. Plus there's the other factor. When the kid gets older. What's going to happen when the kid gets older? What's going to happen when the kid's fourteen and he doesn't want to take his meds? You've got to stop taking care of the kid. And you're not going to have that control. And a lot of kids will go downhill. And it's . . ." Mrs. Chase shrugged.

"I don't know. I think you've got to accept it. It's like I think you have to accept your child as he is. And you have to accept that and make the most of the years you have. And, but I don't want to, you don't want to, deny it.

"You don't have a choice, because it's like the only way to do it, to me. A lot of kids will say, 'Well, what good will it [adhering to the treatment regimen] do?' Well, sure, if you're going to think that, that's what's going to happen. What choice do you have? The only choice you have is to fight it, or else. Things aren't going to turn out right just because you're going to sit there and go, 'Well, let's see what happens.'

"I always try to tell myself; I try to think, 'Oh God, what if this ever happens? How will I ever cope?' And I can't picture and I think, 'Oh my God, I'll never be able to go on.' But then you have to say to yourself, 'Well, when things like these things do happen, they usually just don't happen.'

"It's kind of like a long process that you sort of know you just can't think about. You've got to figure. Well, I guess you know somehow, some day, some way; things, whatever's going to happen, is going to happen. And it'll happen. Some slow. Or the way it's supposed to happen. And I'll be ready for things."

————

Jason coughed on and off over the next half hour. From time to time his mother or his sister would look over to him, but for the most part their eyes just ran over the waiting room, not quite stopping anywhere in particular, until the door of one of the examining rooms opened. As the family exited the examining room, the Chases looked over to the reception desk to see if they would be the next to enter.

The Woodwards

(Individuals mentioned by name in order of appearance)

THEA WRIGHT: Outpatient clinical nurse specialist
ALYSON WOODWARD: Eleven-year-old child with cystic fibrosis (CF)
MRS. IRIS WOODWARD: Mother of Alyson Woodward
AARON WOODWARD: Twelve-year-old well brother of Alyson Woodward
MR. IVAN WOODWARD: Father of Alyson Woodward
DARA: Friend of Alyson Woodward who died of CF
TROY: Friend of Alyson Woodward who died of CF
LEANA LINDER: Friend of Alyson Woodward who died of CF
PEPPER LYONS: Friend of Alyson Woodward who died of CF
WAYNE: Friend of Alyson Woodward who died of CF
SKIP SCHMIDT: Friend of Alyson Woodward who died of CF
SKIP LACHMAN: Friend of Alyson Woodward who has CF
SONIA: Friend of Alyson Woodward who died of CF
TOBY: Friend of Alyson Woodward who died of CF
NELL: Friend of Alyson Woodward who died of CF
KENT: Friend of Alyson Woodward
MARTA CLAYMAN: Friend of Alyson Woodward with CF
BRITT [FOSTER]: Friend of Alyson Woodward with CF
GUY: Friend of Aaron Woodward
MRS. MAY FOSTER: Mother of child with CF
MRS. MIMI REARDON: Parent of child who died of CF
MRS. DOROTHY LYONS: Parent of child who died of CF
PAULINE: Friend of Mrs. Iris Woodward
DR. EVERETT REESE: Pediatric pulmonologist

"What brings you here today?" Thea Wright asked Alyson, who was curled up on a waiting-room chair. The girl leaned her head on the armrest, the color drained from her face. "We didn't expect to see you here so soon."

"She's very constipated. You know?" Mrs. Woodward answered, raising her eyebrows. "We've been down in the emergency room most of the morning. And then they sent us up here."

"Did you have an X-ray?"

"No."

"OK. Let me see what the boss wants here." Thea Wright walked to the back of the clinic area, behind the examining rooms, where the physicians' offices were located. Alyson closed her eyes.

Mrs. Woodward managed a smile and then turned toward Alyson and gently stroked her leg. "Alyson, you know your brother. . . ."

Alyson didn't open her eyes.

"Aaron," Mrs. Woodward continued, "was so worried when we left this morning [for the emergency room]." He kept saying, 'She'll have to come to the hospital and have surgery.'"

"They fight like cats and dogs. 'Well I hate you.' 'You're a pain.' 'Why don't you just go away?' But he really does care for her. He really does worry about her. When she's sick, it's, 'How's Alyson?' I say, 'Wow, for someone who doesn't care, you sure want to know.' He does care. Deep down inside he does care for her. And when they are outside and something should happen; he'd defend her until the end. But when they are in the house it's something different. If it's just the two of them together, they will fight."

"It's scary sometimes," Aaron would explain. "You don't know what's going to happen. Or you go away and she's in the hospital. Then, it's a lot scary. When she has an infection she ends up in the hospital. When she has a cold she usually stays home. When she has a cold it usually gets worse if she doesn't catch it right away. My mom always calls the hospital and asks for better advice; what might increased medicines do and stuff like that. I always hear her on the phone. And then she [Alyson] takes a lot of antibiotics when she gets worse. Because normally she doesn't have to take them as much. But she takes a lot more to get rid of the infection." Aaron paused for a moment and then rushed in, "It's one of the deadliest diseases. You are in the hospital a lot. Your chances of surviving are almost zero. That's a lot really scary.

"Scary. You never know what is going to happen. You wonder about stuff. A lot of her friends die and it's scary." Aaron became very quiet, before continuing. "It's like you are responsible for a lot of stuff. Like yelling at her or getting mad at her gets her real mad and makes her do worse. You wish you didn't do that.

"She can't stand me." Aaron paused and reconsidered. "Well not really. She acts like it, but I don't really think so. Same thing with me. Sometimes I can't stand her, but I really do."

Mrs. Woodward had thought that Alyson would say, "'Oh I can't stand my brother.' But if something is with him, she'll worry too."

In fact, when Alyson would begin to talk about her brother, a big grin came over her face, "My brother! Oh God! He's mean. He blames everything on me. Like if he did something and then he thought that I said something bad, a bad word, because sometimes I have trouble saying this one word, he says, 'Oh she said a curse.' Because he said that. And he tells on me a lot. Then my mom makes us both go to our rooms because she doesn't know who to believe.

"He'd probably say the same about me. He'd probably say, 'She's a brat. She starts everything.' He starts it too. It's not always me." Alyson was emphatic and her tone became increasingly so.

"It's not fair! Why should I have all this stuff and he has nothing? I have three different things and he doesn't have anything. He doesn't have CF. He doesn't have asthma. He doesn't have scoliosis.

"He's lucky he doesn't have CF, but asthma or scoliosis. Why should I always go in the hospital and not him? And when he says, 'Ah-ha, you have to get a blood gas' [a medical test]; then I feel like hitting him. Because sometimes he'll say that and I'll get mad at him. He says, 'Alyson cries for her blood gas.' And he's just as chicken. He never even had a blood test. That's why he's always chicken."

If one were to ask Mrs. Woodward, she would say, "Aaron gets it from his father. He [Mr. Woodward] doesn't like any kind of needles, any IVs or anything. He's a big baby. He's always been and always will be, a big chicken. He just isn't very tolerant of that type of stuff. He doesn't like it. That's why he doesn't come to the hospital a lot. He does not like a hospital atmosphere or doctors and all the things like that. He doesn't like seeing kids, or anybody, being hooked up to IVs or having tubes run in them, whatever the problem may be. His stomach can't tolerate that.

"Alyson understands that the hospital isn't his favorite place to be. And so does Aaron. After all, he's a chicken himself. He had to go for a booster shot and the doctor had to tackle him and hold him down. At twelve years old, he's just following in his father's footsteps. Well, he's never had a blood test or anything like that, or an IV, so to him that's one big fear if he ever had to have it done."

Aaron once remarked, "My mom always talks about that she wishes she could be like Alyson for a couple of months and let Alyson be normal for a couple of months; take her place, so she could stop suffering for a while. I don't like IVs. If you could get around any needles I would do it."

Aaron felt that blood gases and IVs, not to mention pulmonary function tests and losing weight, bothered Alyson too. "My sister gets scared when she is losing weight or when she has to get her blood gas. She's scared of it sometimes—when she's doing bad and she has to take a test, like the pulmonary function, and she knows she hasn't been doing good. She gets scared of that. She's scared of getting the tube through your arm that goes to your heart, the Hardy line. She gets scared of that when you miss sometimes. And it's just frustrating.

"She doesn't like resident doctors. She wants the real ones. She doesn't like the residents to come in and have target practice on her with IVs. Because they stick her a couple of times before they get it. And she yells at them that she wants a real doctor.

"And she got upset when she found out she had that pseudomonas [Pseudomonas cepacia, now known as Burkholderia cepacia]. She got that not too long ago. It's the worst one [bacterial infection]. She got worried because all the people she knows that have died had it. That got her scared."

Alyson would say, "It's pretty scary when other kids die from CF, especially my friends. You're like, 'Oh no! Are you next?' Because there are so many: Dara, Troy, Leana Linder, Pepper Lyons, Wayne. I know Skip Schmidt, not Skip Lachman, Sonia, Toby. That's all I know, I think. And Nell. There's more, though. A lot. I don't know them all."

Mrs. Woodward would note, "She has lost a lot of friends. A lot of them have died; especially in the last two years, a lot of kids her age. She's even said, 'I've lost a lot of my friends. There's not that many left.' I guess it gets them thinking too, 'Hey that could have been me.' I think that kind of gives her more encouragement to try harder.

"She's had to deal with other kids dying since the time she was three. She had seen, she had gotten close. She was like everybody's little sister. They just kind of adopted her, and she has learned to adjust to it. She has seen other kids. She has gotten close to them and they die. And I explain it to her. 'So-and-so was very sick and they died.' And she just always understood, even when she was real young. I think, one of the really close ones, she was five years old, and she said, 'Why don't we send her mother a card and tell her we're sorry?' So she's obviously understood. And she realizes that they get so sick they do die, and then they don't have CF anymore. Then they don't suffer any more. And so she understands that.

"We don't hide anything. Whatever there is to know they both know. I don't believe in keeping it from the kids because I've seen other families where they don't tell the kids everything and then if they hear something else somewhere else it's like, 'What? What's that? Why didn't you tell me?' I haven't been like that. I have been very open with Alyson since she has been little. And there have been times when she hasn't wanted to do this or that, and I explain, 'Look, you have to do this because if you don't this will happen.' So she has always known what the score is. I've never hidden anything from her."

Aaron was also aware of the deaths of others who had cystic fibrosis. "I know a lot that died," Aaron would say, "but I can't remember their names. Well, some I can, like Troy. I was sad when Troy died, because Alyson was like best friends with him. She liked him a lot. I talked to him a lot in the hospital when I came to visit Alyson.

"Alyson always tells me about the kids in the hospital. She tells me who's in the hospital, what is happening to them, how they are doing, and when they're coming out. She tells me all about the IVs: who does good ones and who does bad ones. She tells me about her pulmonary function tests; if they're good, and about her friends' PFTs [pulmonary function tests]. Some stuff she just tells me when she comes home from the hospital and starts talking about it."

Notably, neither Alyson nor Aaron said that she or he talked to the other about Alyson's overall condition or prognosis. According to Alyson, "He knows most stuff because Mom tells him." And according to Aaron, "I try not to talk to her about it so she doesn't get upset. I talk to my mom. Not a lot, sometimes; when I think about it.

"Sometimes I wonder when she might die, how it's going to be. I wonder how Alyson thinks about it; how my mom and dad think about it. I think about it sometimes. It depends on where I'm at. At the mountains I never think of nothing like that. But if I'm home or at the hospital, I'm always thinking about it. And at school, sometimes, because in school all the kids ask me about it, mostly girls. They're more interested in it than boys are. They feel more sorry I guess.

"More girls have CF than boys do. Most of the people she knows are girls that have CF. And she's got friends at St. Chris that don't have CF. She likes Kent. I'm not sure about his last name, but he has something else. And Alyson is friendly with him. She's made a lot of friends at the hospital, a lot. She knows Marta Clayman and Britt, that's her best friend.

"When Britt's in the hospital, for a couple of hours every day Alyson is talking to her on the phone. They are almost best friends; well, from the hospital. Britt doesn't live around here. She lives in Lancaster.

"And they told Britt that she's going to die. I mean half of her life is up already. They told her parents and her parents told my parents and my parents told me, but not Alyson. It was kind of scary, because Alyson's got the same disease, so that it might be half up for her too, but they didn't tell me. That's hard.

"They thought I was asleep, and they were talking about it [Britt's condition], and I overheard it and asked them to tell me about it. And they told me.

"But Alyson is doing better than Britt is. Britt had lavages and that kind of stuff. And Alyson hasn't had none of that stuff. They wash out their lungs and then after that they get real sick for a couple of days. And then they are all right. When you have lavages a lot that means you are really sick lately. But Alyson hasn't had them. She never got that bad yet. They were going to put a Broviac in Britt, I think. And Alyson hasn't had that either.

"Alyson's Britt's best friend. And Britt's always writing me letters. We went to Sesame Place together with Britt and her parents. We went a lot of places together. CF day at Dorney Park, we went there together. And Britt's always coming over our house. And Alyson's gone over their house for a couple of days."

"And when they're together," Mrs. Woodward would describe, "they go off by themselves and they sit and talk. They can ask questions and just discuss anything in general about CF and they understand each other; where Alyson hides it from her friends at school.

"Her real close friends, she'll tell them that she has cystic fibrosis, but she won't tell the other kids. No one really knows what's wrong with her at school. They may know she's in the hospital, but that's all. They don't know why. Only her close friends know that she's in because she has cystic fibrosis.

"She doesn't show it. Like she goes down to the nurse where there's other kids taking medication. They just know she has to take medicine, that's all. But they don't know why. It was her option to carry the pancrease [enzyme capsules] with her, but being's she already had to go for her InspirEase [inhaler with medication] at lunchtime at the nurse, she decided, 'I'll just take it there.' So in the nurse's office, she will take it in front of some of the other kids taking their medicine, but she doesn't want to do it in the classroom or at lunch.

"And Aaron'll tell people that Alyson has cystic fibrosis, but he really doesn't really get into it. It's not like you want to go shouting from the rooftops, 'My sister has cystic fibrosis.' And then have people go, 'What's that?' A lot of people don't know what it is. And rather than go through the whole thing of explaining, if somebody asks, 'What's wrong with Alyson?' he would tell them, 'Well, she has CF,' and whatever."

Aaron would agree. As he said, "When Alyson's in [hospitalized], the kids'll ask me what's happening and stuff like that. I tell if they ask. Otherwise no. Except maybe for Guy, my best friend. I knew him since I was five. We've gone to baseball together and everything. I talk to him when she's in the hospital, how long she's been in."

"And I'm kind of the same way about it," Mrs. Woodward would say. "I don't have many people I really talk to about it except maybe some other parents with CF that I talk to occasionally or write letters to, like May Foster. And I talk to Mimi Reardon. She had a son that died January a year ago. Dorothy Lyons had a daughter that passed away. And my friend Pauline, who has a daughter with heart problems. There's just a few, not that many. They understand what you are going through. Where if you have somebody who doesn't have a sick child at all, they just can't understand and conceive the things you are going through and the things that are running through your head; what you are thinking about or what it's actually like. They can say, 'Oh wow, you must be going through a lot.' But that's all the further it goes. They don't really know how deep it runs.

"The kids may look fine; they may not look very sick, but yet inside they are sick. And no matter how hard you try, no matter what you do, there's no fighting it in the long run. You know you can fight cystic fibrosis for the time being, but sooner or later they are going to succumb to it. There is no cure. That's kind of depressing in a way, but yet you take it day by day and just keep trying as hard as you can for as long as you can.

"You can't give in, though. You can't just say, 'Well there's no hope. Why try?' You can't do that. Well, I'm sure you could, but you wouldn't have your child around very long. I mean, I can't perceive myself doing that. She's my little girl. I love her dearly and I'll do all I can for her. You can't just give up." Mrs. Woodward shook her head and pursed her lips with determination. "Being there for her is number one.

"Like originally I started working as a nurse. I was taking a night course and I was working for three doctors, before we got married. And then when I got married I got pregnant right away [with Aaron], so I quit. I thoroughly enjoyed that [working for the doctors] and it had occurred to me to go on and get a degree and everything; which I would still love to do. But I won't take that time away from Alyson, because who knows how long she may have to live. And while she's here I want to be with her. I would feel terribly guilty for not being there when she needed me. So I just put that on hold until I can. So we are planning on when she gets out of high school, in umpteen years, to go to nursing school together." Mrs. Woodward laughed, enjoying the idea.

"I've had to devote a lot of my time to her. You don't really have time for yourself, really. Like for instance, when Alyson is in the hospital, I just don't totally desert her. Making sure I come down to visit her, talking with the doctors, knowing what her case is, knowing what they are doing. Just if I have any questions I ask them. And I, like, know exactly what the score is and where she stands and what is being done about it.

"And then there's trying to keep things as close to normal at home as possible. Trying to be there for them [husband and son]. When Alyson was little I used to come and stay with her overnight, and Aaron got to the point where he felt left out. So when she was old enough to stay by herself I would come to the hospital during the day and then go home at night and give him equal time. Be home when he was home. So that way he has his mother too. The only time I'm not there is when he's in school. I'm there before he leaves, until he's left, and then I'm home right about the time he gets home.

"And even still, I think he has bad feelings about Alyson's having CF. Because it kind of takes away from time with him. I can't be there too. If I am doing a treatment, obviously I can't be spending time with him. And it has presented some jealousy. 'Well, you do everything with her.' But doing treatments is no picnic. I am not there having fun doing it.

"I think he just uses that as a crutch, 'Well, you always spend time with her.' But there's time that we spend time with him alone too, but he kind of forgets that right away. And I'll say, 'I just spent the whole day with you yesterday.' 'Oh yeah,' he says. 'I forgot about that.'

"But I see that with other kids, though. They get very jealous and they want you all to themselves. I think there would probably be jealousy whether or not Alyson had CF. But being that I do share time with him equally, like when she's in the hospital, I think that helps. It's not as if he's being neglected and not having time too. He has me the whole time he's home. So it's not as if I am taking anything away from him—any time away from him."

"My mom tries to treat us equal," Aaron would acknowledge. "She tries to treat us like there is nothing wrong with us, like there is nothing wrong with Alyson, to keep her attitude up. And sometimes she gets treated a little better because she doesn't have as much of a life. She's going to die young." Aaron looked down for a moment.

"And sometimes she gets out of doing things," he commented, lifting his head. "Take chores. I feed the dog, mow the lawn, and clean my room. And Alyson sometimes does the laundry, sometimes; and feeds the cat and the bird. When I don't do mine [chores] Mom gets on my case about it. And Alyson sometimes just sits around and acts like she doesn't have to do anything and I'm the janitor. When we pack to go to the mountains she just sits in the car and waits 'til everything's done.

"And every time we're ready to go to church she complains she has a stomachache. She gets out of it, because my mom knows she's sick a lot. And my mom knows I'm not sick as much, so she makes me go to more stuff. Once in a great while she may let me stay home because I've been going every time and my sister hasn't.

"In some ways they treat her normal. But some things they have to do special for her. Like they try to keep her doing activities to keep the stuff in her lungs loose. And we have to buy a special little mask when she rides her motorcycle [dirt bike] so the dust doesn't get to her. She can't be around ragweed and stuff like that. And sometimes we have to stop in the middle of something and give her a treatment or a medicine. We try to. Well, for that kind of stuff we give her the spray which eliminates giving her her aerosol, so she doesn't have to worry about that. And she never likes what we cook. She always wants cereal. And mom lets her if she eats good cereal instead of all the sugar cereal. She keeps eating Honey-Nut Cheerios and Frosted Flakes all the time. See, keeping her weight up is real important.

"My dad tries to keep her going when she's losing weight. Like, he'll want to have a race. Or he tries to lose weight and she tries to gain weight. And that's what my mom does too. And Britt and her try to see who can gain the most weight. Like when Britt comes over for a couple of days they see who can gain the most weight. They sit there and eat as much as they can and weigh themselves quick. They eat a bunch of peanut-butter-and-jelly sandwiches and jump on the scale. They gain a couple of pounds that way.

"My mom usually comes up with the stuff to help gain weight and I add on to it. Like if I drink a Sustecal shake, she will. And stuff like that. My mom gets all frustrated sometimes when Alyson loses too much weight. She tries to keep a going type attitude at it and tries to keep Alyson happy so she does better. And she talks her through difficult situations and stuff like that."

"I get reminded to eat a lot," Alyson would declare. "'Eat, eat, and eat.' And when I get sick I usually lose like five pounds. Last admission I lost seven and a half. But I gained it all back, except for one pound. So I've been eating and eating and eating, because I couldn't eat at all. I just puked it right back up. So I just kept on eating. See when you can't eat for a while they threaten you with NG [naso-gastric] tubes. Because once when my liver was getting big and I couldn't eat or anything they couldn't get over my problem that I couldn't eat. My liver was getting real large and stuff, and I couldn't eat or anything. I just wasn't eating at all. I didn't eat at all. I was like, 'Why should I eat?' I wasn't hungry. And so they threatened me with NG tubes, because they thought it was just me that wouldn't eat. And they wouldn't really believe me, the doctors. My mom thought I really didn't want to eat too. She kept on telling me, 'Eat. Eat. Eat. You have to drink Sustecal.' I lost a lot then and gained extra back."

According to Mrs. Woodward at another time, "You have to be kind of a coach. 'Go. Go. Go. Keep on trying.' Because they need somebody there to keep pushing, to give them the encouragement they need, even when things don't really look good. They're really sick and you come into them. You can't go in there crying your heart out, 'Oh I feel bad about it.' You have to keep your chin up and keep a positive attitude and keep them trying.

"I think at times that gets very hard, because you may really feel rotten inside and really feel depressed about things, but you can't let them see that. It's very important, their attitude. Alyson had a period last summer where she had gotten really sick and she just felt so rotten she decided, 'I'm not going to try anymore.' And when they get that kind of an attitude, I've seen kids do that, and sure enough within a month, some of them have died when they get that attitude. They feel sick and they decide they're not going to try. They don't want treatments. They don't want their medications. And it gets very difficult. So as long as they can keep a positive attitude, that's very important. And we're just as responsible to keep that attitude up." Mrs. Woodward paused for a moment. "Alyson's a strong kid. She's a fighter. She's not the type to sit down and give up."

"It's a disease you try to fight for a long time and then you. . . ." Alyson paused and then quickly added, "But my asthma is worse than my CF. So that's good. Because CF is worse than asthma. Because asthma could go away, but CF will not go away. So it's good that my asthma's worse.

"CF's a bad disease. It has to do with your lungs. And when you come in to the hospital you usually have to get an IV. I hate them though, boy, because they have to stay in your arm. Then they give you your medicine if you have an infection. That's what they do to make you better. Because I couldn't get it [the infection] out by myself. They help me do a lot better.

"CF is bad, though. But not as bad as my asthma, because my asthma's worse," Alyson repeated.

"For somebody, if their cystic fibrosis is really bad sometimes, they're in the hospital. When they're in the hospital they don't do as good sometimes. They just pass away. But my CF is good. 'It's mild,' they said. Mine's pretty good. That's all I care about." Alyson let a giggle escape, before she mused, "Sometimes I wonder though. Could there be a cure? Is there such a thing as a cure for CF? But I don't know," she shook her head. "They keep on doing research and research and millions of dollars, but so far they haven't got a cure yet. I wonder what a cure would do, though. If I did have a cure, I wonder what it would do? Just stay the same? Or get worse? Or what?

"I asked the doctors, 'Is there going to be a cure for CF?' Do they know? They say, 'We really don't know.' And I ask them, 'If they don't get a cure, what would happen?' And they said, 'We really don't know.'"

Alyson became quite still. She then stirred and straightened. "I wish for a cure for CF. And that CF would go away and everybody would be cured for everything."

"I know," Mrs. Woodward would later say, "from talking to the doctors that even if they came up with a cure they would not be cured. There is no way of taking their CF away, just to be more tolerant of it. If I had a wish it would be to find a cure where they can live without being sick like they are now; not having to die from CF at a young age."

———————

"Mrs. Woodward."

Mrs. Woodward, startled, said, "Yes."

"They'll take Alyson in X-ray now."

"OK. Thank you."

"And then come back up here and Dr. Reese'll take a look."

"Fine."

"Alyson. Alyson," Mrs. Woodward quietly stroked her daughter's leg. "We need to go to X-ray."

Alyson slowly stood up. Her mother put her arm around her shoulder and together they made their way across the waiting room to the door.

CHAPTER 9

The Fosters

(Individuals mentioned by name, in order of appearance)

BRITT/BRIBRI FOSTER: Ten-year-old child with cystic fibrosis (CF)
TYLER FOSTER: Nine-year-old well brother of Britt Foster
MR. GENE FOSTER: Father of Britt Foster
MRS. MAY FOSTER: Mother of Britt Foster
THEA WRIGHT: Outpatient clinical nurse specialist
ALYSON [WOODWARD]: Friend of Britt Foster with CF
DR. EVERETT REESE: Pediatric pulmonologist
LEE DEWEY: Inpatient clinical nurse specialist
TOBY SPRINGER: Young adult with CF
DR. ABE LELAND: Pediatric pulmonologist
SONNY HOLMES: Eleven-year-old child with CF
SABRINA STAPLES: IV nurse
GRAMMY: Grandmother
KIP: Friend of Tyler Foster
GRANDPOP: Grandfather
DR. MARSHA FREEMAN: Pediatric pulmonary fellow
DR. LENORE HASTING: Pediatric pulmonologist

THE FOSTERS, as they were known, strode into the waiting room. Britt, Tyler, and Mr. Foster headed over to the four empty chairs against the wall facing the reception desk. Mrs. Foster went directly over to the reception desk. "I hope we're not late."

"No," said Thea, the outpatient clinical nurse specialist, looking over the receptionist's shoulder at the appointment book. "You just missed Alyson." At that, Britt came over to the desk.

"Did she have an appointment?"

"No. Alyson was . . ."

"Where's Alyson?" Britt interrupted.

"She's in X-ray. She'll be back in a bit."

"Right!" Mrs. Foster said sarcastically, knowing how long everyone waits in X-ray.

"We wanted to have our appointments together, but I had to come in sooner, since I was just in [hospitalized]."

"Well, now you'll be able to see her."

"Yeah," said Britt, who returned excitedly to her seat.

"Have you thought anymore about what we had talked about in the hospital?" the nurse asked Mrs. Foster.

"You mean the Broviac."

"Well, yes, and . . ." Thea moved over to the side as she spoke. Mrs. Foster paralleled, until they were huddled against the wall next to the filing cabinets.

Mrs. Foster had indeed thought a great deal about the Broviac, as had everyone else. Even before the staff broached the subject with Mr. and Mrs. Foster and Britt, much thought had been given not only to the merits of such a device, but also to how the subject should be handled. At a staff conference when the idea of inserting a Broviac was first discussed, Dr. Reese reminded the team that, "while the Broviac may help things along, the parents will need to know that this is not a terminal event. They've seen others who have had it who have been terminal. And she will probably need IVs four times a year."

One of the pulmonary fellows agreed, "Yes. And we need to look at her overall condition. She will continue to deteriorate."

"Her lung disease is bad," added another.

"I think her parents are interested," Lee Dewey, the inpatient clinical nurse specialist, commented. "Mrs. Foster has expressed some concern this hospitalization about Britt dying."

"I think we need to talk to them," said Dr. Reese.

"I'll see what I can arrange," Lee volunteered.

"Fine."

A week later Lee Dewey came by to talk to Britt about the Broviac. When she entered Britt's hospital room Britt was sitting up in bed, drawing. Her father was sitting in a lounge chair by the bed, a magazine opened on his lap.

"Britt. Would you like to see a Broviac?"

"What's that?"

"Would you like to see a Broviac? Questions you had about the IV. Did Mommy talk to you about it?"

"Yes," Mr. Foster interjected.

"Well, you talk to her."

"OK, but let me tell you a little about it. And then I'll bring it over and you can see. Are you listening?"

Britt nodded.

"OK."

"You tell me, OK?"

"OK. It's a special kind of IV. It's called a Broviac. And it's an IV that the doctors put in. And it comes in usually somewhere in your chest where you can't see it, like where you put your clothes. You really can't see it. And it's permanent; which means, every time you come to the hospital they don't have to stick you with an IV. They hook up the tubing and you are ready to go."

"There's one thing."

"There's probably more than one thing," Lee smiled.

"See, I don't think I need it yet."

"Well, what we are talking about is, number one, you should have it done when you are feeling good. You are starting to feel real good now, and you've started to do better. That's when the doctors want to put it in. You can go home with it in. You can do what you want. You can go out and run around and play." Lee paused about a breath's length. "It will have a cap on it. It will be soft. I will have to get one and show you. It's not very big. It's skinnier than this," Lee explained, pointing to Britt's IV line.

"And it will be soft and there will be a little yellow cap on the end like they used to put on the end of your IV, the yellow ones. I don't know if you ever saw the yellow caps, but it will just be a cap on the end. All you have to do when you are not using it at home is flush it two times a day. That's all. And it has a little bandage on it that you can change. It [bandage] only has to be changed three times a week.

"And it will be sore the first couple of days and then after that you won't even know it's there. And that means no more IV sticks. Ever."

"I don't think I want it yet," Britt replied. "I'm going to wait 'til I have to come in some more, because I don't think I'm gonna come in much this year."

"Well, why don't we talk to Mom and Dad."

"I feel like I shouldn't have it right now."

"OK. Why don't we talk to Mom and Dad more about it and then you can talk and then we can make a decision. Why don't we talk to them too so that they know more about it. Let me show it to you and then we can make a decision. But you have to remember that when you come in [to the hospital] and you're sick, they won't put it in. It has to be done when you're feeling well. So we don't want to wait until you get sick again and go through all these IV sticks. Do you see what I'm saying?"

"Uh huh. I just don't . . ."

"I mean," Lee added, before Britt finished, "you don't have to say yes, but I think you should think about it a little bit more, and wait until you see one and . . ."

Before Lee could finish, Britt asked, "When am I going to see one?"

"When I bring you one. It's really a fake—a fake chest where it's in and I'll show you exactly how it looks, OK? You know Toby Springer, don't you? You know Toby."

Britt shook her head no.

"No. OK. Maybe she's coming in. See, she's got one and you'd never know it. But you might be able to see one in some more people."

"That little girl?" asked Britt, pointing to a very small, jaundiced, multiply handicapped deaf child walking from bed to bed, in the six-bed room.

"She might have one. She isn't one of our patients. Isn't that the little girl . . ."

". . . that can't hear," Britt filled in.

"Yeah. She might have one, or it may just be a central line."

"I think it starts with a B."

"Oh, it's a Broviac. OK. Where does she have it?"

Britt pointed to her chest.

"Yeah. OK."

"I didn't see it, though."

"Maybe she'll show it to you, when we talk to everybody about it, and then you guys can talk to each other."

"I'm scared."

"You're scared?" Lee pulled back. "You have to remember that we're not going to make you do it. OK. It's a decision all you guys can make. We're gonna let you see what you think about it first."

"Do I still have to get blood gases when I come in here?"

"Yeah."

"Then I don't want it."

"You get blood gases no matter what. But what it saves is IV sticks; since your veins are not very good."

"I'm going to wait until I run pretty much out."

"I think you are close to that." Lee looked directly at Britt. "Why don't you think about it."

Britt looked to her legs, "Look how many veins are in my legs."

"Yeah, but they're not good veins for IVs."

"Why not?" Britt countered.

"Because they are very tiny. Any vein that you can see is usually a tiny vein because it means it's way up close to the top. It's a superficial vein."

"What if it's real dark? What about the one on my head?"

"That is also a very tiny vein. And also you don't want an IV in your head. It would hurt."

Just then Dr. Leland and Thea came in. They had begun the afternoon rounds. "Hi," Dr. Leland directed to Britt as he nodded to Mr. Foster.

"We're discussing a Broviac," Lee explained.

"Oh, OK," Thea smiled.

"Britt's showing the items in her head and the veins that she thought might be good."

"Oh, OK," Thea repeated.

"But they're real tiny," Lee explained

"One more vein left?" Thea inquired.

"They are real tiny ones, Britt," Lee reiterated. "They wouldn't last long if they could even get them in there. Didn't I tell you that's why they never use those veins that you can see? That's because they are real tiny veins."

"I didn't know that," Britt replied.

"I talked to Sonny Holmes's mother," Thea commented, addressing Lee. "Sonny Holmes is an eleven-year-old that just had one. Close enough to your age," she said, turning to Britt.

"Look," said Britt, still scrutinizing every inch of her arms, "you can't see that one and it's big."

"Oh, good, OK," Lee replied to Thea.

Britt, knowing that was not in response to her remark, said with more urgency and direction, "Lookit. Lookit." A response was not immediately forthcoming and Britt continued to search. "Dad, this must be a needle my mom gave to me when I was little. Look at that. Daddy, lookit."

"I don't think so," Lee said taking Britt's arm. "It looks like a pimple or something. Those things are no good, Britt, for IVs."

"You've had them all over the place," Mr. Foster remarked.

"Uh hum. But how about if we wait and you talk to your mom and dad about it, and we show you one, and we let you talk to people who have one, and then you can decide. OK?" Lee laid out the plan. "But what I don't want you to do is worry. Don't worry about it. Alright? Because if you decide for it, it's only going to be something good for you. And if you decide you don't want it now, that's OK. Just remember that when you come in and you're sick, they can't do it then."

"OK," Britt sighed.

"Because you will be too sick to have it put in. They always want to do it when you're really healthy. OK?" Lee turned to Mr. Foster. "Do you think she is going to worry about it now?"

"No," Mr. Foster shook his head.

"Some nerve," Britt muttered under her breath as Lee followed Dr. Leland and Thea over to the next patient's bed.

"Say Dad," said Britt after a moment's silence, "say I'm going home."

"No. We don't know that."

"Yes I am."

"We are going to get a pulmonary function test."

Britt whispered to herself.

"I can't hear a word you are saying, Britt."

"I am going home in two days."

"Maybe. Maybe."

"Daddy, you are going to get it. I am going home in two days and that's when I'm going home." At that point Lee passed Britt's bed as she was leaving the room. "Lee," Britt called.

"Yes, Britt Foster," Lee replied.

"Dewey."

"Dewey?"

Britt tried to read Lee's pin that said, "kids are really special." Instead she read, "Kids are really bad. Kids are bad. Kids are bad. Kids are pets of people. Kids are—"

"Let me go find Sabrina," Lee interrupted, "so she can come show you this IV. OK?"

"Who?"

"The girl, Sabrina, the IV nurse, you know her."

"Uh-oh."

"You need a flush," Lee added, looking at Britt's IV and flushing it. "Let's wait 'til it clears."

"Yeah." Then as Lee checked out the IV, Britt continued to feign reading the pin. "Kids are dumb people. Kids are dumb people. Kids are dumb people."

"Is that OK?" asked Lee, again ignoring the pin reading.

"What?" asked Britt.

"Is it OK if Sabrina comes over now, if she is not busy?"

"She's the best. No, she's the second best with IVs."

"Who's the first best?"

"That nurse that put this on it."

"She'll show you the Broviac. OK?"

"OK."

"She has one [demonstration model]. OK. Let me see if she's not busy. OK?"

"Can she come down right now?"

"Well, that's what I'm going to ask her." Just then one of the floor nurses walked in. "I just put a flush in," Lee told her.

"OK."

"Britt, I'll go check and let you know," said Lee. She turned and left the room. Mr. Foster followed her out down the hall.

"She knows a lot," said Mr. Foster, catching up with Lee. "I don't know how she picked up most of it."

Lee smiled.

"Most of it by herself, really," Mr. Foster continued. "We do talk to her about it. We don't feel that we shouldn't talk about it. She'll come in, and talk about it. I know parents that are kind of the opposite, they kind of keep it quiet and I don't think that's right."

"No," Lee replied.

"It's something you've got to deal with, and they should know about it.

And then it has a negative side to it too, because she did say one thing that did bother me; is people feeling sorry for her. Now that happens at school, because everybody at school is aware of her problems, which has its good sides and bad sides. But for the most part it doesn't make too much of a difference.

"I'm not 100 percent sure, but I think Alyson's mother [Mrs. Iris Woodward] is the kind, they don't tell anybody about it, only those who have to know. So I don't know. I don't know if that's good or bad or indifferent. But we've always felt that we just wanted her to be able to talk about it."

Lee smiled and nodded

"For instance, her complaining about the doctors. She knows what's supposed to be done, how it's supposed to be done. Sometimes they don't realize that. She knows what hurts and what doesn't hurt and when it's not going right. And she says things that probably upset people, but she's the one who has to live with it. She has to bear with it. Or if she has a pain or whatever; there is a certain degree of her being right to complain if it's extremely painful.

"Or, well, another thing: We had talked to her about how we don't know what she feels like. Nobody does. I mean other than other CF kids. We don't know what she goes through. She doesn't know what it feels like to be normal. It's something she wonders about."

Earlier that same day, Britt had said in a conversation with her dad, "I don't know how you feel not having it. That's something that I wonder about. What does it feel like not having it? I wonder if you feel different, better. See, I don't know how you feel. I would say it feels—you don't feel it sometimes. But I feel it most of the time at home. I can't breathe, 'cause I can't go to sleep. When I go to Grammy's I couldn't breathe and I couldn't go to sleep because I kept wheezing and it bothered me so much. See, I feel, well, just, it feels so bad.

"And sometimes it's scary. Not much. Only when I'm in the hospital. I don't think CF is that scary. Do you Daddy?"

"Sometimes I think . . ." Mr. Foster began.

But before Mr. Foster could finish, Britt added, "Yeah, I would say. It's so hard to explain."

"When you don't understand some of the things that are going on," Mr. Foster continued. "That not knowing kind of creates fear by itself, I think."

"You know what?" Britt put in. "They ought to have a doctor who has CF. They should have a doctor with CF. Then he'll know how it feels, how it would be. I don't know. It's just, I feel kind of mad with the treatments. That's the worst of things. It's just I don't know the feeling. But it bothers a lot, because of the treatments. And I wheeze at night and stuff like that." Britt was quiet for a moment, but her mouth was pregnant with more to say.

Finally she began, "It's the worst disease in the world, because you have to get treatments every day. Even when you are in the middle of playing, you've got to go home and get your treatment. And then you have to get your aerosol three times a day."

"We are up at five o'clock every morning just to get everything done," Mr. Foster interjected.

"In the morning when we go to school it takes longer for me than for Tyler."

"To get everything in, to do her aerosol, PT, and treatment."

"That takes about half an hour," Britt finished her father's sentence. "And then you have to, well, a while after that, you have to eat. If I don't eat that much, you are not going to get . . ., or something like that. It's that I have to eat pretty much. My brother doesn't." Britt paused. "And you know the one thing that disgusts me?"

"What's that?" Mr. Foster responded.

"Meat. I don't like meat. And that's the one thing that they almost always cook."

"Well, it's good for you."

"Well, it's not good for me. Oh, good for me, but I hate it. And when I get out of the pool," Britt added to her list, "I mostly feel salty and itchy and burny. I have to go take a bath or else I won't feel better. And sometimes I lose oxygen."

"It's more difficult for you to breathe."

"Yeah. My lungs get stuffed up and I have to go to the hospital. It's so easy for me to go in the hospital. See, with CF you have to come in the hospital a lot and you lose all your veins. I mean the veins get smaller and smaller and stuff like that and all. I don't think they are good anymore that much, veins. You need a lot of veins to keep on coming here. I'll tell you.

"And I have to do so much stuff. When I get sweaty, I get sweaty so fast. I have to take a lot of salt and I have to watch my bowel movements. Make sure I have enough pancrease. And it's not fun. And I get hotter than anybody in the house when it's hot. I can't stand it. I hate it.

"And another thing that I hate is I get pancrease before I eat. And then, say I was playing, and then I just wanted to take one little snack; I have to take a pancrease. And I just wanted to munch on it when I went out. And lunch time either you start taking a pill every time you munch on it. You could start on it and then not eat for a while and then do it again, and then you have to eat it all up right then while the pancrease is working. That's what I hate. And there's even more."

Britt's hate list continued. "Another thing is some people feel sorry for you. And you don't know what to do because you don't want them to. I wouldn't say it happens that much, but sometimes it happens. And I hate it when it happens, because I don't want to be CF. I don't want to have the CF." Britt paused for a moment. "You know the best way that my life would be?" she asked her dad.

"No, what?"

"Not having CF," Britt replied emphatically. She looked around the room, from one bed to the next and added, "At least I don't have another disease like cerebral palsy."

Four of the children in the six-bed room had cerebral palsy and were profoundly impaired mentally as well. Britt picked up the crayon labeled "flesh" on her bed tray. "All right," she said with renewed vigor. Almost on cue her dad looked back down at his magazine. "First I will draw a face. This is going to be me. I'm going to draw me first. Draw the nose in me. I've got brown eyes. So you put brown right in here. I'll get black for the eyebrows. I'll tell the colors of the things and everything I'm doing."

Mr. Foster did not look up.

"There we go. I guess I do have blondish brown eyebrows. Shall I put blond eyebrows on me?" Not waiting for a reply Britt went on. "And I drew the hair yellow. And what I'm going to do is draw the neck. I'm going to take an orange and draw the neck orange. And I don't know what I was wearing then, so I'll just draw the crayon top. Naah. My red top I have on. It's darker red. It's this red," she said pulling out another crayon. "This must be like a purple."

"Tyler called," Mr. Foster commented, looking up from the magazine while Britt colored in the top.

"He worries a lot," Britt replied offhandedly while she continued to color. "He worries about me mostly. I don't know why. Here, I'm coloring the shirt in. Sometimes he talks to me about what he worries about. Sometimes, I wouldn't say much, because he doesn't want me to know. He just, well, I can hear it on the phone that he is. At home he says, 'If you don't eat you're going to die.' Or he says, 'You're going to die, BriBri.' He's, I don't know. He's scared. He's heard a lot of CF patients die. He's really scared."

Without skipping a beat Britt continued, "Now, what I'm going to do is first get the red again because I got the purple reddish to outline it. Then I'm gonna get the red to put a little lipstick on her, just for color."

Again without transition or pause Britt said and repeated, "I don't get scared. No, I don't get scared. Tyler gets scared because he thinks I'm gonna die. But I don't get scared, because I know I'm not, because I know I'm strong enough. When I was four years old I fought it off, because I was going to die, but I fought it off. I was only twelve months old or something and I did then too. I don't know how, but I did." Britt shrugged, the crayon never leaving the paper, she never looking up.

"I am a fighter," Britt announced. "Tyler just doesn't understand that I am." Pulling back from the paper, Britt added, "Here I am from the jeans up now, kneeling. And I'm going to put you and Mom in there too," she said to her father. "What socks should I put on there? Any socks? I'll just put their feet in. I'm going to put the Monopoly board here." Britt continued to color and narrate as she drew her family playing Monopoly.

Just a few days earlier Tyler had said, "But I still get worried about Britt. I just know that with CF you could die from it. And you get all skinny. And your lungs fill up with mucus. And you can't breathe. And you die. But she's in the hospital fighting."

And a week later, the week before Britt was discharged from the hospital, Tyler would say, "I'm going to be a scientist when I grow up—a real good one, a scientist that knows everything. Kip [his neighbor and friend] and me, we are going to make a medicine for CF. But I am sure it will take time to make them better.

"I think about it so much. It always comes into my mind, that cystic fibrosis. I think about it all the time. I think about it at school. I think about it when I play. I always think about it. Sometimes when I play I'm always thinking there is something else and I think about it. I never really think about it when I'm playing, except when I am playing with Britt, I think about it. But I still play. And most of the time we fight. Britt starts the fighting anyway."

Britt would agree. "Sometimes we play some together and then we start fighting. Always whenever we play we start fighting. I know that. Only sometimes we don't start fighting, but most of the day we fight."

And several months later according to Mr. Foster, "I will fight with Britt too, sometimes deliberately. I will deliberately argue with her. I don't know if that makes any sense, but I will do it just because sometimes she thinks that she can get away with things."

"Which she can, and Tyler can't," Mrs. Foster added.

"Yeah, right."

"But, I will deliberately argue with her. And nine out of ten times, she will [argue back]. She's a tough cookie when it comes to a fight, an argument. She'll be stubborn as all heck."

"And we let her get away with things. Tyler, we usually don't. And, we're not the only ones that let her get away with things, because Tyler also says he lets her get away with things."

Mr. Foster nodded in agreement.

"It's like three of us. And she, I think she . . ."

"She's aware of that."

"She is."

"She's very aware of how to get her way, sometimes."

"And like I said, Tyler will go and get her things. She'll ask him, 'Do this for me. Do that . . .' And my father lets her get away with things that he doesn't let Tyler.

"Yeah, definitely."

"Definitely."

"No doubt about that. That was the problem I felt when we were living with her parents. When we were living there, Tyler was kind of there whenever anything happened."

"And Tyler got the blame."

"He got the blame for it. I mean, regardless if it was true that Britt did it, Tyler got the blame for it. Now, I didn't think that was right, but that was how it was. How should I say this? The situation that we were living in was over-crowdedness; two families trying to live in one house, and May's mom and dad are super people. I mean, they are really. Nobody could ask for better in-laws than they are. They'd do anything for us anytime. And we've never had a real problem there for the year that we did live there. I mean, there wasn't an ongoing conflict all the time, but grandparents tend to spoil grandchildren. And we're trying to teach them some kind of discipline and some kind of direction, I guess. And grandparents just have a natural tendency to spoil or cater, and sometimes they would override it. And the kids knew it, because when we would say 'No' to something they'd run to Grammy or Grandpop."

"Yeah," Mrs. Foster agreed.

"And that was creating a problem, too."

"But, Tyler always . . ."

"But, Tyler always got . . ."

"Yeah."

"If anybody was going to get hollered at, it was always Tyler."

"And if Britt would, if Tyler would get punished for something, if Britt would do the same thing Tyler did, she would . . ."

"The punishments were not the same," Mr. Foster clarified.

"And even with us, too. We seem to go easier on her," Mrs. Foster admitted. "It's like everybody's afraid to punish her. They don't want to."

"Well, that's something I've been more aware of, I think, in the last couple of years. And I've been trying to be . . ."

"We've tried to be as . . ."

"Tough with her; especially in front of Tyler. Because I want him to know that she's getting the same thing. But Britt will go into a . . ."

"Yeah."

"She'll really make a big fuss about it. But, I try to stick to my guns with her, and usually she'll come around," Mr. Foster noted.

"And my parents, too. If I would yell at Britt or try to punish her they would get very upset. So I just didn't, and it just seemed to carry on."

"Britt still does that to this day," Mr. Foster pointed out. "Her mom's over here, and there's something going on or she can't do something she wants to, she'll go, 'Ah, Grammy rah, rah, rah.'"

"Britt'll call her up on the phone, 'My mom won't let me do this.'"

"Oh, yeah."

"And then my mom gets on the phone with me and lets me have it." Mr. and Mrs. Foster laughed.

While Thea and Mrs. Foster chatted by the file cabinets, Britt walked by on her way to the pulmonary function lab for her first pulmonary function test since she had been discharged from the hospital. The scene was not unlike that of three and half months ago, when Thea and Mrs. Foster had been standing and chatting there while Britt searched the file drawers for recipes. "I never have an appetite," she said then as she flipped through the files.

"You're telling me," Mrs. Foster acknowledged. "Here I am chasing after Britt with Tasty-Kakes and Tyler's begging her for some, and he's overweight. And I'm hyping on him about 'Don't eat, cut down.' And he grabs."

"We've also taken him off sugar, because he's so hyperactive. He shouldn't be eating candy because he's hyper; not only because he's gained. I won't let him have the candy. But the more I'm on him about cutting down, the more he wants."

"Mom, you need this," Britt proclaimed, pulling out a booklet that dealt with nutrition.

"Thanks dear," Mrs. Foster answered absently as she continued her conversation with Thea. "I wasn't too happy about the PFT [i.e., having to have the pulmonary function test]."

"We didn't have time for PT [chest physical therapy] this morning," Britt put in.

"But you gained two and a half pounds," Thea encouraged.

"Britt, could you come with me," said Dr. Freeman as she approached Britt. "I need you to cough for me," she added, holding out a flat covered dish.

"OK." Britt followed Dr. Freeman back to her office.

"You look worried," Thea opened.

"Yeah. She's had this dry cough, and she was clear. I'm afraid it will get worse. And I think I might be bringing Tyler down. I want him to see somebody for his problem. With Britt it's physical, but for him I think it might be greater because it's mental.

"Tyler's teacher said we should give him more attention. But it's hard, because I worry about Britt when she's in the hospital. I stay there all weekend and he gets shifted around. It's not a normal family life. He tells me he's OK and not to worry about him. He knows I worry about her. When I explain things to him he pats me on the back and tells me not to worry. But I know he worries too. Sometimes at dinner or something he'll say something like, 'You better eat or you'll die.' And then she gets all mad and says, 'No, not from that. No, I won't die from that.'" Mrs. Foster smiled and chuckled lightly, recalling these interchanges.

"Last year," she continued, "when Britt was in the hospital, she wrote him a letter and told him how much she missed him and what she was making for arts and crafts. He uses it as a book mark.

"And then I was so worried about her failing in school I brought her books every time I came to the hospital and studied with her. Report cards came out and she got all 90s. And Tyler, who usually does better than Britt, had an F. I just wasn't paying enough attention."

This was not the only time the subject of attention would come up. "When Tyler was a baby," Mrs. Foster recalled, "it was right at the time that Britt was diagnosed. And everything was Britt. I left him cry. When Britt was a baby as soon as she cried I was picking her up. Tyler, I fed him when I had to feed him and that was it. Tyler was an infant in the crib and I was rocking Britt in the rocking chair. It seemed like, I don't know. I just felt that he's fine, he'll be all right.

"Britt was a terrible baby. She cried and cried and cried and cried and cried. She never slept. If she slept, she slept for three hours at night, then she'd wake up again. I was constantly walking her, rocking her, up with her. And at that time I had to give her six treatments a day. I don't know why they had me giving her six. It may be because she had pneumonia at that time. And at that time this was serious. I had to do it. Dr. Hasting was the doctor then. I mean, 'You better do it or you're an awful mother.' And every time I came to clinic, 'Are you giving her the six treatments?' Oh, and at that time my husband [first husband] wasn't home that much, I really didn't have any help hardly at all from him. So Tyler, I gypped him of a lot of holding, handling, holding, loving. And I really feel bad about that now. All I can remember of him as a baby is I would just stick the bottle in his mouth. I wouldn't even hold him to feed him. And I wonder if that somehow didn't affect him."

And then again, three days before Britt's most recent hospitalization, Mrs. Foster brought up the issue of attention. Standing in the waiting room, she said, "I want to give Tyler more attention. He needs it. He wants to show it, but he can't. He should. It's hard."

Tyler, who had been playing nearby, interrupted her conversation and asked, "It's hard for me, what? I should do what?"

"You feel like more," Mrs. Foster called back. "You want some of the attention."

"No. I don't want most of—I know Britt has CF and she needs all the attention."

Earlier that same day Tyler had said that he wanted to write a story about his sister and dictated, "My sister has cystic fibrosis and I hate it. I wish there was a miracle; that they could have a medicine for cystic fibrosis." When asked if there was anything else he wanted to add to his story, he said, "That's the only thing I can think of. That's the thing that always comes into my mind. That's the thing that always ever comes into my mind.

"When I have to write something, I usually write about my sister, and just like these two sentences. These are the sentences that I usually write. Those are the sentences I do write."

In fact, nine months later, Britt and cystic fibrosis figured into one of Tyler's homework assignments. Asked to write a sentence for his three spelling words: treatment, sickness, and illness; he wrote, "My sister gets three treatments a day. My sister has a sickness. Cystic fibrosis is an illness."

When Britt heard her mother read the sentences aloud as she checked Tyler's homework, she became quite upset. She stormed into the kitchen. "I don't want him to write about my CF." With that, Tyler and Britt started arguing.

Later that day Mrs. Foster said, "Britt is constantly disagreeing with everything Tyler does. And she's always trying to get it through his head that the things he is doing are wrong, just because she doesn't view things the way he does. And he gets real aggravated because he feels he's the one who's right and she isn't. And then they start fighting and screaming at each other.

"Tyler seems to let Britt go with a lot of it. Sometimes he gets to the point where he will just scream right back at her. But in a sense he lets her get away with things. He'll fight a little bit, but he'll always, he's the first one to give. For an example, one time they were fighting over a sleeping bag. She wanted it, she really wanted it. And it was his turn to use it. And she just kept going on and on and on. I don't know what her reasons were, but it was his turn. They had one sleeping bag and I had said that they had to take turns with it. Well, he let her. He gave in.

"And if we tell Britt to clean this or pick up the books or something, put it away; she'll be moaning, 'Oh I don't feel good. I don't feel like doing it.' And he'll end up getting up himself and he'll do it for her." Mrs. Foster shook her head. "He just seems to. Maybe because she's a girl, cater to her a little bit. Or she'll ask him, 'Oh could you please go get me some pretzels.' He'll go up and get them, but she won't. She would never do that. I shouldn't say that, maybe sometimes she would. But he would more than she." Mrs. Foster smiled.

"And they stick up for each other. Yesterday Tyler came home crying because the bus driver yelled at him and told him that he's going to have to kick him off the bus. Because Tyler's loud. Well, Britt saw this. And Tyler didn't think he yelled at the bus driver. And Britt just kept screaming, 'Yes you did. You yelled at him.' The bus driver said, 'Where were you?' And Tyler instead of saying, 'I was doing this;' he'll go, 'What do you mean I was . . .' He'll say it smartly. Now Tyler kept insisting that he didn't yell at the bus driver and Britt kept arguing with him that he did. She's really trying to help him, get through to him what he did, and he gets all aggravated and mad at her and then they start fighting. But really they do so care about each other. I think this fight [over the homework] was because Britt's at the point of not wanting people to know that she has CF. She's thinking of changing schools so kids don't know. The beginning of this year she was saying she doesn't like the way some kids treat her special. They won't want to play with her, or sometimes they're afraid that she can't do it."

"They become overcautious," Mr. Foster remarked.

"Tyler's protective too," Mrs. Foster added.

"Yeah, in a way, I guess."

"Tyler's always saying, 'Why don't you go down and get your treatment already? Do you want to die? Go down and get your treatment.' And she'll argue back about the treatment or something, and he'll go, 'Go already. Do you want to die?' And then she's all huffy."

"Tyler will make comments like that when Britt's resisting treatment or something like that," Mr. Foster said.

"He'll come up with ideas of how to get her to exercise. He'll go, 'Oh that'll be great for her.'"

"Of course Britt doesn't think it's so great."

"Tyler knows it's important for Britt to exercise, to cough up all that junk. He knows it's important for her to eat. He'll try to concoct ways of getting her to."

Mr. Foster nodded in agreement.

"We went through a period," Mrs. Foster continued, "where she just really didn't want her treatments and I just yelled at her. She didn't say, 'What's the use?' But I sensed that's what she felt. And I yelled at her. I said, 'I wouldn't be giving you these treatments and yelling at you and trying to get you to try harder if I didn't feel there was any hope.' And it seemed that kind of perked her out of it.

"I have stressed to her that there is hope, that they are very close to finding a cure."

"And maybe that's why she doesn't feel it's [death's] an immediate threat," Mr. Foster added.

"Tyler thinks when kids die it's because they didn't take care of themselves. And I always try to tell him that there's different severities. And I'm always telling Britt that she doesn't have such a severe case. But I just don't want her to worry so much.

"Britt knows just about everything she would have to know," Mrs. Foster uttered heavily. "But I think she still feels there is hope."

"I don't think that part of it [death] is reality to her."

"I think, I don't know what the word for it is, but I think it gets her mad."

"She gets mad," Mr. Foster shook his head.

"Yeah," Mrs. Foster agreed. "And that comes out in different ways. But she won't come out, she would never, she has never said to me that she was mad or angry that she has CF. She'll just get frustrated with other things, but I can tell it's that [CF]."

"Well, she's already said that. I've heard her say when she was mad, 'Why do I have to do this?'"

"But not too often."

"No. That's only been maybe once or twice in over four or five years or something like that. And that was probably her frustration."

"When she's sick."

"Not particularly CF."

"When she gets sick she gets really crabby and everything."

"We can tell."

"Everything. She picks about everything, from her cousins to her brother. Everybody."

"She'll fight with everybody."

"Everybody's against her."

"She'll get crying; like crying jags."

"Yeah," Mrs. Foster agreed.

"Whining type things. That's usually a foolproof sign that she's getting sick. That's probably one of the first things. Kids will have bad days and be like that, but when it becomes two or three days in a row, which usually it is, she's not feeling good. And that's her way of showing it, I guess."

"And I think I'm a little like that too," Mrs. Foster added, "especially when she's sick. I'm worried about her and yet it comes out in different things. Like my hair. I'll cut my hair." Mrs. Foster laughed. "And I'll clean like crazy. I'll worry if the furniture looks right the way it is. I'll worry. I do weird things when I worry."

"She's a worrier. When she worries it comes out in strange ways. Like she says about the scissors—cutting her hair. When she's worried or something is bothering her, her hair never satisfies her. No matter how good it looks, she doesn't like it. I even hid the scissors on her and it didn't help. We had too many scissors." Mr. and Mrs. Foster laughed and continued to, as Mr. Foster recounted how "our house is always clean, spotless. And then when she worries she gets on a cleaning jag where she doesn't want to stop."

"Yeah," Mrs. Foster smiled.

"I mean to the point where it's eleven, twelve, one o'clock at night and she's still cleaning. And that aggravates me sometimes. Either relax, or go to bed, or something. Not to be cleaning all night long. Because the house is never dirty. She keeps it spotless."

"I get nervous, upset, worried."

"And Tyler's a worrier too. I think he gets that from his mother. He worries. Particularly when Britt's in the hospital. He worries, but he doesn't express it and doesn't say it. Even though he's never said he's worried or anything like that."

"He gets his worries out in strange ways too."

"He seems like he's off somewhere, especially with his schoolwork," Mr.

Foster began to explain. "I think it's hard for him to concentrate when Britt's in the hospital. And the fact that sometimes he gets trucked all over the place at those particular times, that doesn't help things either. I think that is a problem too. We've talked about this ourselves. And when she's in the hospital we have to still maintain this house for him and not put him at her mom's or my mom's or somebody else's house. I think, that's not good for him when she's away. And I think he still needs the stability of this house. So that's why we kind of thought really good about it when Britt was home on the IV. I think that helped. That seemed to be a one hundred percent better situation. Even though it was a lot of work. Well not a lot. It was our inexperience more than anything."

"I think it was actually easier," Mrs. Foster commented.

"Yeah," Mr. Foster nodded.

"Than running back and forth to the hospital."

"If you come home three-thirty, four, you try to grab something to eat, run to the hospital. You're there till nine-thirty, ten o'clock at night. Then it's two hours to drive home again. If you don't get the proper rest, you're not rested for work. You come out of work, you're still tired; and you turn around and do the same thing. And then that's it. It really wears you down so much. And then we get irritable with each other, and with the kids or with Tyler or whatever."

"We all get real irritable."

"Everybody does. It really gets weird."

"Well . . ."

"It's an exhausting type of thing that you really don't realize and don't have time to think about, because you're so busy. It wears you down."

"That's why I felt bad about the time that I just exploded in the hospital. I said, 'I'm leaving this hospital.' It just comes over you." Mrs. Foster shook her head. "Anyway I think being at home was good for Tyler because he seemed to be a part of helping her, being that he was home. He hardly sees her at all when she's in the hospital, because he doesn't like the drive and we just leave him with my mom."

"Yeah. He's not big on drives or rides anywhere."

"But with Britt being home, he was able to help. Maybe give her a treatment. And he was more a part of it. I think he felt he was doing something or helping."

Mr. and Mrs. Foster looked at one another, smiled, nodded, and became quiet. Mrs. Foster's declaration pierced the silence, "It's a terrible disease. It's just such a slow, torturing," she continued. "I can't even think of the words for it." Mrs. Foster sighed. "I think it's just slow. And to have to watch the pain, the suffering." She halted with each phrase.

"I don't know. It's always there. I'm always tense. I'm always watching her. I'm always listening to her breathe. She comes home from the hospital and she's fine. And then, before you know it, she's getting sick again. And each time she comes out there's more and more damage there. Every time. And every time there's more, there's more hurt. It just takes a little more out of you every single time she's in. Because it just seems to creep more and more. Damage. And I guess I try, we all try, so hard to keep her as clear as we possibly could. And it's just impossible. It's what you go through: getting her to exercise, doing her treatments, trying to feed her." Her weariness was audible.

"You get so frustrated. You get so frustrated to the point that you wonder, 'Is this really doing any good?'"

"Try so hard," Mrs. Foster shook her head, "and it doesn't seem to do anything."

"You work so hard giving her treatments, and trying to make sure she eats, and watching the weather for days that could be bad for her, where she could pick up a cold or something, or . . ."

"Keeping her away from people who have colds," Mrs. Foster continued the list her husband started, and then picked up again.

"Keeping her away from kids that have colds, that are sick. And everything that you go through when you beat yourself down; day after day after day after day. And then she crashes and gets sick anyway and you think.

"And then when you go in and she's on antibiotics, you want so much for her to be cleared up, just as good as she was before she got sick. And it's always never as good. Always there's more infection, more damage in there. You can't win." Mrs. Foster smiled wryly and repeated, "You just can't win. But you keep doing it, because we want. We want for a year. We want."

"You want to give her as much time as she possibly can have," Mr. Foster finished.

"Sometimes I get mad and say, 'Oh what's the use?'"

"Frustrated," Mr. Foster interpreted.

"And I'll get mad at her when she doesn't do her treatment and I'll say, 'All right then. If you want to get sick; then the heck with it.' And then . . ."

"'Cause she's . . ."

"I'll go down minutes later and I'll say, 'I'm giving you your treatment.'" Mr. and Mrs. Foster laughed.

"See," Mr. Foster continued, "she fights it. And that comes sometimes at a time when we may feel frustrated about doing everything and not accomplishing anything. By the same token Britt is fed up with the treatments and everything else. So she's fighting and resisting. When the two things happen at the same time, then all hell breaks lose. Because you're trying to do the best you can and she's not cooperating. And that becomes very frustrating sometimes too. You holler and you holler, because you have to holler. I can understand her just being sick and tired of treatments and all that, everything else that goes with it. I can understand that, but it has to be."

"You have to do it. You just want to hang on as long as you can. And then they're so close to a cure, which I don't know. You get your hopes up about it. But then it just seems hopeful. But it . . ."

"It depends," Mr. Foster picked up, "on who you listen to; as far as that goes. I don't know. I really wonder how close they are [to a cure]. And if they are close, is it in time to do any good for Britt?"

"But," Mrs. Foster added quickly, "there's always that hope in there; no matter what anybody says to bring you down. Not to bring you down, but to make you feel like there's no hope. You still have that. You still have that hope." Mrs. Foster paused, prayerfully determined, and then her visage changed.

"I feel frightened. I keep wondering what's coming up ahead. This is why Gene doesn't want me watching this movie [*Alex*], because then I start thinking. I keep thinking I don't want her to suffer. I don't. One mother told me that her son really fought it. He was really angry when he found out he was dying, that he was going to die. I keep worrying about that. I worry ahead." Mrs. Foster giggled nervously. "And I shouldn't. I keep thinking to myself, 'Take it day by day.' But I don't. I'm really ahead all the time. I don't want that to happen, but I think about it."

"For a while there you had a time where you thought about it pretty much, not a whole lot."

"Yeah. Depends. Sometimes I go through . . ." Mrs. Foster didn't finish. "This year wasn't too bad?"

"Ah, no."

"I think so."

"I think a lot of that has to do with how Britt is doing."

"Yeah, " Mrs. Foster agreed. "It depends. It was for a long period of time. Now it's like for maybe one night or a week I'll dwell on it more. I think it was the last time she was sick. Usually when she's sick I'm constantly on it. Or before, if I feel she's starting to get sick. It's day after day, like that's all there is, that's all I think about."

"Well, you had a really, really extreme period there when she was really sick and got that vasculitis."

"Yeah."

"I mean that was a really bad time for you."

"Usually when she's doing good, I'm pretty, pretty good." Mrs. Foster paused. "I think we're pretty busy during the days. A lot of times it's at night when you sit down and say, when we just think about how busy we are. During the week I'm pretty good because I'm tired and I fall asleep. Maybe Saturday night I'll dwell on it more. I'll talk to him and it makes me feel better to talk about it. Plus, I don't know, I'll ask him, 'Do you think she's doing pretty good now?' And he says, 'Yeah.'"

"I think the worst time you had was when Britt was in the hospital with the vasculitis and her veins collapsing," said Mr. Foster bringing up the vasculitis again.

"Yeah," agreed Mrs. Foster, this time following up on his mention of it specifically. "They don't know what caused it. I think maybe just her veins. How many antibiotics did they pump into her veins?" Mrs. Foster shrugged. "Maybe they can only take so much.

"There's nights when I toss and turn a lot," said Mrs. Foster, returning to the subject of when she thinks about CF.

"She can't fall asleep."

"Yeah. And that's on my mind. But during the day, not so much. It's usually at night. And when I can, when I think."

"Before you started working I think it was worse."

"Yeah."

"When she was home all day, there were times when I'd come home from work and you'd be a total wreck."

"Yeah."

"Well she wasn't working. She just started working," Mr. Foster added.

"It's about my third year now."

"Right."

"That I'm working."

"But three years ago when she was home all day, it was a lot harder on her. I think you had too much time to think," he addressed his wife.

"Yeah. And boy my house was clean then." Mr. and Mrs. Foster laughed. "I mean people used to hate to come to visit me. They were afraid to come in here, everything was so spotless."

"But who cares about company?" Mr. Foster joked.

"What are you going to talk about [with others] anyway?" Mrs. Foster replied more seriously. "When you talk to other mothers with normal children, they're thinking about the future: college, cheerleading, 'I want my daughter to do this.' When they talk about the future, it's hard. You don't have anything in common. You're living in a more day-to-day life; where a lot of people aren't. We're in a way enjoying each other more because we are taking it day to day." Mrs. Foster looked at her husband and smiled.

"We don't, I don't worry," she restarted, "worry about her suffering at the end and things like that. But we seem to take it, to enjoy each day, to enjoy her." Mrs. Foster paused. "One thing about CF, though, is when she is feeling well she enjoys life. And I thank God for that."

"We don't plan for the future, like a lot of parents do. No, not a whole lot."

"And with daily-life things, it's like a lot of mothers are involved in different sorts of things. Say for instance . . ."

"School," Mr. Foster filled in. "They put enormous amounts of pressure on parents. I don't know, maybe under different circumstances, that wouldn't bother us so much."

"Or . . ."

"Me," Mr. Foster began, before Mrs. Foster could finish her sentence, "it aggravates sometimes because they have a hundred million things they want you involved in. We don't have time for that kind of involvement."

"Well, like my sister-in-law," Mrs. Foster tried again.

"But you try and tell somebody that and they look at you," Mr. Foster finished.

"My sister-in-law is going to college now. She has spare time to do these things. She also has two children. But I feel like I think because Britt's life may be limited, I would feel guilty to do something like that. I want to be here with her, I want to spend time with her. I think if she didn't have CF, things would be different. I think I would be thinking more of myself. I would be doing things for myself more. I would go to college. Or maybe I'd get involved in different things. Right now, we all go to CF meetings, talk to parents that have something in common with us—people that will relate to what we're going through.

"I feel guilty to leave all the time, even on a Saturday night or a Sunday night. And I think I get mad at myself for not doing it and I'll start picking at Gene like, 'Why don't we go out?' or 'Why don't you take me out, already?' When really I know he would take me out if I wanted to go out. But I don't want to go out." Mrs. Foster chuckled. "And then he's says, 'Let's go out.' And I don't really want to go out. I don't. I feel I should do this with the kids, or I should do that." Mrs. Foster looked at Mr. Foster and sighed, "To have a child with CF I don't think is a normal life."

"It's hard. It's frustrating in a way that we can't do things like other normal families do."

"Yeah," Mrs. Foster agreed.

"Even as far as going places or doing things. You've got to get home to give that treatment."

Again Mrs. Foster nodded.

"We may have to leave or something like that because we have to get home and give Britt a treatment. Or another way it affects us—it's not like a normal situation in the morning. Some people can sleep late and their kids can get up, get themselves something to eat, go watch television. They can get up and go, if they want to get up and go. But we, when we get up, we have to get breakfast, get the aerosol mixed, give Britt a treatment; and you don't realize how much time is gone. The morning's half shot by the time you get it all in; by the time you get things organized." Mr. Foster laughed. "And those are little things, but they're the little things that you take for granted.

"We're into a routine where we do this every morning, but then when she gets really sick there goes the routine. Then there's the running back and forth to the hospital, and coming home from work and running down there, and running back. You don't think about how tired you are, how run down you are. You're just thinking about if she is getting better. Is she feeling better? Is it helping? Your thoughts are on her and how her health is and not on yourself. And that creates problems where we get edgy with each other. It kind of disrupts every darn thing. It's just devastating. It's rotten. It's basically a home-wrecking disease.

"I don't know. I, you, have really mixed emotions about it. I really, really worry about how it's going to affect May. Or if that's going to change her when Britt should die. I think that's constantly on my mind because I don't want her to go, but I don't want anything to happen to May.

"And I'm so afraid. When Britt had vasculitis and she was real sick, she really had herself convinced that Britt was dying then. And all she kept talking about was that she wants to go with her. And that scared the hell out of me.

"It's a very strong concern, because sometimes I think maybe they are too close. I don't know if that's good or bad. And since they are very close, it could be more of a problem. Right now it's nice, but in the long run . . ." Mr. Foster just stopped there.

Mrs. Foster looked at him and tried to manage a smile. "I'm closer to Britt than to Tyler," she began, "but now I'm starting to feel a little more closer to him. There for a long time, however, I would go to hug him, like just this last year, and he'd back off, back off. He's just so fidgety. He didn't want to be held. It's just this year, I finally, he's finally letting me hug him at night, kiss him. And he would never let me scratch his back. Just this past month he's letting me scratch his back. I could never feel a closeness with him that I can now. It's still not there. Not like with Britt. Britt, she's cuddly. She always wants to cuddle with me. I mean touching, just holding, this type of thing. And Tyler isn't. He's started a little bit, but not as much. No."

———

Britt passed her mother on the way back from the pulmonary function test. "One twelve," she called out as she passed with a huff.

"That's not good?" Thea called to her.

"One thirty's better. It's because I'm coughing a lot."

"Would you excuse me?" asked Mrs. Foster.

"Sure, " replied Thea.

"Britt," called Mrs. Foster, crooking her finger, "Let's go back to the PFT lab."

Britt followed her mom.

CHAPTER 10

The Baileys

(Individuals mentioned by name, in order of appearance)

MRS. EVELYN/EVIE BAILEY: Mother of Casey Bailey
CASEY BAILEY: Eight-year-old child with Cystic Fibrosis (CF)
LEE DEWEY: Inpatient clinical nurse specialist
DR. SHELBY TRENT: Pediatric pulmonologist
LEANA LINDER: Child who died of CF
THEA WRIGHT: Outpatient clinical nurse specialist
DR. EVERETT REESE: Pediatric pulmonologist
DR. MARSHA FREEMAN: Pediatric pulmonary fellow
EVAN BAILEY: Nine-year-old well brother of Casey Bailey
RITA THORNTON: Pulmonary social worker
MRS. PEARL GREY: Mother of two children with CF
GAVIN BAILEY: Eleven-year-old well brother of Casey Bailey
MR. HARRIS: Health teacher
JOSE: Friend of Casey Bailey
DOLLY BAILEY: Wife of Mr. Bailey's brother
GRETA: Teacher of Evan Bailey
JORGE: Friend
MR. GILBERT/GIL BAILEY: Father of Casey Bailey
MR. MOREY: Teacher
MYRTLE: Friend
PHYLLIS COKER: Hospice nurse

MRS. BAILEY bore Casey out of the examining room. She would not be making another clinic appointment. He would not be going home. Instead, Casey would join the other CF patients on the third floor of the hospital. Like two of the other children with CF already there, Casey was dying. Unlike the other two, eventually he would go home to die.

———

"Casey, are you scared?" Lee asked.
    Without turning to look, he nodded yes.
    "Why?"

"I don't know," his gaze fixed on the window.

"Does the oxygen scare you?"

"Yeah," he answered as it bubbled away over his bed.

"OK. I understand." Lee stood there for a few moments trying to make eye contact with Casey. "Casey, there won't be any shots."

Casey turned and looked at her.

"Casey, if there is anything you want just let the nurses know."

Casey nodded his assent.

"And don't worry. The doctors will tell you how you are doing. I'll be back in a little while."

Casey closed his eyes and Lee left the room. She was met by the house staff assembled behind Dr. Trent, the pediatric pulmonologist assigned to the inpatient service that month. "He's scared," Lee greeted them.

"He's got a right to be," Dr. Trent replied and turned to the residents to give them a brief update on Casey's medical condition. Most were familiar with his history from his last admission in the spring, when a great deal of time was spent discussing the pros and cons of surgically inserting permanent lines for supplementary feeding and/or antibiotic therapy. The update was sprinkled with medical as well as nonmedical terms. "His PFTs are piss-poor. He's hypoxemic. He's growing cepacia. And he has that Leana Linder look.[1] He's too young to be having disease this bad. And too young to have an 'I'm going to give up now' attitude."

"Mrs. Bailey is concerned too. She feels that Casey is fearful and is giving up. We've tried to set some goals with the nurses. They've told Casey that he has to eat," Lee reported.

"Has he seen other kids die?" one of the residents inquired.

"Yes," Dr. Trent replied.

"He wants to see his brothers," Lee continued, "so one goal is that his brothers can come if he eats."

"OK. Let's go in and see him." Dr. Trent led the way.

Ten days passed and Casey's condition did not improve. At the weekly inpatient X-ray conference Lee remarked, "It looks like he's throwing in the towel. He's sleeping a lot."

"Remember, this is the kid who's usually off the walls," a pulmonary fellow noted.

"What about the eating?" another pulmonary fellow asked.

"Some, but not really. We've told the nurses not to push. Why have food be the only thing?"

"Yeah. Right," came the nods and voices from around the table.

---

[1] Reference to a child with CF who for several weeks before her death appeared pale and malnourished.

"What about the brothers?" Thea inquired.

"They've been in. His dad said he really perked up when he saw them."

"Well, what do you think here?" Thea asked, turning to Dr. Reese.

"I think he's climbing up the gutters."

"He's been in the fetal position since this morning," Lee commented.

"Look at that X-ray. Bad news. Look at the heart. Marsha, do you want to score it?"

Marsha, one of the pulmonary fellows, looked up at the X-ray, mumbled a few numbers out loud, and then clearly announced, "Nine. I'd say it's a nine."

"Right. And he was a twelve on admission. Nine out of twenty-five, folks. And he's bringing up green sputum with specks of blood."

"And he's had that persistent low 'temp,'" added another member of the team.

"What's that?" asked a new medical student rotating through pulmonary.

"That's short for this child may not leave the premises."

"As in, may not live," one of the fellow's translated.

"Do the parents know?"

"I don't know. They seem anxious to talk," said Lee.

"The parents know," Dr. Reese replied. "Let's see what the story is this afternoon.

As the team made their way toward Casey's room, Mrs. Bailey was coming out the door and down the hall in their direction. "I wanted to show you this," she said to Lee as the others proceeded to the room. "It's a story Evan wrote at school."

"My Family," he wrote. "What a wonderful family I have. We all stick together. We have sad days and happy days. The saddest day we had was when my grandfather died. That really had us down. Especially my mother, because he was my mother's father. The happiest day of our lives was when my mother and father said that we might go to Kentucky this summer. I told my brothers, 'Just think, we can climb trees, climb mountains, and ride our bikes over dirt hills. We can go for hikes with Dad, go on trails, and walk through the woods behind the house.' We were all very excited about the trip until last week when my little brother was taken to the hospital again. His name is Casey and he is 8 years old. He is special because he is my little brother. He has a disease called Cystic Fibrosis and he goes to the hospital whenever he starts losing weight. We might not go to Kentucky after all. I said, 'Well, maybe next year. We have to worry about Casey.'

"I used to think that nobody cared about me, but now I can see why Casey is getting all the attention. It's not because he is better than me. It's just because he needs more of the attention than my brother and me. My parents are doing their very best for us all. I know our family will make it through the good times and the bad, if we just stick together."

As the doctors filed out of Casey's room, Mrs. Bailey looked to Dr. Reese. "He's still not eating that much."

"I know. He's not really any better then he was two weeks ago. I think we need to discuss what we should do—how aggressive we want to be with the antibiotic, if we want to feed him through his vein and so forth." Dr. Reese paused between each issue, giving it time to "sink in," he would later explain.

Mrs. Bailey just nodded.

"I'd like to talk to both you and your husband."

"Yeah. Sure. Of course."

"What time's good?"

"Well. Uh, I guess . . . Well, he's usually here in the afternoon, when I go back home."

"OK. About three or so?"

"Yeah. All right."

'We'll come by for you," Lee volunteered.

Not long after three, Lee and Rita, the pulmonary social worker, came up on the floor to get Mr. and Mrs. Bailey and take them to Dr. Reese's office in the pulmonary clinic. Mrs. Grey, a mother of two children with CF, saw them leave and remarked, "When they come for me, I'm not going. I'll know by their coming [what they have to say]."

The Baileys were on their way to what the staff called "the come to Jesus meeting," or more specifically, "the come to Jesus meeting, chapter one." With the two clinical nurse specialists and the social worker in attendance, "We'll talk terminal care with them. In the second chapter, we'll tell them what it's really like when they die," Dr. Reese explained.

And in fact, at the initial conference Dr. Reese did lay out the various options—which came down to home or hospital death. Mrs. Bailey thought, "We should go home and talk to Gavin and Evan. When Gavin was here he said, 'Casey was real sick.' And Evan just watched the oxygen and the TV the whole time."

"I think Gavin knows," Mrs. Bailey continued, "but Evan doesn't."

Dr. Reese explained that "different members of the family can react differently. One can cry and the other can look callous. It's a time of great stress."

"I think it's going to be hardest for Gavin and Evan," Mrs. Bailey predicted.

Dr. Reese did not rush. There was time for silence, to collect one's thoughts, to ask questions.

"You know," said Mrs. Bailey, breaking one such silence, "he asked me, 'Am I going to die?' I told him you don't have to, but you need to fight.'"

Thea gently but authoritatively explained how "sometimes people need permission to die. After a while there's no need to fight. He's not just throwing in the towel. His body's exhausted; it's giving up."

"He will ask about dying. Or he may simply tell you," Dr. Reese posited. "These patients know."

"They do," Thea agreed.

"We will not treat him as aggressively—not push eating. And he will notice that."

"The nurses on the floor mentioned that Casey didn't want to be moved," Lee interjected.

"This is not uncommon," Dr. Reese reassured. "They all know about that back room. It's hard to get well patients to stay there. He's been here when patients have died. He knows the score. He also probably wants to stay where he is because he has company."

"No, he definitely does not want to be left alone," Mrs. Bailey added. "He wakes when he's sleeping."

"You'll see a pattern of sleeping days and waking nights," Dr. Reese affirmed. "Because with night sleep he worries he might die in his sleep."

"I see."

"We'll try to make him comfortable. But some of the things that we need to do to make him comfortable will compromise his lung function."

As Dr. Reese began to explain the effects of increased oxygen, Valium, and morphine, Mr. Bailey, who had been basically silent throughout the meeting, began to cry.

"It looks downhill," Dr. Reese seemed to be directing his remarks to Mr. Bailey, "but the picture could change." Then looking back to Mrs. Bailey, where he had been focused most of the meeting, "Yet again, it's unlikely. And even if it does, these are issues you will have to confront at some point. And there's no reason not to begin thinking about them now."

"I want to take him home," Mrs. Bailey burst forward.

"You don't have to make a decision now. We are not asking you to make a decision now."

It would be another ten days before Mr. and Mrs. Bailey took Casey home. They were quite concerned about taking him home with an IV. At a meeting with Rita they went back and forth. Finally, Mrs. Bailey said, "We'll wait."

"That's what I wanted too," Mr. Bailey sighed, "but I was afraid to say it first because I thought you wanted Casey home."

"I do. But I'm not sure how we'd manage. Gavin says he wants to learn how to do the IV. I told him that if he wanted to help he'd have to go to school and then he could help later. And they both offered to do jobs if Casey could come home. But still."

Arranging for Casey to go home with an IV also posed problems for the pulmonary staff. If Casey were sent home with an IV the Baileys would need some nursing assistance, and that was hard to come by. Casey was on medical assistance and they had difficulty finding a hospice or home-care program that would provide the home care Casey required. For a while it looked as if Thea and the graduate nursing student she supervised were going to provide the care.

Aside from the medical issues, Mrs. Bailey also struggled with getting Gavin off to school in the morning, and Evan back to school after leaving and then coming home crying before he even got to school.

Mr. Bailey said, "It's hard to get Casey to talk to his brothers on the phone when they call, but he's always glad after he does. He seems to rally then."

Casey also began to experience more pain. Lee promised him more pain medication. She told Dr. Reese of his needs and her concerns.

"There's no reason for him to be in pain. There are things we can offer. I also want another CBC [complete blood check] before taking him off the antibiotics." Once he was ooff the antibiotics there would be no need for the IV, thereby removing what Dr. Reese saw as the major stumbling block to Casey's going home. "I'll talk to Casey later about going home."

"It's bye bye!" Dr. Reese saluted, trying to lighten the heaviness he and Lee shared.

Lee did not return Dr. Reese's attempt. She just stood there.

"To take him home is to accept that there is nothing more to do," Dr. Reese added, returning to his previous demeanor. "That's hurdle one [referring to the meeting he had had with Mr. and Mrs. Bailey]. Hurdle two, logistics."

"I know. Thea and I'll work on that."

"Fine. Let's try to get him home by the middle of the week."

"In case they want to bring him back."

"That wasn't my reasoning exactly, but OK. Yes, they should know they can bring him back."

"I guess it's time for chapter 2."

"Thea and Rita will do that."

Thea and Rita met with Dr. Reese about "how to handle things." Thea saw this as "reality talk—meds, post, funeral, the whole bit. If Reese can't be there at 9:30, Rita and I will start. But we won't do the post—that's for the physicians. They can better explain why it's needed.

"I'll talk about the meds—Valium for stomach pain, Tylenol with codeine for chest pains, and morphine sulfate if all else fails. I'll tell them about the problems with morphine and explain that if the child dies after they give it, it is not because they gave it, it's just part of the dying process.

"I'll also tell them the signs of impending death—continued sleep or bed-wetting or not coughing. Once the child stops coughing, death usually follows in about twenty-four to thirty-six hours. I'm usually hesitant to tell them this, though, because sometimes when parents know this they keep the kid coughing. And this could happen with Mr. Bailey.

"In all, I think their chances of managing at home are pretty good, if Mrs. Bailey stays home from school," Thea emphasized.

"And what a homecoming it was!" Mrs. Bailey recalled. "Gavin and Evan put Casey in his red wagon and off they went. They charged up the street. Gavin pulled the wagon and Evan carried the oxygen. There he was, in his own golden chariot.

"It was real hard at night. We're already exhausted and it's only been one night. Casey didn't sleep all night. As soon as we stop, he yells, 'Keep rubbing.' We're taking turns sleeping.

"He wouldn't let his brothers do anything. Finally, I said to him, 'Look at the couch. See your brothers, crying. They want to help too. Let them.' He said he was sorry, and Gavin and Evan got up and sat on the bed.

"Gavin wants to buy Casey a toy with the money from his paper route, and my friend's coming over with Chinese chicken wings and a Transformer—anything if he'll eat.

By afternoon the Bailey house was packed with people: Mrs. Bailey's friend was there with the promised chicken wings and Transformer; Mr. Harris, the health teacher, brought cards from classmates and friends; the neighborhood bartender and two of the regulars had come with Go-Bots, and Jose, Casey's friend from down the street, came with his mother and sister and a card. Casey presided from the head of his bed with oxygen running into his nose and toys at his feet. Gavin went out to the kitchen before he left to do his paper route.

"Mom," he asked, "if Casey rolled over on his oxygen could he be killed?"

"No! It's the disease that's killing me, not the oxygen," Casey bellowed from the living room.

Gavin moved closer to his mom and lowered his voice. "What will happen when Casey won't eat anymore?"

"We'll give him Sustecal and Polyviocase?"

"And then when he won't take that?"

"Well, as long as he takes fluids he'll be OK. Now you go do your paper route," said Mrs. Bailey, steering Gavin toward the door.

Gavin turned around. "Can I have a piece of fruit?"

"You have to ask Casey. It's his fruit."

"Oh, well," Gavin replied as he headed into the living room. As he left, Mr. Harris came in.

"Thanks for coming."

"Oh, it's OK. You may want to look at these," said Mr. Harris, thrusting the cards at Mrs. Bailey, "before you give them to Casey. One girl really cried when Gavin told her that Casey was home and what was happening."

"I'll look them over. Dolly, my husband's brother's wife, wrote Casey one that I won't show him. It's too teary."

"And then another girl couldn't understand how a child could be dying unless he was shot."

Mrs. Bailey shook her head. "Look, I know Evan's been in some trouble at school. The principal said that under the circumstances he would try to be understanding, but not forever. He said that Evan couldn't act this way for long, as it's creating a problem."

"Oh."

"Would you ask Greta to go easy on him?"

"Sure."

"And would you please tell Jorge not to keep calling here with questions about the home and school association. Number one: I'm no longer involved. Number two: Casey will not be coming back."

"Mom!" Casey yelled from the living room.

"OK. I'm coming."

"I'll go see what he wants."

"No. It's OK. I should go. I'm just exhausted and I was just on the phone with the pharmacist. He said he didn't want to make it [the morphine sulfate] up. I told him he didn't have to; it came made up. Then he said he didn't carry it. Maybe the neighborhood. Who knows? But you know, when Casey needed Ceclor he didn't even want to sell it to me. He said it was very expensive and medical assistance took too long to pay. The hospital finally had to call him."

"Really? That's awful."

"Finally, I said, 'We just brought our son home from the hospital and he probably isn't going to make it.' That's what you have to do to get them to do anything." Mrs. Bailey pushed her chair away from the table with what appeared to be renewed energy and determination and went back into the living room.

"Casey had a good weekend," Mrs. Bailey noted four days later. "We all went to Gil's parents in New Jersey for their fortieth wedding anniversary. Gil's brother came and got us in his van. We laid Casey out with his oxygen and all. He really liked it. I'm even thinking of starting back to school tomorrow.

"Gavin still doesn't want to go. I convinced him to go though. I just told him, 'If something were going to happen, do you think I'd go to school? And I'm going.'

"And then he comes home from school and Casey won't let him or Evan play with any of his toys. He [Casey] just spent his entire savings—forty dollars—at K-Mart and he won't let them play with anything he bought. He said he'll let them play with them sometime.

"Evan picked up a Transformer and Casey yelled from his bed, 'No!' So Evan just sat there.

"It's real hard for them. He won't have anything to do with them. He gets really mad if they even try to come over, or rub him, or do anything for him. It has been very hard for them, Gavin especially. Casey even hit him when he tried to sit on the bed."

"Mom! Mom!"

"Coming Casey."

"Now!"

"I said I was coming." Mrs. Bailey went out to the living room.

"What is it Casey?"

"Rub me! Rub me!"

"OK," said Mrs. Bailey, taking over from her husband. As she silently rubbed Casey's back Gavin came in.

"Did Mr. Morey talk to you today?"

"Yeah. When I'm at school I shouldn't think about Casey."

"Shut the door! It's cold!" Casey yelled.

"That's right. There's a time and a place for everything."

"Shut the door," Casey repeated.

"It's cold," Mr. Bailey interjected. Gavin turned and went back outside, shutting the door behind him.

"I'll take over," Mr. Bailey said, rising from his chair between the bed and the door.

"Thanks."

"No!" Casey yelled.

"Come on, Casey. Aren't you feeling hurt because I won't do it? How do you think it makes your brothers feel when you won't let them do anything?" Casey didn't reply.

"Well, I need a break. Maybe a cup of coffee." Mrs. Bailey went into the kitchen and fixed herself a cup of instant and sat down at the table. "He's been asking about heaven: if he'd see his grandfather; if he'd have to take his pills. I told him that in heaven he wouldn't have CF and he'd be all better.

"We've tried to explain to Gavin and Evan about how Casey loves them very much, but he knows he'll be going soon, leaving soon, saying good-bye. And it's hard for him to be close to them because he knows he'll be leaving.

"And we told Gavin we'd been told what to look for. But I'm not going to tell him, because when he'd come down to go to school in the morning he'd see Casey as having those signs.

"At school he had his computer privileges taken away for not concentrating. The teacher didn't know what the situation was. So I called the principal, and he saw to it that Gavin got them back."

The next day Mrs. Bailey left for school as planned. As she bent down to kiss Casey good-bye he pulled away. "Why are you leaving me?"

"I'm not leaving you. I'm going to school."

"Why are you going to be a nurse? You can't help me anymore."

"But I can be your mother and love you." Mrs. Bailey gave Casey a hug and a kiss as the doorbell rang. Mrs. Bailey went over and answered it. "Casey, it's Myrtle."

Casey turned toward the door and eyed the large white cake box. "What's that?"

"Strawberry shortcake."

"I don't like that," Casey retorted and turned back over.

"That's real sweet of you, Myrtle. Gavin and Evan'll like it."

"I only brought three pieces. I thought one for you, one for Casey and one for Gil."

That was Mrs. Bailey's only day at school that week. By evening Casey seemed weaker. By Friday he was not coughing or expectorating any mucus. He was sitting up to sleep. Mrs. Bailey called around to several funeral homes to see if one could handle the viewing and cremation as well as bring Casey's body to the hospital for the autopsy.

Casey's brothers were not with him at the moment of death. According to Mrs. Bailey, "He waited to die, until the boys went out of the living room. It was about one o'clock. Gavin went downstairs to lift weights and Evan went upstairs. He had been pulling on me and yelling, 'Help me! Help me!' And all I could do was give him more morphine. It was horrendous." Mrs. Bailey paused, "But in a way it helped me to let go.

"Before that he slept a lot. And then he began to hallucinate that there was smoke. We just kept swooshing our hands through the air and telling him, 'We're clearing it away. We're clearing it away.' I think he knew he was hallucinating because he said, 'I'm silly, Mommy. It's the medicine.'

"And then in a very clear voice, different from any other the whole time he was sick he told us, 'It's OK.' Gil took it as a sign, and he started crying. I told him not to. He said he would. And then out of nowhere Casey piped up, 'You will soon.'

"Friday he let Gavin rub him, which was good. And he called Evan over and asked him to give him juice. He couldn't even lift the Tommy-Tippy or suck it up from a straw. It's like Phyllis [the hospice nurse] said, 'He finally got his act together.'

"After we gave him the last morphine we told him it was OK to go to sleep. And then the funeral director called. I had been trying to reach him since Friday. And then while I was on the phone with him, I heard him [Casey] gasp. I dropped the phone and ran over. 'Hold me,' he said. 'Hold me.'

"I called up to Gil. He had just gone upstairs for something. Gil came down and picked Casey up. Casey turned to him and smiled. He died in his dad's arms at 1:30 [Sunday afternoon]."

Not long after Casey died, Evan asked his teacher, "Do you think I'm cold-blooded? I just couldn't stand him that way—just laying there with his oxygen in his nose yelling, 'Rub Me! Rub Me!'"

Casey's plaints of, "Rub me! Rub me!" echoed in Gavin's mind as well. "He kept calling, 'Rub me! Rub me!' I tried going over to him to rub him, and he told me to go away. He like pushed me away."

Part Three

CONTAINING THE INTRUSION

Parents' Responses to the Care the Ill Child Requires and the Concerns the Child's Condition Engenders

OVERWHELMED. The word that I heard repeatedly as parents described the year following diagnosis of cystic fibrosis (CF) was "overwhelmed." Parents spoke of being overwhelmed by the diagnosis, what they felt they needed to learn to do in order to care for this child—who in their minds was a dying child.[1] There were also the other children to consider—the well siblings. Parents wondered when to get them tested and what to tell them about their baby brother or sister. All of this was added to the daily tasks that could not be ignored: cooking, cleaning, looking after other children, and earning a living.

How do parents manage? How do families deal with it all? In this chapter I examine six fundamental issues that parents of children with CF confront and the strategies that they adopt as these issues arise. The issues are not unlike those that all parents of chronically ill children must deal with, namely: the tasks of care, information about the disease and the child's condition, reminders of the disease and its consequences, the child's difference from other children, competing needs and priorities within the family, and the ill child's future. The strategies that develop in response to these issues in families of children with CF are, respectively (1) routinization of CF treatment-related tasks; (2) compartmentalization of information about CF and the child's condition; (3) avoidance of reminders of CF and its consequences; (4) redefinition of normal; (5) reassessment of priorities; and (6) reconceptualization of the future.

In the first part of the chapter I define the issues and describe how the strategies develop and change over the course of the illness in response to the care the ill child requires and the concerns the child's condition engenders (see Table 2). In the second part of this chapter I consider how the strategies contribute to the sense of normalcy and control one observes in these families for long periods of time (Lewis and Khaw 1982: 636; Norman and Hodson 1983: 242; Fosson, D'Angelo, Wilson, and Kanga 1991: 309; Binks 1982: 43; Angst 1992: 11–12; Eigen, Clark, and Wolle 1987: 1512).

---

[1] This sense of being overwhelmed is also characteristic of parents of newly diagnosed children with other chronic life-threatening illnesses. As Weyhing (1983: 127), mother of a child with muscular dystrophy, writes, "When we saw several professionals close together in time, their separate recommendations sometimes seemed overwhelming. We had the feeling that we could not carry them out even if we devoted our total time to trying."

TABLE 2.
The Strategies Parents Adopt over the Course of the Illness

Periods in the Natural History of the Illness

Strategies Parents Adopt	I		II		III		IV		V		VI
	Diagnosis	*First Annual Examination*	*Years Post Annual Examination*	*First Exacerbation*	*Recovery From First Exacerbation*	*Increased Hospitalizations*	*Development, Increase in Complications*	*Conference With Dr./ Team*	*Increased Deterioration*	*Conference With Dr./ Team*	*Terminal Phase*
Routinization of CF treatment-related tasks	●	⇒	⇑	▲	⇑	▲	▲		▲		■
Compartmentalization of information about CF and the child's condition	●	⇒	⇑	▲	⇑	▲	▲	▲	▲	■	
Avoidance of reminders of CF and its consequences			●	▲	⇑	⇑	▲		■		
Redefinition of normal			●	▲	⇑	⇑	▲		■		
Reassessment of priorities			●	▲	⇑	⇑	▲		▲	■	
Reconceptualization of the future			●	▲	⇑	⇑	▲	▲	▲	■	

Key: ● = Begins ▲ = Changes ■ = Ceases ⇑ = Intensifies ⇒ = Continues

1. ISSUES AND STRATEGIES

Tasks of Care / Routinization of CF Treatment-Related Tasks

In the weeks and months following the diagnosis the parents must learn how to give their children chest physical therapy (PT) as well as various medications including pancreatic enzymes, and in some cases, bronchodilators and antibiotics. Tasks like PT are difficult. Many parents do not feel they have mastered it until late in the first year after diagnosis, and even then questions remain.[2]

> Every once in a while I ask somebody at the clinic to brief me on clapping [referring to PT] because I forget. [Father eight years after child's diagnosis.]

Neither is it easy to administer pancreatic enzymes, especially to an infant.

> But it seems like I'm constantly feeding her enzymes and giving her a bottle and trying to get those enzymes in her mouth. Chasing those beads down her chin, those little things. There's more under her neck than there are in her mouth. It's real nervewracking. [Mrs. Daley]

The care is demanding and not necessarily easy to manage.

[2] In Part III, Chapters 11, 12, and 13, I sometimes characterize behavior as typical of a "majority of parents," "many parents" or "some parents." These words stand for an approximate range of percentages: "majority" is 80 percent or greater; "many," less than 80 percent but greater than 50 percent; "some," less than 50 percent but greater than 25 percent. I do the same with siblings' behavior.

Virtually every point I make in Part III is illustrated with an example, most commonly quotations from participants in the study. Some of the examples the reader will have already encountered in Part II (Chapters 2–10), others are new. In those instances where I thought that seeing the remarks or actions in the context of other remarks and actions would be helpful in understanding the more general point, I drew the examples from Part II. In instances where I thought this was less necessary I used material not found in Part II. Taking examples from portions of my field journals and transcripts not included in Part II also allows the reader to become familiar with more of the individuals in the study and the various ways that individuals present themselves and their approaches to the illness.

When a point is illustrated by a quotation that also appears in Part II the pseudonym used in Part II is given either before the quotation or in brackets at the end of the quotation. If the illustrative material does not appear in Part II then only the category of person (e.g., mother, well sister, ill brother) is given. In order better to protect individuals' identities, a few of the individuals quoted or mentioned in Part II have been given another pseudonym in Part III. For the same reason, a few of the individuals who are quoted or mentioned only in Part III have been given more than one pseudonym in Part III. In all instances individuals have their own set of names that does not overlap with anyone else's. No individual is a composite.

To locate the context of examples which also appear in Part II use the speaker's last name. Chapters in Part II are titled by surname; for example, the context of a remark by Mrs. Sherman would be in Chapter 3, "The Shermans."

It was really hard in the beginning. It really was. I spent from early morning to midnight doing things. I got to sit down about midnight. There were just so many things you had to mix. You had special formula; you had to make that. You had to boil the water. Then you had to wait for the water to cool. And then you had to mix it. And you'd have to mix that every single day for her all the time. The hours you spent feeding her when she first got home.

We used to take two and a half hours for therapy [PT should take approximately forty minutes per session]. She would cry, so I'd pick her up and hold her for a while and then Madeline [well sibling] would be running around and getting into things. So I'd have to stop and get her off the counter or out of the windowsill. So it was two and a half hours. And by then it was time to do it again. There wasn't time for anything else. [Mother six years after child's diagnosis]

Parents need to find a way to meet the requirements for CF care and at the same time manage a household, care for other children, and earn a living; "to get it all together," as several commented.[3]

It took a while to get into the swing of things. You can't, like a normal person, get up in the morning and say, 'I'm going to take a shower.' I have to get up in the morning and say, 'Three and a half enzymes. Point three of vitamin E.' You have to click into gear as soon as you get out of bed and think of what you have to give him right away. [Mother nine months after child's diagnosis]

Through a process of trial and error parents learn how to work the tasks of CF care into everyday life. As two parents whose child had been diagnosed seven months prior to the interview explained,

FATHER: There's tons of things that we're still trying to do. Plus fitting in Devin's treatment. And you're thinking about OK, now I've got to get the enzymes, and now I have to do this. You're more . . .
MOTHER: And juggle when I'm going to run the vacuum cleaner, and give treatment. The way the morning goes is he [Father] gets up and usually gets the baby [Devin] up. Today was a nice day because Devin was up at what a quarter to seven, and he got him up and gave him his bottle. Right?
FATHER: Uh-hm.
MOTHER: And so then, when I got up, a quarter after seven, then I was able to get the girls [two well daughters] their breakfast, get the baby dressed. Sylvie gets herself dressed. And, eat breakfast myself. Then he gets out of the shower. I go in the shower while he's eating breakfast and then he leaves at ten of eight. And then Sylvie has to be on the bus by twenty after eight. And then in between I can get dressed and get maybe a few dishes washed up or I choose between

[3] "To varying degrees all families having children with CF must reevaluate their goals as well as their strengths and weaknesses in order to reschedule their daily lives to accommodate the needs of the child with CF" (Denning and Gluckson 1984: 467).

washing the dishes or getting Avrie dressed. And then I come back in the house about twenty-five after eight, give Devin his aerosol, and then he plays for a little while. And then I can make the beds or something. And then usually at nine o'clock I start the chest clapping [PT]. So everything runs smooth.

But if the baby doesn't wake up until quarter after seven, then it's a mad rush, because I don't get to take a shower, because I have to give him his bottle. And then it's bad if like Avrie and I had dentist appointments last Friday at ten o'clock in the morning. And I had to be in Burlington at nine thirty, which is a twenty-minute ride. And so then I'm trying to give him his chest clapping at my mother's house, before I go to the dentist. So I said no more to morning appointments. It just makes things too hectic.

Parents reported that their ability to juggle CF tasks increased over the course of the first year. Statements from parents like, "It was real hard to get things organized that first year, but once that was over we made it through," were not uncommon. Parents would tell the physicians about their increasing mastery of PT. One mother claimed that she had "found a way to hold a book on [her] lap and do PT. You learn to do a whole lot of things you didn't think you ever knew how to do or you'd ever figure out how to do."

Throughout the first year following diagnosis and over the entire course of the illness parents are engaged in a process that I refer to as the *Routinization of Cystic Fibrosis Treatment-Related Tasks*. This process involves the integration of the CF tasks in such a way that they become a part of everyday life. Care requirements become chores like any other—part of what needs to be done in the course of a day. For example, one mother, in recounting her daily routine, began, with no particular emphasis,

I do my beds and while he is getting his mist I dust. Then I give him his PT.

By the end of the first year, and certainly by the second, parents typically see these tasks as "part of my life," "how I live," "what I do every day," "like brushing your teeth," "a habit," "second nature."[4]

It's part of our lives. You clean the equipment every day. You do that bit. You do all the other stuff. You incorporate it all into your life. It becomes a routine like any other routine. Like anyone else with children, you get up at a certain time, you go to your job. We do the same here. It's just that there is another part that is incorporated into the morning. [Father]

There is a sense in which a task like PT becomes, in the words of one father, "a ritual."

---

[4] Indeed, these tasks have become so much a part of parents' lives, so "second nature," that even after the child's death some mothers report going "to the cabinet to pack the meds" before leaving on a trip, and "looking in amazement at a mother who doesn't give her baby enzymes before she feeds her."

Outpatient visits to the CF center also become routinized.

Clinic visits are an absolute routine. The night before we make up a list of the medications we need and I ask the doctor some questions—equipment replacement and so forth. And then on the day we go we try to get there as early as we can. Celine [wife] goes more often than I do. And they [center staff] have their routines of course. [Father]

Just as some families divide the tasks of care at home so do they divide the tasks of the visits. One father, for example, explained to me that "My wife goes with [the child] for the X-rays and I go for the PFTs [pulmonary function tests]."

With the first major exacerbation, the illness dramatically intrudes into the family's life and activities. Well-established routines are broken as more therapy is required and the child returns to the hospital. On recovery from the first major exacerbation, therapy that had in some cases slacked off after the first annual examination, when the child was doing relatively well, begins again with new zeal.

We got right back to it. It took some getting used to, but we got back to it. It's sort of like riding a bike, I guess. We fell off and then got right back on. [Mother]

Routines again develop to cover all that needs to be done. Provisions are made for changes in the daily schedule and trips away from home. For example, Mr. and Mrs. Reynolds noted,

"So, whenever we get ready for a trip the last thing we say, 'Do we have Carl's enzymes?'"

"If we have his enzymes and medicines we can do without everything else."

"And money," Mrs. Reynolds laughed. "Sometimes we add money, but . . ."

"Well we like to take our credit cards," Mr. Reynolds joked back before Mrs. Reynolds could finish her thought.

"Enzymes—always—if we're going. After you've packed and you're kinda going through your mind, 'Do I have this? Do I have that? Do I . . .' As we get in the car, as long as we have the enzymes we kinda . . ."

"And his mist machine [nebulizer]."

"And even that, you can always pound him."

"Yeah."

There are routines for interruptions.

Now when we go somewhere I just reach up into the cabinet and grab the basket. Last year I got a basket. I have everything in there. We just grab the basket and put it in the trunk and off we go. [Mother]

PT still gets done, but not necessarily at home.

If we are shopping in the mall and it gets late, we just do the PT in the car on the ride home. I can see how families would get into problems if they didn't do things because they had to be home to do the PT. [Mother]

Any change in the child's condition, however minor, is taken into account in the reintegration of the CF tasks into everyday life. For example, in scheduling Carl's therapy Mr. and Mrs. Reynolds took into consideration his tendency to vomit after coughing.

"You have to try and work the eating with the coughing," Mrs. Reynolds would explain.

"With the treatments, an hour before eating, which we don't always wait. An hour after the therapy. We don't always wait an hour, but we never pound him after he's eaten."

"No, and after he eats a big meal we try to make him be quiet for twenty minutes or so."

"Yeah, go over and play with his cars or something."

"Play quietly instead of racing around, because that sometimes will make him cough."

Other events in family life, not related to the ill child's condition, can have an impact on the routinization of CF treatment-related tasks. Several mothers in the study told me that when they separated from their husbands the patterns of care changed. However, the sense of therapy as part of the daily routine did not.

After we separated, I went back to work and my mother switched to part time. She was working it so that she could give Darcy a lot of her treatments. I was giving her one a day and then my mother was giving her ones in the afternoon and then I was giving her the nights. [Mother]

After the first major exacerbation physicians often bring children into the hospital for "tune-ups." During such "scheduled," periodic hospitalizations the children receive more aggressive PT and intravenous antibiotics. Just as the scheduled and periodic clinic visits and the events surrounding them become routinized, so too do the periodic hospitalizations or tune-ups and the events surrounding them. For example, when a mother of two children with CF was told that both of her children's PFT scores had dropped she interrupted the physician's explanation of the scores with, "OK. You don't have to tell me. Just are we going to be admitted? Because if we are I want to get a few things done and come back. This will be their summer admission. We come in every summer so let's just get it over with. I want the usual four hour passes for fun. I'll be here to take them out on the weekend. Their grandmother will come down during the week as usual."

It is important to note that just because parents are able to integrate the tasks of CF care into everyday life does not mean that they no longer see the orchestration and performance of these tasks as a problem. Many parents commented that even years after the diagnosis, and with their child doing reasonably well, they found that "fitting it all in is still a problem."

> Every day, it's just how are you going to fit this in. We have to fit in his chest PT. If you have something different one night you have to go somewhere you have to think, "OK, you've got his meds. You have to get the machine. You have to make sure you take them."
> I've had all the mistakes happen to me. You take the machine, but you forget the medicine, or you don't bring it and then you end up needing it. It's a lot of stuff like that. [Mother]

As the complications of CF begin to develop new treatments are required. More care is needed. It becomes increasingly difficult for parents to integrate the tasks of CF care into everyday life so as to make them part of everyday life and not life itself. While the daily routines are not abandoned, there are often cutbacks on PT treatments.[5]

> There is just too much to do. We can't seem to do it all and have any kind of a normal life—so we skip some treatments. At least that way we do the others. Otherwise it is too much and we wind up doing nothing. [Mother]

However much one does or does not do still must fit into everyday life, with all of its other demands. As the parents of an eleven-year-old daughter, who had been struggling with several complications of CF (Burkholderia cepacia, intermittent oxygen use during frequent hospitalizations) explained,

> FATHER: We are up at five o'clock in the morning, just to get everything done. To do her aerosol, PT, and treatment takes about half an hour to an hour. I usually get up at five and then I get myself ready for work and then I get Avril [child with CF] up, give her aerosol and PT. Then Norine [wife/mother] gets up and gets her dressed and packs their [two children] lunches and gets their books and everything ready and then she gets herself ready for work.
> So from five o'clock til about eight when the school bus comes it's a little hectic.
>
> MOTHER: Then the kids get in at five after three—they leave themselves in—and then he [father] comes in at three thirty.
>
> FATHER: No, normally about a quarter after, twenty after.
>
> MOTHER: Yeah. You were late today.
>
> FATHER: Well, I knew you were home. So I didn't rush out of work, like usual.

---

[5] The difficulty in getting the child to do the treatments contributes to and reinforces the cutbacks.

MOTHER: And he gives Avril her treatment right away when he gets home. And then I'll be in maybe four and I'll start supper, and then we start doing homework with them. They usually don't do it by themselves. They usually have 'I don't understand this.' And we help.

Then by the time we're finished with the homework, the snack time—she has to have a snack for the calories and all. Then Avril has to get another treatment, and then it's time for them to eat dinner and go to bed. And you know how kids are, trying to get them to go to bed.

FATHER: And that's a normal day, when we don't have anything else going on. Half the time this calendar, these blocks, are filled in with things we have to do. The school and the practices for confirmation and little league. There's never any rest. We just get up the next day and start all over again.

Following the development and increase in complications there is increased deterioration. The child is "sick more often." Also, as the child's condition deteriorates, the tasks of CF care not only increase, but also become more complex to manage. There is an even greater need for more aggressive home therapy as well as more frequent clinic visits and hospitalizations. The routinization of CF treatment-related tasks becomes increasingly difficult. As one parent remarked, "When she gets sick, there goes the routine."

As the child's condition continues to deteriorate, reestablishing former routines as well as making new ones is difficult. Not all CF tasks find their way back into the daily routine with the same intensity. For example, while PT is still "required," it may diminish as care for the oxygen equipment and catheter takes its "slot" on the daily to-do list. There are sheets on bulletin boards to track night feedings and the phone numbers of home-care services are there beside that of the CF center. Blocks on calendars are filled with notations about equipment deliveries and pickups as well as more frequent clinic visits. Nebulizer cups share space on the kitchen drainboard with pieces of equipment for newly recommended treatments.

Information about the Disease and the Child's Condition / Compartmentalization of Information about CF and the Child's Condition

Just as parents try to manage the care the child requires so too do they try to manage the information that they receive about CF and the child's condition. At diagnosis and through the first year, parents are bombarded with information about CF. Professionals, family members and even strangers—are all telling them what to do and how to do it.

FATHER: There is just so much to learn to do. They tell you so much, in regard to the care and lots of different things.

MOTHER: It's confusing. And everybody has their own way of doing things.

Parents learn, for example, how to recognize when a cough merits the doctor's attention.

The nurse down there [at the CF center] said that "You have to learn to judge the coughs, too." There's a good cough and a bad cough. And all that, so that you can tell if he's really sick and you need to call or if he's not really sick. [Father]

Parents begin an intensive quest for information.[6]

I have a bulletin board in my kitchen. Every clipping I find with something about it [CF] I put on there. There must be three, four articles up there now. [Mother]

In reading the pamphlets you tend to find out more, like about sinusitis. You can find out what some of the medications are and why the vitamins are important and that sort of thing. [Father]

They read all that they are given and ask for more.[7]

I read a lot about it. I read all I can. Then when I go to the clinic I base my questions on what I have read. [Mother]

There are lectures, presentations, groups, and books on everything: How to do PT while whipping up high-calorie recipes for your child; how to have fun with your spouse and well children while coping with a chronically ill child. Mrs. Sherman explained that,

My way of coping in the beginning was sort of finding out everything and writing about it, or going to conferences. That sort of thing was helpful to me. When Katrina was first born [Katrina was diagnosed at birth] I did a CF parents' newsletter. The foundation ran it off for me, and we sent it out to all the parents. We also started a parents' group around the time she was born.

One subject that concerns young parents is the genetic nature of the disease. For parents who have other children it raises the question of getting these children tested. Two months after her daughter was diagnosed one mother remarked,

We haven't had our other child tested yet. I am afraid to even kiss him.[8]

[6] Bearison and Pacifici (1984: 271) noted the same behavior in parents of children with cancer.

[7] Interestingly, many view the information that they receive at this time as the most credible.

[8] Children with CF secrete large amounts of salt and therefore often taste salty. German folktales tell of "the baby who tastes salty will surely die."

For some couples there is also the question of whether to have more children. As with all information that they receive at this time, the issue is mulled over, sorted, and assigned a place in their thinking about the illness. The process is captured in this conversation between a husband and wife.

HUSBAND: You know, we, I, pretty much understand the genetic part of it. It's a genetic disease and, you know, the possibilities exist that if you have any more children. And there was a very remote. . . well, there was a very real chance that we weren't going to have another child.

WIFE: I would just as soon get it all taken care of and . . .

HUSBAND: Yeah. I think she would . . .

WIFE: . . .and that would be it. But I can't persuade him to do that. I don't want to have any more children. I'm a definite, where he is a question mark.

HUSBAND: I'm a question mark because I would like to see what happens . . .

WIFE: Three years down the road.

HUSBAND: I definitely would not want even to think about having a child in the next couple of years.

WIFE: Yeah. I could never take that chance. And I never want to. I have two healthy children. . .

HUSBAND: Yeah, I think as time goes on I might. I think I might tend to be more her way. It's risky. I know I'm not prepared to take that risk again.

WIFE: I think that's the hardest thing for young couples. You're afraid. And really, that's what it comes down to. If I ever got pregnant now I would be scared to death. I would be scared to death. It's a chance. And I think as soon as anything would happen, I would just freeze up because I'm so afraid. I just don't want to, you know. Next time I would just like to and have that decision. I just want it over with. Not to have to worry about it because I look at Phoebe Dalton and there are three in the family [with CF] and to have one of your brothers die must be horrible.

HUSBAND: You have a sick child and you know it's going to have an effect on the kids.

WIFE: Yeah. That's one of my main things.

HUSBAND: I don't know if I want to bring in another. You would not want to take a chance of having another child having cystic fibrosis. And having to go through it all over again. And I don't know. But then, you never know. I mean realistically, she could get sick tomorrow, and not make it; or in the next couple of years. That's a possibility too. And then, that could affect how you think in a way—well, geez, "Do I want to have another child?" I don't know. You go back and forth. (Pause) I'm a little mixed up right now, but I don't want to seal off all my options.

WIFE: I do.

HUSBAND: (Laughs)

WIFE: Some day I just might sneak myself in the hospital and get it all taken care of. (Laughs) And end it. That seems like the easiest thing to do.

HUSBAND: I would lean her way right now, probably. I don't know if I want to go through this again.

WIFE: No.

HUSBAND: It's very hard.

WIFE: For everybody, it would be hard. Horrible.

HUSBAND: Yeah. It would be tough on everybody, yeah. I mean right now you wouldn't even, I wouldn't even want to think about it, because number one, you wouldn't have time too. You wouldn't have time to do everything that would be involved if you ever had another child. And, you know, the other thing is the financial end of it.[9]

Parents also are faced, often for the first time, with the costs of medical care for a chronically ill family member.

FATHER: There is some cost involved.

MOTHER: They say "expense."

FATHER: You know.

MOTHER: We didn't realize. And we're just finding out. We're over our limit on medications. Five hundred dollars would be covered. But we're over that, so now it's out of our pockets. And it's a big thing.

FATHER: Yeah. It is a big thing. We're in an HMO, but we're thinking about another plan.

MOTHER: We're waiting right now.

FATHER: I can't do anything until the open-enrollment period, which is sometime in November. Before then I'm going to sit down and really weigh it. Look at all the different plans. Right now it's just the medication. It's expensive. It's about a hundred bucks a month. And we're not eligible for the State program. I think they said sixteen hundred dollars. So, you live with it.

MOTHER: Dr. Ziegler gave us all these samples, that was nice.

FATHER: Yeah.

MOTHER: When I needed, I went in to ask. But, some of them do and some of them don't. But I think if they knew we were paying out of our pocket.

FATHER: Well, I hope the next year it changes a little bit. It's about a hundred dollars a month and at the end of the year you get reimbursed for five hundred or so. Maybe you spend a thousand dollars a year. But, what can you do?

MOTHER: Yeah.

FATHER: You know. You do what you have to do. And, you just, I think, just thank God that you probably have the means to do it.

MOTHER: Yeah.

[9] The decision to put off the decision about having more children is also found in discussions of parents who are thinking about adoption or insemination with donor sperm.

FATHER: We're not wealthy, but we're not . . .

MOTHER: We're not poor.

FATHER: We're not in poverty, either.

MOTHER: Yet.

According to the parents the biggest issue that they have to deal with is the prognosis. When the child is diagnosed and throughout most of the first year parents see the child as a dying child. "I think about it, the dying, all the time," was a common refrain among the parents of newly diagnosed children. Some felt that they did not want "to get too attached." "We will lose her." Several spoke of picturing themselves at the child's funeral. They are concerned about the impact of the child's death on the other children.[10] As Mrs. Daley remarked,

When I think of Darrell and Erika [well siblings] having to face death I get upset.

In short, in the days, weeks, and months following the diagnosis there is a great deal of information that parents must process. The information is not without an emotional charge.

It probably took me a good year to smile. Once I saw her walking around and doing things like all the other kids, that's when [I started to smile]. I don't know how long it took for him [referring to her husband], maybe a few months. I think he felt OK about it a few months after [she was diagnosed]. But me, at least a year to get used to it. I was numb. To everything, I think.

It was on my mind constantly. That was all I ever thought about—CF, CF, CF. Why didn't I know about it? Why did it happen to us? There were so many things to think about all the time. There was the therapy and the medication and what to do when she got sick.

And I was afraid at first, because I thought the first year she was just going to die. That's what I thought. I thought that she was going to die. I didn't think she was going to live. [Mother]

In the first year following diagnosis parents report struggling with the place that treatment regimes, protocols, symptoms, acute crisis, the potential for cure, and terminal prognosis would occupy in their minds. Between approximately eight and sixteen months following diagnosis parents begin to engage in a process or strategy that I refer to as the *Compartmentalization of Information About CF and the Child's Condition.*[11] Information is processed and sorted in such a way that particular kinds of information are kept from

[10] For further discussion of the parents' view of the child as a dying child see the section "The Ill Child's Future / Reconceptualization of the Future."

[11] While all parents begin the process within the first year, they do not all begin at the same time. As is evident in the preceding quotation, even within the same family the parents report the onset of the strategy at different points in the first year following diagnosis.

immediate awareness. Decisions, however conscious or unconscious, are made about where various kinds of information will be stored in their minds.[12]

It is helpful to consider compartmentalization of information as a filing project. In each parent's mind there is a large cabinet marked CF with many files inside: files on genetics, the cost of treatment, chest physical therapy, prognosis, research leading to a cure, research to improve the quality of life, child's physical condition, etc. Each bit of information parents receive is placed in its appropriate file folder. Some file folders are more accessible than others. Early on in the illness parents keep the research files more accessible, but the prognosis files less so. The less accessible files might be stored in the back of the cabinet or in a bottom drawer, with inactive or temporarily inactive files. Each file can be retrieved at any time, but an attempt is made to keep files like the prognosis file, where they will not interfere with current operations.

In the first year following diagnosis parents endeavor to push information about the fatal prognosis to the backs of their minds, to the back of the file cabinet. There they will not be forgotten, but neither will they be the focus of attention.

> Of course, you always have in the back of your mind it's a chronic disease and it's a fatal disease. But I don't spend a lot of time worrying about that at all. [Father]

Parents try to give more attention to advances in medical research and the potential for cure.

> First thing I think about is they have to find a cure. That's the first thing, a cure. [Mother]

> I think about it medically a lot. I think about the medical aspects—physiology and the scientific aspects. And then I'll think about the interpersonal relationships. And some days I'll think about one more than the other. If I feel down then, when I think about the interpersonal aspects, then I'll think about the advancements and things that are going on. Then I won't think that things are so bad. [Father]

The possibility of a cure being found continues to receive primary attention in the ensuing years, when the child is doing relatively well. As Mrs. Sherman, the mother of an eleven-year-old who had never had an exacerbation, commented,

> It's more important to me now that they find some cure for it, because she's just getting into her teenage years, doing nicely, and I would want them to come up

[12] A fuller discussion of the consciousness or unconsciousness of compartmentalization of information and other strategies may be found in the second part of this chapter.

with something. I hope they can come up with something that will control it at least. I'm sort of interested in all the research and stuff. I don't know whether it's going to be soon or if they'll find something or what.

"Worries" persist, but "threads of optimism" also surface. As Mr. Sherman's discussion revealed,

> "In addition to being a background worry like that, it's also a race, because you can see the National Institutes of Health working on it, and the hospitals. And you can—I don't think it's entirely just imagination—imagine that something good can come of this, fairly soon. And so you say, well, it's just a question of how soon can they get there; before lung involvement takes place with my child. And so it's that as well. And it makes you really aware of that whole side of things, the research end of it.
>
> "And then, also, it makes you aware of the fact that a lot of work is being done, but an awful lot is not understood. And doctors can mention a whole lot of different ways of that. So I'm just saying we don't know this, we don't know that. Some of them say it in a much more elegant way, but it's the same message. And at times you feel you know almost as much as the doctors know about it."
>
> Mr. Sherman hesitated and then burst forth excitedly. "But by God, there should be some way of solving this thing. When you think of all the fronts they're working on: genetic, pulmonary, and just medications; amazing things, brilliant things. In fact, therapy itself is pretty brilliant considering it's free and it does have a lot of effect in many patients." Mr. Sherman settled. He became quiet, reflective again.
>
> "There's that kind of thread of optimism. It works through, I guess, all parents. If that's the word for it. Optimism or hope, I guess is all that it really is. But that, the fact that CF for many patients like Trina lurks rather than manifesting itself, makes it a very strange thing to live with."
>
> Mr. Sherman paused and added, "I used to think, well, of course death is lurking as well. So it's not as though they won't lose a life, no shadows at all, but it's a medically discernible problem and it is threatening. I think it's sort of hanging over our heads and all."

Regardless of how well the child is doing, parents continue to think about the illness. As the mother of a thirteen-year-old diagnosed relatively late in life, but doing well two years after diagnosis, remarked,

> It's always there, a little cloud is always walking over top of you. You still laugh and you still play, but it is always there. It doesn't go away.

Concern about when the disease "will progress" or "worsen" remains constant over the course of the illness. It is as Angst (1992: 90) notes in her study of the parents of children with CF, "what parents think about most." There is a difference, however, between the way in which parents think about the illness when the child is doing relatively well, and when the child was diagnosed (and as is discussed later in the chapter, when the child's condition begins to deteriorate). When "bad thoughts" do occur, parents find they do not dwell on them as they had when the child was diagnosed. As one couple whose ten-year-old daughter had not been hospitalized since her diagnosis at ten months described it,

> WIFE: Well it's always on your mind, but you don't dwell on it.
> HUSBAND: It's like bad news hanging there. You just never know when this thing is going to let go.

Parents reach a point where they can hold onto several views of the illness at once. They can look at each of the possible outcomes from premature death to cure, or at least control, as "real possibilities." On one occasion they can take up one of these views and on another put it aside.

> I don't dwell on it. I don't think to myself, "I wonder how many days it's going to be before he is sick or something." But I don't have false hopes. Like just because he's healthy for two and half years doesn't mean that he's not going to get sick again. [Mother]

At this time and for years to come the difficult issues CF raises emerge in dreams, in reactions to movies, on birthdays and special occasions, as well as with advances in the child's development.

> I imagine her choking to death, coughing to death. [Father]

> My husband's birthday is always a hard day for me. It was the day Malcolm was diagnosed. [Mother]

> I don't like birthdays. Another year closer to when we won't have him. [Mother]

At these times parents find themselves "thinking about it all over again."

Information moves back and forth triggered by particular events, or a different sounding cough or even a turn of phrase.[13] However, unlike during the months immediately following the diagnosis, such thoughts are fleeting, not lingering.

> Occasionally I think about it. Like if Luke [well brother] will say "Oh, when me and Trevor get married" or, "When me and Trevor do this" and "When we're as big as Daddy," then, sometimes the thought just runs through your mind like a wind.

> I don't know if Trevor will ever get to be that big, or get to do that, because he may not live to be that old. But, I don't dwell on it. In the beginning I did. I pictured myself at his funeral, and, you know, all the natural feelings that you have. [Mother]

With the first major exacerbation requiring hospitalization and in every succeeding hospitalization thereafter the process of compartmentalization of

---

[13] Noted by Angst (1992: 89–90) as well.

information begins anew. Information about the course of the disease, lung deterioration, and the prognosis, carefully tucked away while the child was doing well, comes to the forefront of one's mind. Parents speak of "it all coming back to me," "having to think about it all again."

New information acquired at the time of the first exacerbation is processed and sorted. Parents formulate a view of the illness as "something we can live with." While the chronic character of the disease comes more to the forefront of parents' minds it is balanced by a sense of CF as "something we are going to live with."

> It's funny, but recovering from that pneumonia convinced me that the first time that she got sick wasn't going to be it. [Father]

Advances in genetic research and alternative forms of therapy continue to occupy a prominent place in parents' thoughts about the illness. Several parents after the first major exacerbation remained firm in their conviction that a cure would be found. One mother of a child with advanced disease suggested that I go and talk to two other mothers whose children had been hospitalized for the first time and were now at home "doing quite well," "to see how differently they see it all."

> You ought to go talk to Mrs. Dixon. She told me that this was Kelsey's first and last hospitalization, because "there's going to be a cure," she said. She's not worried, because they will have gene transplants soon. And Mrs. Barrett isn't worried now either. She was when she first came in, but not now. Then [when her child was first admitted] she was crying all the time and talking about having to face it, but not now.[14]

After the child recovers from the first exacerbation the "difficult thoughts" about the course of the disease remain, but as in the period of relative health that preceded the exacerbation, parents do not dwell on these thoughts.

> It's like you're thinking about him being sick, but you're not thinking about what's going to happen. I mean, it's in my head all the time that he has it. It's just I don't think about what's going to happen or what could happen. I don't like to think about that. [Mrs. Farrington]

Yet, as Mrs. Farrington herself points out, and others agree, thoughts about the prognosis emerge again with movies, on special occasions, and in dreams. Acute episodes of sickness or changes in the child's condition are also catalysts. Several parents remarked on how "it's only when he's [or she's] sick that it really comes up."

[14] Interestingly, the staff made the same comments about the Dixon and Barrett families. The staff also noted how parents of children who had experienced only one exacerbation and recovered, frequently talked and asked about the new research and studies that were being conducted at the hospital and other CF centers.

As the number of hospitalizations and exacerbations increases many parents find that it takes less and less to stimulate their thinking about the negative aspects of CF. Mr. and Mrs. Reynolds, parents of five-year-old Carl, who had been hospitalized five times, but as yet had shown none of the complications of the disease, noted:

"Or something will come that will remind me of it," Mr. Reynolds added. "Or he'll do something funny and I'll think, 'Well how many more years is he going to do something funny.' But I kinda lock things out of my mind. And I just go day to day, don't think too far down the road. Now she's not like that."

"No, I don't. I'm worse when he's [Carl's] worse. When he's sick, when he's starting to catch a cold, then that's it. Then I start thinking, 'Geez how many more colds? What so far has happened to your lungs and to your heart to make the progression worse?

"I try not to dwell on it. I don't want to or I'll make myself a basket case."

"She'll lay at night and just think of this and that."

"Yeah. My mind just races from one thing to another. I've already pictured him laying in a casket and thinking, 'Oh God! How am I going to handle that?' I guess I do look ahead if I think, 'How am I going to handle that?'"

Even as the number and frequency of hospitalizations begin to increase parents still feel that it is important to try to give the possibility of cure a prominent place in one's own thinking about the illness. One mother in reviewing the information that she had about CF and her daughter's condition went on,

First you find out that you have CF. Then you go in the hospital and find out that you have allergies. Then you go in the hospital and they say well you might be a borderline case of diabetes. Every time there's something new. Well when you add all these things up in your mind, what do you have? No wonder some of these kids go bad. And you have to keep trying the reinforcement, saying, "It's going to be OK. They're going to find a cure."

Parents feel that is reasonable to stay focused on the cure given "changes in CF care." They speak of all of "the hope that there is now, with the new research."

As the number of hospitalizations increase parents find it more difficult to maintain the "somewhat optimistic view" that they had after the child recovered from the first exacerbation, as well as to control the frequency with which they think about the course of the illness; but they do try. Mrs. Chase's remarks reveal the thoughts of a parent whose child has been hospitalized several times, but has not developed any complications.

"And I think the big thing you always think about are all the little things—the infections and the pills and this and that. But I think you could cope with all that. But the big thing that you always have in the back of your head is the prognosis. And I think you suppress it a lot. But I don't think there's a day that goes by that you don't think about it. And I think that's how it is for everyone.

"And I think you think about it all the time. And I think if they could control the disease like they can control diabetes or something like that, I think it would definitely change a lot of things.

"When someone is sick at the hospital, really sick, like when someone dies; oh God, then you think about it all the time. No, you think about it. It's not that you don't think about it. I mean it's not like you think about it every day, but it crosses your mind every day.

"You just can't imagine sometimes how you'll ever cope. And you think about it when you think of the future. Like I think when you get married and you have these kids and you have all these goals of what your life's going to be like and then you tend to think of the future and it gets pretty hard." Mrs. Chase began to cry.

"I'm a crybaby," she declared with a smile, wiping away her tears. "But then you have to think that you don't know—that's the thing. It might turn out fine. You have to think of the positive. You have to think of yourself in those statistics that are like the sixty-four-year-old grandmother [with CF]. There's a sixty-four-year-old grandmother, I think, or something."

Mrs. Chase articulates what many of the parents are doing with the information that they have at this time. They are well aware of the prognosis, but they are trying to push it back, "to suppress it" as she says, and emphasize "the positive." Parents want to keep the prognosis from immediate awareness and find it difficult to do so.[15]

By the time the children begin to experience complications from the illness, the place given to hope for a cure is given to hope for the discovery of a means to control the illness. A mother of a child who had developed Burkholderia cepacia (at this CF center it is regarded as a "complication of CF") was very angry when the mother of a child who had been hospitalized only once, spoke to her about a cure for CF,

She said, "I just know there is going to be a cure and I don't want to talk about anything else." Well, yeah, you can believe in miracles, but how often do you see them? I believe it might be controlled. But I'm not looking for a cure. If somebody could control it that would be much better from my point of view.

In the face of ever more frequent hospitalizations and complications parents claim that while they still do think about the consequences of CF, they do not dwell on these thoughts.

[15] Angst (1992: 89) also found that "most parents tried to keep these thoughts ['negative realities of the disease'] more distant, and for the most part were able to master this strategy. However, when their child was ill or exhibited increased symptoms, or when parents were unoccupied or exposed to knowledge of other children who were not doing well, these thoughts came to the forefront." While I agree with Angst's description of parents' thoughts, I do not agree with her characterization of the process as "mastering a strategy."

It's all the little bitty things that add up. You can't go to bed at night with a window open, you're afraid they're going to catch a draft; or simple little stupid things like that. It becomes part of your life and it's taken on a daily basis, but you don't dwell on the worst. [Mother]

The continuing ability to think about, but not to dwell on the progression and outcome of the disease, may in part be possible because even in the face of increasing complications there are still times when to use the words of parents, "your child is not sick."

When they're good you don't think about death. When they're not in the hospital you don't. Then they're going to be one of the ones that lives to be one hundred and five years old. They're going to outlive everybody. And then when they're worse. . . [sentence not completed; mother]

With further complications and exacerbations the child's condition begins to deteriorate markedly. When this point is reached parents (at the CF center where this study was conducted) are informed that the disease is now "severe" or "advanced." Parents' thoughts turn to the prognosis. But unlike in the years following the first annual examination and even through the initial exacerbations and hospitalizations that follow, parents now find it increasingly difficult to separate the terminal prognosis of CF from their own child's condition. The terminal prognosis for CF merges with a sense of the very real possibility that one's own child could die. The prognosis is increasingly personalized in a way that it was not when the child was doing relatively well. Consider these two statements, for example—the first by a mother of an eight-year-old, diagnosed at four, who has not had a major exacerbation; and the second by the mother of a ten-year-old, diagnosed in infancy, who now required oxygen and for whom a central line was being considered:

I really don't believe Neal's dying. I really don't. I mean I know he will, but it's dealing with the disease now that I think about.

I used to think about other children dying from CF. I knew children died from it, but I don't know. Now I'm really worried about Dorrie dying. I never saw anyone die. I never had anyone die.

Given that along with the possibility of a premature death, parents still hope that a means of controlling, if not of curing, the disease will be found, it is not surprising that those who for a time had shown no interest in research begin to ask about gene therapy or transplants. In their zeal for these therapies, it may appear that they no longer realize how great are the possibilities that their child will die sooner rather than later; but in fact they do. For example, the staff was quite concerned about Mr. and Mrs. Foster when they wanted to take their daughter to another institution which offered heart-lung transplants and experimental therapies not available at this center.

The staff wondered "how realistic" these parents were. The parents' statements indicate that they knew of the realities. In fact, their awareness motivated their actions.

"You just want to hang on as long as you can. And then they're so close to a cure, which I don't know. You get your hopes up about it. But then it just seems hopeful. But it . . ."

"It," Mr. Foster picked up, "depends on who you listen to; as far as that goes. I don't know. I really wonder how close they are [to a cure]. And if they are close, is it in time to do any good for Britt?"

"But," Mrs. Foster added quickly, "there's always that hope in there; no matter what anybody says to bring you down. Not to bring you down, but to make you feel like there's no hope. You still have that. You still have that hope."

Even as the child's condition begins to deteriorate, thoughts about the toll the disease has taken on their child's physical well being and the probable outcome, retreat somewhat when the child is not acutely ill. As Mr. and Mrs. Foster went on,

Usually when she's sick I'm constantly on it. Or before if I feel she's starting to get sick. It's day after day, like that's all there is, that's all I think about."

"Well you had a really, really extreme period there when she was really sick and got that vasculitis"

"Yeah."

"I mean that was a really bad time for you."

"Usually when she's doing good, I'm pretty, pretty good." Mrs. Foster paused. "I think we're pretty busy during the days. A lot of times it's at night when you sit down and say, when we just think about how busy we are. During the week I'm pretty good because I'm tired and I fall asleep. Maybe Saturday night I'll dwell on it more. I'll talk to him and it makes me feel better to talk about it. Plus, I don't know, I'll ask him, 'Do you think she's doing pretty good now?' And he says, 'Yeah.'"

"I think the worst time you had was when Britt was in the hospital with the vasculitis and her veins collapsing."

As the deterioration progresses the prognosis file is brought forward and looked at more frequently and the files on cure and even control of the disease are filed far behind it and seldom if ever looked at again. This does not mean, however, that parents constantly dwell on the terminal aspects of the illness, or that they even apply it consistently to their own child. For some parents, not until the physician tells them that the child is terminal do they begin to combine the two files ("disease has a terminal prognosis" and "my own child's death"), and bring them forward together. For others it comes before their conversation with the physician and other members of the CF team about planning for terminal care. As one father remarked to a friend at his son's funeral,

> The docs prepared us and all. They talked to us about Bruce dying and what we needed to be prepared for. So we knew a few weeks ago. Libby came to it though, five months ago, before they told us Bruce was terminal.

Reminders of the Disease and Its Consequences / Avoidance of Reminders of CF and Its Consequences

When the child is first diagnosed parents begin to build up relationships with other parents of children with CF. They attend support groups for parents of newly diagnosed children. They speak to each other on the phone with some regularity, and in some cases with parents of children who were diagnosed many years ago. Parents see these relationships as essentially "helpful."

> It's nice [to be in contact with other parents of children with CF] because you have something in common. But at the same time it makes it hard, because like Alana [another parent's child] has been in the hospital four times. And then you feel bad for saying that yours is doing good. Or I might say it was nice because when I was really feeling down she was too. It's more nice than bad, but you just kind of have to watch what you say, because I know how I would feel if the shoe was on the other foot. [Mother]

Toward the end of the first year following diagnosis and certainly by the end of the second parents begin to question whether or not it is "a good idea" to be so involved with other parents of children with CF. There is concern not only about how much time activities and conversations with these other parents take, but also about the impact that such activities have on their everyday lives. For example, one father did not want to continue in the heavy fund-raising activities that he and his wife became involved with shortly after their daughter was diagnosed, lest CF become the center of their lives.

> It's nice to do all this stuff, the basketball marathon, the walkathon, and the bowlathon, but there are other things to do. I don't want our lives centered around cystic fibrosis.

He was not sure that his wife's continued involvement in these activities as well as her calls to other parents and visits with adolescents with CF was a good idea.

> They're nice people, but I think Anita is getting too emotionally involved with other peoples' situations. And I think that's bad. I think it's bad. And I've told

her this. I think that you have enough to deal with your own and you just have to draw the line a little bit and see.

His wife was also beginning to question these activities citing the impact that they had on her. She, like many parents, found that contact with adolescents with CF and other parents raised difficult questions about her own child's future, their relationship and the course of the disease.

There's this bind. I like to talk to some of the other mothers and the older kids, to see how they deal with it and what it will be like. I guess I like to see how they cope. But then I see how some of them treat their mothers and wonder am I going to have that with Leah. They all rebel; I know that. But then what happens when they rebel against the treatment? It gets me thinking. And then I wonder if it's such a good idea to get involved.

See, when I was at the hospital I got friendly with the older kids because I wanted to see what they would be like. And then I started thinking that with some of them the end might be near. And that's hard. The way they are dying; it's so slow in the end. There is a part of you that doesn't want to know. And if you talk to them then you know. Then, there is also a part of you that wants to feel good when you talk to them.

In the months and years after the first annual examination, when the child is doing relatively well, parents begin to distance themselves from things associated with the disease and its consequences. Whenever possible parents avoid activities or situations that could lead them to confront, think about, or otherwise deal with the negative aspects of CF. I refer to this process as the *Avoidance of Reminders of Cystic Fibrosis and Its Consequences*. Individuals, in this case parents, engage in behaviors that allow them to establish or maintain distance from the disease and its consequences.

For the majority of parents the distancing occurs "quite naturally; almost unnoticeably." They stop going to parent support groups, reading about the disease, and participating in fund-raising activities.

I got less interested in that and more interested in just dealing with her usual, the normal school problems. I just didn't want to focus on CF. I think it was because she was doing well and I started to realize that I couldn't go on being this involved forever. [Mrs. Sherman]

For some parents the change in their behavior is quite deliberate. They say that they do not want to talk to other families, in "parent groups," in the waiting room, or anywhere else for that matter. Talking to other parents raises issues that they would prefer not to think about or deal with.

There are these meetings [parent groups] on weekdays and I can't make it. To tell the truth I don't want to go just to hear their problems. I know what's going on. I know I have a child with CF. What they do and what I do—to each his own. It just adds to more of your problems if you go and listen to other peoples'. It just adds on more questions and problems and worries. I don't want to go. [Mother]

Parents feel that they know "what is going on," can find out what more they might need to know, and that they need not be reminded of what can happen over the course of the illness. One father, speaking at length about his position on attending parent group meetings and being involved in fund-raising, reflects the attitude of many parents.

> Well I don't like to go to those things because all you do is hear the worst stories. I don't need that. I don't want that. The way I look at it, if there's anything we should do medically, going to the Clinic [outpatient visit at CF center] every three months, they're going to keep us up to date on it, what's going on. And we really haven't had to deal with any real difficult psychological problems as far as I'm concerned.
>
> Maybe if she were worse we would feel like we would need parents, other parents to compare notes, but not now. I don't need to go over there and listen to the horror stories. I just don't need it.
>
> Sometimes I feel a little guilty about not trying to help more with getting money. But we did it for a long time though. And Gretchen was a poster child. But then we started getting all these calls and there were some real horror stories and I didn't need that.

There is also a marked shift in parents' waiting-room behavior, from the socialization with other parents so prevalent in the year following the diagnosis to a kind of civil inattention in the ensuing years when the child is doing relatively well. By the end of the second year following diagnosis parents are no longer seen talking to one another about their child's treatment. One mother summarized the sentiments of many parents when she said of herself, "I don't want to hear their stories."

For other parents, the ways in which they distance themselves from the disease and its consequences are quite noticeable. Some begin to miss clinic appointments. And of those who keep their appointments, many do not tell the physician about changes in the child's condition. Others do not ask the doctors about troublesome symptoms, or for test results that point to the more long-term consequences of the illness. For example, children can be doing well, without exacerbation, yet laboratory studies indicate that there are changes in liver function that could lead to or point to problems later on in the course of the illness. These children are regularly tested and carefully monitored for further changes. It is not unusual for parents not to ask for the results of these studies.

> This thing with the liver, what can I do about it? I have never heard back on the ultrasound so I'm figuring if anything were really bad we would have heard.

Besides, she is doing so well in every other way. If there were anything that really needed to be reported on I'm sure they would have called me. I'm sure. [Mother]

In general, parents would prefer to avoid discussions about the long-term prognosis, especially with the CF team. For example, one father who asked the doctors many questions about CF, but assiduously avoided questions about his son's prognosis explained that,

I never ask the doctors about how Neal is doing. Maybe because I really don't want to know, but maybe because also they don't want to be pinned down. I think sometimes there may be a problem with Neal, but I don't say. He's just one of those kids who punks along till something really gets him. And when it does they'll tell us and we'll do what ever we need to.

At the clinic, one is also struck by the lack of dialogue between husbands and wives. As one couple explained,

WIFE: We don't talk while we're here. Sometimes we talk afterwards and sometimes we don't.
HUSBAND: I bring work and I don't do it. I can't focus. Coming here makes you think about too many things.
WIFE: Yeah. I get real anxious before a visit. It brings up all this stuff that I usually don't have to think about.

At this time, and for a long time to come, discussions about CF are rare at home as well.[16] "We don't talk about it much. We don't talk to each other about it that much," is a common refrain among parents. This is in marked contrast to the months following diagnosis when "CF was the only thing that we talked about."

He [husband] comes home for lunch and we talk about it at lunchtime. We talk about it at dinnertime. We talk about it at bedtime. [Mother seven months after child's diagnosis]

Parents of children with mild disease, two or more years beyond diagnosis, told me that the interview was the first time that they had talked about the prognosis since the first year.

When the child is doing well there is little talk about the disease beyond what happened at a visit, or what treatments are needed.

---

[16] Angst (1992: 79) also found that "CF was not a topic that children or families commonly discussed." Similarly Burr (1985: 30) noted that Obetz and others (1980) found that "parents of children in long-term remission of leukemia (more than four years) reported that they had difficulty talking with each other about the illness or discussing it with the child."

The issue of communication amongst parents and children about CF and the ill child's condition is discussed in Chapter 13.

We'll talk about a new medicine, but not the other things. I would never say I'm really scared that Gideon's going to die. I don't think I'd say that. I don't think he'd [husband] say that. And we don't talk about when Gideon will have to go into the hospital.

Two days ago I said, "Gee would you mind getting up a little earlier? I'm sick to death of doing therapy." He said, "Fine! Great!" Well it turned out we needed milk, so he had to run down to Wawa and I just ended up doing the therapy. But just to have him say, "Yeah, great," that was enough. But that's all that gets said; nothing else about the disease or the treatment. [Mother]

Parents feel that whenever one begins to talk about the disease or illness beyond what needs to be done in terms of care and treatment, the risk is there that issues that "may have been put to rest, at least temporarily" will reemerge and "envelope"; i.e., remove the distance that they have tried to establish.

With the first major exacerbation, whatever distance the parents have managed to establish by the way in which they have handled their contacts with other parents, their conversations with one another and their clinic appointments dissolves. With the first hospitalization "it all comes back again." Through observation of other children and conversations with other parents and clinicians parents are again reminded of the course of the disease and its consequences.

Upon recovery from the first major exacerbation parents again try to establish distance from the reminders of the disease and its consequences.[17] Many of the behaviors first observed when the child was doing well, before the first exacerbation, reemerge. Many parents continue to absent themselves from parent meetings, have little if any contact with other parents and remain uninvolved in fund-raising activities. As one mother explained,

I'm not interested in talking to parents of other kids with CF. Maybe if they had older kids [with CF], maybe then.

Some parents are reluctant to have their children participate in studies, lest it raise issues that they would prefer to avoid. Recall, Mrs. Farrington was undecided about whether or not she wanted Cody in the prednisone study, because of what participation might conjure up.

Once you do it [enroll the child in the study] then you start thinking about it, the bad parts and all. I don't like to think about it.

In time, without further exacerbations or hospitalizations some begin to miss appointments again. As the mother of a fourteen-year-old who had not been hospitalized since he was ten said in response to questions from staff about her irregular clinic attendance.

[17] Kathy Charmaz (1991: 157) found a similar pattern of behavior among the chronically ill adults whom she studied.

I can't deal with coming here. I can't bear to see some of the children and what's happened to them.

Outpatient visits to the center continue to raise issues that parents would rather not address.

It should be noted that some of the parents who contemplate cutting back on outpatient visits to the center ask the physicians before they do. When parents ask, staff tell them that they understand that they may not want to come as frequently, but that they would prefer that they did not cut back on their visits. Staff members are concerned that, given parents' reluctance to ask questions and report changes in the child's condition, "things could get out of hand really quickly if they come in less frequently."

Many parents also continue to try to maintain distance from the disease and its consequences by avoiding the possibility of hearing at an outpatient visit what they do not want to hear. For example, when the nurse practitioner asked the mother of a child who had had several tune-ups if she had any questions for the attending physician before she left, the mother responded, "That's OK. I don't need to ask him this time. He's doing so much better. I'll deal with it another time."

As the number of exacerbations and hospitalizations increases parents are often reluctant to go to the CF center any sooner than they absolutely have to. For the parent, visits to the center raise the possibility of hospitalization.

Once they have us there I know they're going to admit him. And from the looks of his PFTs we'll probably have to stay. I wanted to see what was happening first, if it would resolve itself. That's why I've been waiting for this appointment [rather than calling for one sooner]. [Mother]

If outpatient visits can serve to reduce the distance one has established from the negative aspects of CF, how much more so hospitalization, with its intensive therapy, medication, and tests.

Every time I go to the hospital I think that this time could be, well, you know. [Father]

Hospitalizations also put one in contact with other sick children, many of whom "were like the way mine is now. And now they are sicker. You can't help but think, 'Is this the way it goes?'" Seeing severely ill children reminds parents of what they had learned at the outset was a major characteristic of CF, progressive deterioration. It is an aspect of the disease that they try to keep from dominating their everyday thoughts and lives.[18]

When you see some of the kids here that have to have oxygen tanks and they always have to have that. I don't want him to ever have to have that. If he can't

[18] For further discussion of this point see the preceding section on compartmentalization of information.

live and be like he is now, I don't want him to live like that. I think that would tear us apart more than if he would just get sick and die. Of course that's easy to say now. [Mother]

The impact that contact with other children with CF has on parents cannot be minimized. Ill children are stark reminders of the negative consequences of the disease. In their presence parents' thoughts often "jump to what is yet to come." As Mrs. Reynolds had elaborated on one occasion,

> And sometimes when I do see the other CF kids that are here [in the hospital], it scares me a little bit 'cause I think, "Oh gee, I don't want Carl to have to be on oxygen." Or if I see the older kids and they're not doing well, then that brings me down a little bit. [Mrs. Reynolds]

Parents vividly recall their encounters with other ill children, and the effect that these meetings have on them. One mother recalled how, when her daughter was diagnosed, a child with more advanced disease stopped by the room while the mother was out getting dinner from the cafeteria. When she came back to the room, her daughter introduced her to the visitor.

> "Mom, this is Candy. She has cystic fibrosis too," she said. Well that was like one more slap in the face all in one day, because even though I had taken in the diagnosis, I was not ready to stay in the room and say that my kid was like this kid.

It is not surprising that parents look for ways to avoid hospitalizations. If hospitalization cannot be avoided, then at least the place that reminds them of the disease's outcome can be. Several parents who had been willing to have their children hospitalized at the CF center hospital when the child had to come in for tune-ups, began to request hospitalizations at their local hospitals when the number of hospitalizations increased. While all of these parents mentioned how the local hospital was more convenient and less disruptive to family life, many added that it was also easier to go to the local hospital because "there aren't so many really sick kids there."

Another way in which parents try to avoid the issues that hospitalization raises and to maintain some distance from CF and its consequences is through home IV therapy. As the complications of the illness begin to develop and intensive therapy becomes more necessary parents often request home IV therapy. For example, one mother whose child had been admitted over the weekend had asked several of the doctors if she could take her son home.

> I don't understand why he had to stay here. I hope that they'll let us take him home. I don't know why he has to stay here. We could manage the oxygen and

all [referring to IV medications] at home. He's been on IVs at home before and there's not much to the oxygen, really.

At home, not only does one avoid seeing other sick children, but also one does not have to deal with the staff on a regular basis. Difficult questions can be put aside.

Hospitalizations, exacerbations, and complications are constant reminders of the progress of the disease and its outcome. With the development of further complications requiring hospitalization it becomes impossible to avoid reminders of the illness. As one mother said, "Where can we go? How can we escape? It is everywhere."

Despite this, parents do try to escape through various activities. As one mother of two children with CF quipped,

> When the going gets tough I go to the casinos to forget it all. That's my escape. Some people smoke, some people drink, I hit the casino. I don't bet a lot, that's not the point. I just take out my frustrations on the machine whether I win or lose. Then I like to eat. I use eating as an excuse. But nobody's hurt by those things.

The overwhelming sense of being unable to escape may in part explain why, once the complications of the disease increase, parents no longer resist contact with other parents; in some cases, they even seek to reestablish contact. Review of the waiting-room observation reports indicated that parents of children who had begun to develop some of CF's complications began talking to one another. This is not to say that they always wanted to talk to other parents. As one mother of a child who had within the last two years developed Burkholderia cepacia put it,

> There are days when I want to talk about it. And there are days when I just want to push it away.

Even when parents do talk to one another in the waiting room, conversations are often brief, as several parents observed.

> Something you notice [in the waiting room] is how people don't look at each other and talk to each other. There's very little conversation. Once in a while you'll hear a mother say to the other, "How are they doing?" If they say, "Oh, they just got out of the hospital," you don't hear any more conversation. That's it. That's the end. [Mother]

Parents of children who have developed complications are often aware that parents whose children are doing well do not want to talk to them, lest issues come up that they do not want to deal with. One mother's view of parents whose children were doing relatively well ("new parents" as she called them) as compared to mothers like herself (whose children had already begun to develop complications) brings into bold relief the difference in the way these two groups of parents deal with reminders of the disease.

> New parents don't want to talk to older parents, 'cause they're afraid of what they're going to hear. Parents of children that are doing well don't want to talk to you if your child's been hospitalized. They don't want to hear it. They want to bury their head. This is not going to happen to me. And if I don't hear about this then I won't know about it. The only time a parent will call you is if they think you know the answer, and they can be reasonably safe you're not going to tell them anything bad. Like if they want to know about a medication. But they'll never call you and ask you, "Does your child have this?" or "Does your child do that?" Because if you give them the wrong answer, and they interpret it the wrong way, and they don't realize that every child is different, they don't want to hear it.

Many parents whose children have experienced complications know that other parents desire to maintain distance from reminders of the disease and its consequences. They feel that there are certain topics that they can talk about only with particular parents at particular times. They draw their distinctions on the basis of their perceptions of where other parents are in the illness trajectory. For example, as is illustrated in the statement below, this mother of a child who has had numerous complications feels that now she can talk to parents of children who have died, but that they may not want to talk to her. Similarly, she feels that she cannot talk to parents of children who are doing well because they would be frightened by her situation. However much talking there may be at a clinic, the death of a child is certainly avoided, or at least couched in other terms.

> The parent who's lost a child doesn't want to sit with a mother who's losing hers, because that's pain going through again. I know a girl that was in the hospital with my daughter when she first went down [first major exacerbation requiring hospitalization], about five, six years ago; her name was Agatha. And I've seen her mother four times now and we don't talk. We used to. We knew each other well, before this [her child's death] all happened. I knew friends of hers. She knew friends of mine. She cannot look at me when we see each other now. And I understand that. Maybe it's the pain coming back.
>
> I think she looks at me as "Well, I buried that, now I want to forget. I don't want to talk to you 'cause I'll have to remember. You might bring up my daughter's name." That's how I feel about it.
>
> And I don't hold it against her. I don't even try now, to talk to her. No, if she would nod, I would nod. A lot of parents are like that.
>
> Mrs. Brock is still in the clinic because of Noah, her son. But she too doesn't want to talk about it [the death of Noah's sister Mona] too much. I don't think about Mona. I didn't when mine wasn't doing too good. It was after Mona died,

and I was talking to her, and she broke up. See, you don't want, you don't want to tread on somebody else's cemetery lot.

You can't be helped by somebody who has lost a child because they're still grieving. You can't be helped by somebody's child who's good, because they don't understand and they get scared. So they're not going to come near you. It's almost like having leprosy.

And at clinic, if somebody dies, it's, like the wake. Because everybody is saying, "Did you see so and so? Didn't you know? Did you see . . .? Didn't you know?" It's not, "They died." It's, "Didn't you know?" Well right away you know they died. They don't come out and say, "Oh, they passed a—[did not finish the word]." It's "Didn't you know?"

Parents do not want to be reminded of their child's condition any more than is necessary. For example, some parents do not like it when friends and family, however well meaning, ask them how the child is doing.[19] A mother of a sixteen-year-old who developed Burkholderia cepacia and was now frequently hospitalized for difficulty breathing said,

My father gets on my nerves, terrible anymore. He'll ask me every day, "Well, how do you think Alyssa looks?" Well, day by day she looks terrific. But tomorrow she could up and take an attack and have to go back. I can't stand that. I'm very short on patience with that anymore. And it's not because I don't want to face it. I just don't want people to ask me how she is day by day. You can ask me once a week. Fine. But he can ask me two or three times a day, come to think of it. I can't take that.

This is in contrast to the first year after diagnosis when parents often become annoyed and angry with people who fail to ask how the child is doing.

No more than parents want friends and family members to ask them repeatedly how their child is doing do they necessarily want to ask the doctors how the child is doing.

I don't ask the doctors about how she is doing. I know to the best of my knowledge that things aren't going all that well for her. But I'm not going to walk up to any doctor and say, "Sit down and tell me." I don't believe in that. I know what's going on. I don't need him to confirm it. We go to the hospital enough. [Mother]

To ask the doctors about the child's condition is to risk losing whatever distance remains between their own child's experiences to date and the negative outcomes of the disease.

---

[19] This is not to say that parents do not want to be asked, rather they do not want to be asked too often or in a way that they see as prying.

> I'm not one for conferences [with the doctors]. When you know you are not going to hear anything good, you don't want to hear. I am not so blind as those who will not see. I see. [Mother]

As we saw in the previous discussion on compartmentalization of information, by talking with physicians one risks having to face information that one is not ready to confront.

As the deterioration increases parents are less able to establish and maintain distance from CF and its consequences. Children require more frequent trips to the CF center as well as more complex and frequent therapy regimens. The reminders of the disease abound at the clinic, hospital, and even home.

> We can't get away from it. It is everywhere, all over our house [referring to supplies and equipment]. [Mother]

Parents take the few remaining opportunities to avoid the negative aspects of the illness. For example, after the pulmonary fellow had examined Avril, she told the parents that they could wait and talk to the attending physician, he would be free shortly. "No, that's OK," they responded in unison. "The last time we did that we wound up getting admitted." They left before seeing the physician. Three days later Avril was admitted for what turned out to be a long and complicated hospitalization. At the time of her admission Avril's mother said, "I knew we were going to wind up back here, but I wanted to avoid it all a little longer. And we had such a nice day planned [referring to the day of the outpatient visit when they had left without seeing the physician]. How could a few days make much difference anyway?"

A potent reminder that many parents, regardless of the child's condition, wanted to avoid, but were not certain that they could, or should, was the television premiere of the movie *Alex*, based on the book by Frank Deford. While parents could easily avoid reading the book, dealing with the movie was another matter, if only because other people would be sure to ask them about it and they felt that they would need to be able to respond.

> When the movie *Alex* came on, I wanted to watch it. I mainly wanted to watch it to get it over with, because I was so sick about hearing about it and getting information on it and having all my friends telling me it was on. I just wanted to get it over with! Plus I knew my friends were going to be looking at me the next day. And I knew they were going to ask me about the movie. So I was going to watch it.
>
> Armen [husband] said he wasn't going to watch it. "Fine" I said. "I'll tape the movie. And watch it." He said, "Fine." So we put the movie on. And, we're both sitting in the family room . . . and I hit the tape player. "OK, you can go upstairs now." He's reading a magazine. And I said, "You know, I'm going to watch this now." "OK. Fine. I'm just going to read a couple pages."

Well, the movie started, and the magazine was on the floor, and we watched the whole thing together. [Mother]

Some parents also felt that they should watch so that they could answer any questions that their children might have as a result of their friends seeing the movie and asking them about things that the parents had not discussed with them as yet (e.g., course of the illness, prognosis).

I knew a lot of my friends were going to watch it, so I figured their kids would too. And then their kids might say something to Reed [well brother] and even if he didn't ask me I should know what he might have heard. So I thought I should watch to know. [Mother]

Once having seen *Alex* parents found ways to distance themselves from the difficult issues it raised, most notably Alex's death at age eight. They commented on "how late she was diagnosed," that "she had a worse case," "how young she was when she had her first pneumonia [exacerbation]," "how scarred her lungs were." In short, parents focused on those aspects of her illness that were different from their own child's and "how unusual her case was."

The Child's Difference from Other Children / Redefinition of Normal

In the first year following diagnosis parents are acutely aware of how different their child with CF is from other children. The differences appear marked and profound. Even as basic a human activity as eating requires consumption of medication to insure digestion and absorption of nutrients. Attention also must be given to intake and output. Days punctuated by rigorous treatments to maintain vital lung function are not part of the usual repertoire of child-care tasks.

Parents long for a "normal life" and wonder if it will ever be possible. At a meeting of parents of newly diagnosed children the mother of a child diagnosed ten months prior said in discussion,

I wonder if things ever go back to normal again. I guess it'll never be the same. Sure we do normal things like family outings and stuff, but we worry about Maxine getting sick, what we have to take for her, what we need to do.

Despite the burdens of care and the constant concern for their child's health and well being, parents want a "normal life," "as normal life as is possible with CF," for themselves and for their children. One father of a newly diagnosed daughter echoed the thoughts of many parents when he said,

I don't want to hide it 'cause I know it's there and I accept it, but on the other hand, I don't want to build my life around it and I don't want to build my kids' lives around it. I really don't. I want them to lead as normal a life as possible. And I want Bea [wife] to lead as normal a life as possible.

Toward the end of the first year following diagnosis parents grow increasingly concerned that others will label the child as different.

> When people say something about him being sick, I'll say, "Well he's not sick. He's only sick when he gets sick." Sure he has a disease and you have to watch it, but it's not like he's always sick. That's what really bothers me. I don't want people to think of him as a sickly little boy. He's really not. [Father]

Some parents deemphasize the negative aspects of the illness in conversation with others.

> I find that when I am talking to other people about it I'm always trying to emphasize the positive. I'm always, "We're so close to a cure." I always say that. I just overemphasize those kinds of things, just so they'll realize that Derrick's OK and he's not mentally retarded, really different. [Father]

Others feel that the best way to avoid having the child labeled as different is not to say anything at all about their child's condition. They do not even tell other people that their child has CF.

> We haven't told many people about Adrianna. There's really no need to. She's a normal looking child. [Mother]

In the months and years following the first annual when the child's condition has stabilized and the child begins to enjoy a measure of "relative health," the parents' desire to have others see the child and family as "normal" intensifies. For example, one mother, in response to my request to include her family in my study, said,

> I don't know why you want to observe us. We're just normal. Jordan's [child with CF] normal. He and Ross [well brother] fight like any brothers would.

Several parents of children who were doing well could not understand why I would want to study them, "normal people," "just like any body else's family."

After the first annual examination, when the children are doing relatively well, parents begin to engage in a strategy that I refer to as the *Redefinition of Normal*. This process involves expanding the realm of normal to encompass the ill child's condition and the family situation. When the child is relatively healthy and the differences in appearance and activity level between a well child and a child with CF are not great, parents minimize the role of CF in their child's life.[20]

Parents make light of differences between the ill child and other children.

---

[20] Angst (1992: 82), in her study of parents of school-age children with CF, found that "All [parents] tended to minimize its presence."

Differences due to therapy, medication, and diet were presented offhandedly. Many parents' descriptions of their child's condition resembled this mother's.

> It's [CF] no big deal now. She does everything everybody else does. The only thing is that we have to do therapy a couple times a day and she has to take medicine before she eats. Other than that, she is totally normal.

Joking is also used to establish the child's condition within normal limits. For example, rather than intimate that the disease was a cause of their child's voracious appetite, parents would joke, "She eats me out of house and home." "He's just a big eater."

Parents focus on aspects of the child's medical history that are like other children's. Parents emphasize the asthma many of the children with CF have over the CF.

> Her problem is her asthma [not her CF]. Lots of children have asthma. We all have allergies. [Mother]

The child's ability to fight off or resist infections easily is also put forward as an indication of how well and not sickly or different the child really is. Exposure to infection without succumbing is eagerly reported at an outpatient visit.

> Trevor's great. He was around people with bronchitis and he didn't get it. And here he is with a lung disease. [Mother]

Similarly, when the child is thinner than the medical staff would like to see, parents attribute it to factors other than CF, to problems that any child might have. For example, in response to the doctor's question about the baby's lack of weight gain the mother responded,

> Her appetite's down. But I think it's just her age. She eats, but only what she likes. She's getting picky. They all get that way eventually.

Other parents noted their own "short stature," "small bones," "baby's teething."

Parents call attention to the aspects of the ill child's life that are like healthy children's—music lessons, scouting, athletic activities—and thereby establish a place for them in the world of normal and healthy children.[21] When I tried to set up appointments to come and visit with the family, parents often told me that I was more than welcome, but I should know that a lot of time would be taken up with the child's extracurricular activities.

> We're happy to have you, but I don't know how much you'll get to see, CF-wise I mean. The girls [child with CF and well sibling] have soccer practice and scouts in the fall. They're so active. Maybe spring would be better. But then they're outside playing all the time. It's hard to get them to come in. [Mother]

---

[21] Bossert, Holaday, Harkins, and Turner-Henson (1990: 58–59), in a study of parents of children with a variety of chronic illnesses, also found this to be the case.

Parents stress not only how active the child is, but also how much more active than their other well children.

> Emma's [child with CF] real active. She runs constantly. Polly [well sibling] is worn out and Emma's still going. [Mother]

Parents report that they do not treat the ill child any differently from the way in which they treat the well child. To do otherwise would make them different and "they aren't really that different, at least not now."[22]

> Ava gets her lickin's like any kid her age. She has her punishments. She has her periods when she's grounded. I holler at Ava just like I holler at Orin [well brother]. How is she going to grow up normal if I don't? [Mother]

Parents claim that they expect them to "pitch in," "help out with the chores, just like anyone else in the family." Interestingly, of the parents who did admit to treating the child differently, the reasons that they gave were not unlike reasons that parents of healthy children would give for treating one child in the family differently from another. They spoke of the child's being "the youngest," "my baby," "the only boy."

Parents try to minimize the occasions where the child would be singled out as different. For example, many of the parents did not want their children going on outings designated for "sick or handicapped children." After her child went on such a trip, one mother said,

> I'm not going to let her go on things like that again. It was singling these kids out as a group of sick kids. And they had nothing else in common at all. For her in her condition since she's in very good health, I couldn't see the advantage of it at all. I think it's better for her to be with regular kids.

When their children enter school many parents ask that the children be allowed to keep their enzymes with them and not go to the school nurse when they need to take them.[23] Otherwise the child would have to go to the school nurse every day before lunch and snack. Parents explain that in going to the school nurse time would be lost from class or play and the child would be singled out as different. Besides, having the child responsible for the enzymes poses no risk to the child with CF or other children. Nothing would happen if the child accidentally took too few or too many. Also, if another child took them they would not be hurt either.

Many parents also instruct their children not to call attention to their illness at school.

---

[22] Whether or not the parents do in fact treat the ill child in the same as they do their well children is discussed in greater detail in the following section and in Chapter 13.

[23] Some school districts have a policy that requires children to go to the school nurse for any medications.

I've been trying to get her not to make too big a deal out of it [CF], especially at school. Because I think she has used it in the past as a sort of way of getting attention. And I don't think kids always appreciate that. So I've been trying to get her to take it in stride and say, "Well, I have to take these pills."

But I know the gym teacher said, "Is there anyone who has any illness, who shouldn't do this sport?" And she immediately went up and told him she had CF. And I said to her afterwards that having CF didn't mean she could get out of doing sports. Although he needed to know about it, it wasn't anything he needed to know.

So I'm trying to persuade her just to sort of take it, try and take it in stride a bit more. Just cope with it as she goes along, without her always thinking of herself as this person who is sick or has a handicap or something. [Mrs. Sherman]

When the child is doing well little needs to be said or done to define the child's condition within the realm of normal. As the child's condition begins to change the process becomes more complex. The first major change to be accommodated is hospitalization. Hospitalizations are not typical of childhood, a fact of which parents are acutely aware. Parents manage to incorporate the first hospitalization within the parameters of normal as they have defined them.

They address the first hospitalization in much the same way as they have addressed other aspects of the child's condition before the hospitalization. They minimize those aspects of the hospitalization that point directly to the CF. For example, they would, like Mrs. Farrington quoted below, talk about the hospitalization primarily in terms of improving weight gain rather than improving lung function and treating infections. The latter are presented as secondary reasons for hospitalization.

When he did go in the hospital it was mostly his weight, his lungs weren't in trouble. He wasn't that sick. They just wanted to get some more weight on him, because he started losing weight. And so they put him in mainly for that, and to clean out his lungs completely with IVs and all. And it wasn't too bad. Like I said, he wasn't really sick, it was mostly his weight. So I knew that his lungs weren't in trouble.

Upon recovery from the first hospitalization parents renew their efforts to establish their situation within the realm of normal. They once again call attention to the ill child's athletic ability and achievements.

Gillian [child with CF] plays on a girls' soccer team. Her brothers play on the traveling team. She was asked to try out for the traveling team, but I didn't want her to. On the team she's on now she has a position that is very active during the game. But the fact that she was asked, that she's tough enough to play on the boys' team, that's something. [Mother]

Parents also continue to minimize the number of occasions when the child could be seen as different. For example, after the first exacerbation, when the child is again doing relatively well, many parents will not permit their children to appear at telethons for CF or to be poster children. They do not allow them to participate in events that would distinguish them from healthy children or call attention to their illness. The child is only sick when symptomatic—coughing, feverish.

> It doesn't seem like she has a lot of lung involvement. She had the episode of viral pneumonia when she was real small, around when she was diagnosed, and then this last episode that was pretty bad, real bad, and landed her in the hospital. But we just came to the conclusion that she's sick or she isn't sick. If she isn't sick, she doesn't cough up a lot of stuff and doesn't appear to be having a problem. [Mrs. Campbell]

As the number of hospitalizations begins to increase parents still endeavor to define them within the realm of normal. As with the first hospitalization they attribute hospitalizations to problems that are not necessarily associated with CF.

> She's been in the hospital a lot, but I think a lot of it's due to the fact that she has asthma now on top of her CF. When she was about five years old they finally diagnosed that. I think that's her main cause of a lot of hospitalizations— her asthma primarily. [Mother]

For as long as possible parents endeavor to attribute the hospitalizations to something other than the CF per se, to something other children might have and be treated for in a similar way.

> Last time Bianca went in [to the hospital] the doctor said something about how it was for asthma. She [Bianca] got all, "No I don't." Well I said, "Do you want to have bad CF?" I thought it was great to have asthma. That was my thinking. I said, "This is nice. You have asthma. That is why you took that attack. Lots of people have asthma."
>
> I didn't want to think of it as a bad CF attack, I wanted to think of it as asthma. And then she got better with Preventol, like lots of other people with asthma." [Mother]

A similar approach is taken when the child is not hospitalized, and problems related to CF occur. They are not attributed to CF, but rather to factors that are common to well people. For example, increased salt intake was not because the child needed it, but rather because the child "liked it," or was "used to a lot of salt, because we all use it."[24]

---

[24] Because children with CF secrete large amounts of salt, as noted, physicians often recommend that the children increase their salt intake, especially in the summer months when they play outdoors.

Parents also try to put the issue of the child's weight gain or loss within the realm of normal. After several hospitalizations many children have difficulty maintaining their weight where the physicians would like to see it. Parents try a variety of techniques to get them to eat, but do not describe them as such. One mother whose daughter liked cheesecake baked several for her in the hope that she would eat them and gain back the weight she had lost when hospitalized. In describing her cheesecake baking to the social worker, however, she did not mention the goal of weight gain. She simply said that her daughter had developed a "passion for cheesecake." The social worker said, "So she's really trying to gain weight." "No," the mother replied, "she just likes cheesecake." As in the period when the child was doing well, without hospitalizations, parents view their child's appetites not only as sign of health, but also as an indication of how much like other children they are. How many times do people say in response to a parent's report of a teenager's hearty appetite, and large consumption, "he's a growing boy"?

> He's [son with CF] doing great. He eats a lot. He eats constantly. He might not eat big meals, but he eats constantly. [Mother]

As in the period when the child was doing relatively well without the need for hospitalization, in the periods between hospitalizations parents stress with the child the importance of remaining active, doing what other children do, not using their illness as an excuse, and thereby not calling attention to their differences.[25]

> He wasn't going to go out for baseball, but I signed him up. He said, "I don't want to do it." And I said, "Why not?" And he said, "Because I won't be able to run so fast." And I said, "So." Then he went on about his pills, and the heat, and not being good, and this and that. And I told him how we'd deal with all that, and that the CF was no excuse." [Mother]

Parents are pleased when between hospitalizations others remark on how well, "unsickly," and hence like other children the child looks.

> There are plenty of people that say, "Well he doesn't look like anything is wrong with him. He looks all right." And that pleases me, because he does look perfectly fine and we don't put a sign on him. [Mother]

Even as complications of the disease begin to develop parents still strive to define their situation within the realm of normal. They are reluctant to attribute changes in the child's activity level to the disease. One day in the clinic, for example, I said to Cato, "You look really tired." His mother quickly put in, "He's sore from skating. We all went skating yesterday. He

[25] Angst (1992: 139), in her study of school-age children with CF, found that "parents encouraged children to participate in a variety of activities and spoke of their efforts to minimize their children standing out as different."

stayed out when we all came in." Whenever possible parents call attention to how much the child is like other children. They continue to point out the child's interest and involvement in numerous extracurricular activities, often alluding to how much more active they are than their healthy siblings.

> Lilah likes to do just about anything. At school she has the intramural sports, she plays the flute, she joined the chorus. Any kind of outdoor activity—swimming, she likes to do. She collects stickers. She's in the Girl Scouts. Right now she's doing the MS Read-a-Thon. She is reading—she was reading—a lot of books; anything to keep busy. She does not like to sit around and watch TV, like her brother [who does not have CF]. She is not that type of person. She'd rather be kept busy doing something, even if it's just playing with a friend. [Mother]

The realm of normal is continually expanded to accommodate the child's condition and treatment. Like therapy and enzymes before meals, when home IV therapy becomes part of the regimen it too is fitted into the realm of normal on the grounds that it allows one to continue to do what others do. If one does what others do then one is like them, not different. In hospitalization there is greater difference.

> The care [with home IV therapy] was pretty full time here. We survived and everything went on like it had done before. If he had been in the hospital two weeks, I said, "Eight hours a day I would have been spending at the hospital." And at that time all I did was sit and twiddle my thumbs or help him with his homework. At least we were home here. He could help me cut up string beans, and he helped do things here. His friends were around. But he wasn't allowed to go and play, really play, but he could go and visit with them.
> And he'd mow the yard, like he usually does. He sat on the tractor and mowed. He just wasn't supposed to be very active so we put him on the tractor and all he did was sit and ride around. [Mother]

Similarly with diet—if one eats what others eat one is not different. One mother, whose daughter's diabetes was being managed with oral medication and diet, changed the entire family's diet to match hers. In that way the ill child was still on a "normal diet" (i.e., like everyone else's) "and besides everyone is better with less sugar." The definition of normal is extended to accommodate the child's changed condition, and in a way that did not draw attention to the diabetes, but rather what was in the best interests of everyone's health needs.

As the disease progresses many children have difficulty maintaining their weight with a "regular diet" and take nutritional supplements. Some parents take their child's weight maintenance "with just regular meals, no supplements" as an indication of how "normal" or at least unlike other children with CF, their child is. For some, like the father quoted below, the act is quite conscious.

> We keep things as normal as possible. See that woman [pointing to the nutritionist standing on the other side of the waiting room]? She wants us to mix up all these concoctions for Les. No way! He eats what we eat. We eat right. We have a garden that we eat a lot of vegetables from.

As complications begin to increase the realm of normal is expanded to include the population of other ill children.[26] The realm of normal is not restricted to a diverse sample of well children. Their lives are defined as "normal for CF." As one mother of two children with CF and two who did not have the disease explained,

> It's funny but having a sick child becomes normal. It's just normal to get up; it's normal to hear them cough. It's normal to hand them pills when they're younger and they're not able to do it themselves yet. It becomes normal. It becomes like brushing your teeth. It's normal to pay hospital bills and to have therapy. Normal to shield them from colds, and what not.
>
> And I remember when people used to come in, they used to see the machine. And Robin had a mist tent. And people would get scared. They would actually be afraid of the kids, afraid to be in your house, afraid to be in your car—unless they knew you. And, I know myself, and a lot of other people think, "What's wrong with them? This is normal?" (Laughs) But it wasn't normal for them, but for us it's normal. Our way of life is normal for us.

Eventually there are changes that cannot be incorporated even in a definition of normal that includes illness. These are the changes that come with increased deterioration—regular oxygen use, restricted activity and mobility. No amount of restructuring of the definition of normal can accommodate the changes that have now taken place. As the illness becomes more and more the focus of everyday life and thoughts there is less and less evidence of the redefinition of normal. Parents cease trying to make the situation appear normal. For as several parents remarked, "What is left that is normal?" One parent went on quite specifically, "Even the hospital isn't normal anymore."

In some sense normal has to do with the familiar, and what was happening to their children at home, let alone in the hospital, was no longer familiar. As noted in the previous section, when the child's condition begins to deteriorate the house is often filled with equipment. Also, hospitalizations that come in the wake of increased deterioration are different from the hospitalizations for tune-ups, exacerbations, or singular complications. There is a

---

[26] This is not unlike what Maine (in Strauss 1984: 122) describes for persons with diabetes. "She [the person with diabetes] has come to realize that she cannot be normal like a non-diabetic; she can only be normal as a diabetic."

sense in which in the words of one parent, "nothing could be made normal again."

Competing Needs and Priorities within the Family / Reassessment of Priorities

Over the course of the illness parents report difficulty in balancing the needs of the well child against those of the ill child. At the time of diagnosis and for a year or more thereafter, parents find themselves giving preference to the child with CF. Recall Mrs. Foster's discussion of the difference in the way that she treated Tyler and Britt when Britt was diagnosed.

> "When Tyler was a baby," Mrs. Foster recalled, "it was right at the time that Britt was diagnosed. And everything was Britt. I left him cry. When Britt was a baby as soon as she cried I was picking her up. Tyler, I fed him when I had to feed him and that was it. Tyler was an infant in the crib and I was rocking Britt in the rocking chair. It seemed like, I don't know. I just felt that he's fine, he'll be all right."

Parents recall the time of diagnosis as a time when the well child "got lost in the shuffle," "forgotten about," "ignored," "overlooked."

In the year following the first annual, when the child is doing well, parents endeavor to redress the balance. They strive to treat the children equally, not to give preference to one over the other. Parents begin to engage in a strategy that I refer to as the *Reassessment of Priorities*. Parents examine competing needs within the family and now give priority to decisions they thought could be deferred. For example, when the child with CF is doing well the needs of the well child are not deferred and are at least on a par with those of the ill child. Parents feel that this is as much for the sake of the ill child as for the well. As one mother said in comparing the way her husband used to treat their daughter and the way he did now that she was doing well,

> Sometimes we give her a smack, because you can't say, "Well I'm not gonna smack this kid, because she could die tomorrow." You just can't live your life that way. They have to know that they have to live and die under the same regulations that everybody else does. And that I think was probably one of the hardest things we had to deal with, because her father was at first constantly giving and constantly doing to one point of really spoiling her, and putting her there like up underneath of a wing. Then I said to him, "You can't do this." Then he went to the point where he hollered at her all the time. (Laughs) You have to have some kind of happy medium.

Exceptions are made for illness-related matters, like outpatient visits to the CF center, which, notably, well siblings do not attend. For example, in the year following diagnosis several parents reported that they had spent more on a gift for the ill child than they would have if the child had not had CF. They claim that they ceased to do that in the years following the first annual and through the recovery from the first exacerbation and tune-ups. "Special treats," "extras," come only in relation to care and treatment.

> Extras only come on clinic days. It's a long day for them and I think they deserve something special for putting up with it all. It makes me feel better too. And then when we do go, Neal [child with CF] will buy something for Ira [well brother]. [Mother]

Some parents also gave the children "treats for gaining weight."

When the child is doing well, keeping that child well is a high priority. Parents try to avoid situations that they see as putting the child's health at risk. Many parents asked friends and relatives not to come to the house if they had a cold. Others would not visit people where they thought some would be smoking; some even walked out of restaurants or family gatherings when there was smoking. One mother, recalling the family's Mothers' Day celebrations, explained that family members' smoking forced her to leave:[27]

> On Mothers' Day we got together as a big family. Three of my relatives started smoking. And I really got aggravated. And so we left. And I said to my mom, "You know if they were Maggie's kids [mother's cousin]," because it was Maggie's family that was smoking, "they wouldn't be doing that." My mom said, "I just don't think they realize." I said, "What? They think that because he looks so good, because he's doing so well the smoke's not going to bother him?"

Several parents were reluctant to allow the well child to have friends to the house for fear that the children might be carriers of infections. Some parents spoke to their well children about the importance of staying well themselves so as to decrease the risk of the ill child becoming infected.

> And we may be a bit overprotective in our household, but we do not permit other children to come into our home who may be ill or who have been exposed, like to chicken pox or something. We figure we have enough in here without asking for more. I know this is an area where Brooke [well sibling] gets upset because I think I told her when Chloe [child with CF] was small that "you must try to protect yourself from getting things so you don't bring them home to the house." [Father]

Concern about infection was frequently mentioned by those parents who chose not to place their children in nursery school. As one mother said,

---

[27] This should not be interpreted to mean that parents who were smokers necessarily stopped smoking. While they felt that it was important for their child not to be around smoke, several found that they could not give it up. These parents smoked outside the house.

> I didn't put Yvonne in nursery school because I think that's a place where you can pick up pretty many germs. Dr. Hasting said that from the beginning that nursery school is not good for a CF child. [Mother]

Two sets of parents, citing concern about infection, delayed entrance to school altogether. Mr. and Mrs. Farrington did not send Cody to kindergarten when he was five, because they worried about his getting sick. They waited until he was six before they sent him to school.

> And then I kept him out of school a year too because of that. Because all I could think of was, he's going to come home every day and he's going to be sick. Or every week he's going to get a cold. So we kept him out a year. He should have gone to first grade, and we just put him into kindergarten. We just figured, "Well, we can't keep him out again. We have to send him." He'll be behind, but Holly is too. She had to be put back and repeat kindergarten.
>
> But it was scary because all I could think of is, "Geez! He'll come home with everything! He'll get sick, and we're going to have problems." And it wasn't that bad. I was surprised. It wasn't as bad as what we thought it was going to be. I mean, he got colds and all, but he didn't get so bad that he had to be hospitalized for pneumonia or anything. And that's probably what we were afraid of. Even my husband was afraid to put him in school. Because that's all we could think of—"He'll be sick *all* the time." But it wasn't like that.
>
> I just kept him out a year because that's what we were thinking about, him getting sick and being ready to deal with all that. After having him do so good, for six years, and then go putting him in school and having to deal with him getting sick and going in the hospital. We didn't want to deal with that. Then we put him in this year and he did good. Yeah. He didn't do bad; not as bad as we thought. Of course, he did get more colds than if he wasn't in school. But it wasn't as bad as we thought it would be.

While parents were pleased when the children fought off infections that other well persons had succumbed to (see section on redefinition of normal), they did not want the children exposed to infections if they could in any way prevent it.

With the first exacerbation the challenge of maintaining a balance among the children's competing needs returns. For example, one mother was torn between visiting her child with CF in the hospital and continuing to nurse her well newborn.

> I thought I might wean her, but then I thought that wasn't right, so I just kept running back and forth.

Upon recovery from the exacerbation, parents once again try to balance the needs of the well child against those of the ill. They feel that this is possible because the child with CF is once again doing well. As Mr. Campbell, whose daughter was doing well two years after her first major exacerbation, explained,

> We've always tried to raise her just like the other two [well brothers her age]; the same kind of treatment and not show favoritism or anything else. And fortunately she's remained fairly healthy so it's a lot easier to do that. If she was real sick, then I think it'd be another problem with what we would do.

As before the exacerbation, special consideration is only to be given in illness-related matters. For example, visiting the ill child in the hospital takes precedence over a well sibling's activities. Parents feel that the visit is necessary if the child's condition is to improve, or at the very least stabilize. As one mother of two daughters, who now had developed many of CF's complications, described her choices when her daughters began to be hospitalized more frequently,

> It was about five years going, the disease got a better hold, or whatever; when they started being hospitalized more often, because up until then they weren't. The boys were being shipped to my mother's, or as they got older, being left alone. I was going down [to the hospital] on my one free day, on Sundays, to the girls, knowing the girls needed me at that particular point, for encouragement, to get better, and yet realizing that the boys were suffering because even though they weren't home, even though the kids went out to play I still wasn't there. If they had softball games or something like that, I still wasn't there. I was with the sisters.
>
> That to me is the top of the line. You were always weighing something. You had to be with the girls, but yet you knew that the boys were lacking something.

As the child experiences more exacerbations parents are increasingly concerned about what the ill child may "miss out on in life."[28] They try to address the issue at the family level. New priorities are established within the family. In the wake of several exacerbations it is not unusual to see families taking more vacations than they had before the child was diagnosed or in the years immediately following diagnosis. Parents feel it is important to "spend more time together as a family"—and make efforts to do so.[29]

> MOTHER: It's more important to us to do something as a family than to go and buy something.
> FATHER: To spend time wisely.
> MOTHER: We want to spend our time together.

[28] Parents' views of the child's future are discussed in greater detail in the following section on the reconceptualization of the future.

[29] Angst (1992: 97) found [but period in the illness when the behavior occurred is unspecified] that among the parents of children with CF "a philosophy that surfaced was one of urgency or of 'doing now, before time runs out.' Three mothers and three fathers spoke of their tendency to take advantage of opportunities and time with their children because of the uncertainty of future time and events."

After their child is diagnosed, many parents talk about the need to "get their priorities in order," "to live every moment as if it were the last," "do it now, not put it off." They often do not act upon that philosophy, however, until the number of exacerbations and hospitalizations begin to increase.

As the child becomes sick more frequently and complications begin to develop, family vacations assume an even higher priority.

> We save so we can go on vacations. That's a priority with us. We don't go out to dinner or buy everything in the store.
>
> Vinnie has a lot of miles behind on him now, in more ways than one. That's why we go on all these trips. [Mother]

Other priorities are also reassessed, notably the material desires of the ill child as compared to those of the well child. Increasingly the ill child's desires take precedence. One mother of six (two children with CF and four who were well), discussing the car she bought for her daughter with CF said,

> I give to the kids [referring her children with CF] more now, maybe more than I should. It spoils them, but really, what difference does it make? It's not like they are going to buy cars when they are older. They may not be able to.
>
> I am not sure what the others [well siblings] think of my doing this. I guess they're jealous, but that's it. It's easier for them to earn money.

While parents are aware that some of the things that they do to compensate for the ill child's condition may create jealousy they feel unable to do anything about it.[30] They want to give the child as much as possible in the short time that remains.[31] What the ill child wants often cannot be met in a way that benefits the entire family—through family vacations, for example.

Some parents report that they are far less demanding of the ill child, "more lenient," than they had been before the complications of the disease began to develop. They report allowing the ill child to "get away with more," especially in the social arena. One mother, in describing what she was like now that her daughter had begun to experience some of the complications of the disease, said,

> I used to be real strict. My god if you were sixteen you had to be in by eleven and all this. Now I close my eyes to a lot of stuff. I overlook a heck of a lot of stuff.

As the child's condition worsens and the disease advances, parents further reassess their priorities. The ill child's needs are more often than not given

---

[30] For further discussion of this point and its implications for well siblings' relationships with their parents and the ill child see Chapter 13.

[31] A similar statement is made by Angst (1992: 91). "Because of the uncertainty of their child's life expectancy, many parents wanted their child to experience as much joy and happiness in life as possible."

precedence over the well child's. For example, one well brother was over-weight. The counselor had advised the mother not to keep high-calorie snacks around the house (e.g., cupcakes, ice cream, chocolate bars). The mother felt that she could not do that because these were among the few things her child with CF would eat, and "she needs to gain weight." The mother thought that her son could "exercise some self-discipline and just not eat those fattening things."

As the ill child continues to deteriorate and the demands for care increase, his or her needs and desires come first.[32] The immediacy of the ill child's needs over all others is reflected in this mother's brief statement about her life with her severely ill son,

> When he calls I come. I drop whatever I'm doing. To hell with everyone and everything else.

The Ill Child's Future / Reconceptualization of the Future

In the United States, children are thought to have a boundless future—without limits, without end. Children are those who will become. When children are diagnosed with chronic and terminal illness, opportunities are immediately diminished. Time, the future, is suddenly cut short.

For parents, receiving the diagnosis of CF is like receiving a "death sentence."

> When he told us the diagnosis the first question I thought of was, "Well how much time do we have?" I only knew that they [children with CF] died. You see the poster child and that type of thing and that's all we could really associate with cystic fibrosis was that they died, and they were poster children. [Mother]

There is a sense in which the clock is ticking, time is not on their side. One mother commented on her son's first birthday,

> I was happy and I was sad at the same time. I thought a year's gone by and he's had this disease for a year. And they have found the chromosomes and the marker, but there's no cure. That's one year out of his life that's gone.

Parents' thoughts of the immediacy of death are reflected in their actions. Several parents remarked that they approached the child's first Christmas after diagnosis as if it "would be the last." They did things for the child that they would otherwise not do. For example, one child, diagnosed at age nine, regularly entered the 4H club competitions at the county fair. The year she

---

[32] Charmaz (1991: 79), in her discussion of chronically ill adults, comments that "as people become immersed in the illness, the structure of their lives changes and immediate concerns inundate them. Priorities change."

was diagnosed her father spent "extra money" to buy her a pig he felt "sure would win. Because there's no telling if she's going to be here to win again."

After the initial diagnosis and for several months thereafter there would often be comments in the chart by the social worker and other staff members about how "concerned," "upset," "frightened" parents were about the future. Until the diagnosis many parents assumed that they would have more children. After the diagnosis they are not sure whether to have more children, and if they do, whether they should adopt or use donor insemination. As noted in the discussion of compartmentalization of information in the year following diagnosis, having more children is no longer the given it once was. Similarly, several parents thought that they would continue their educations. At diagnosis, they no longer see that within the realm of possibilities.

> Everything suddenly changed. I had been planning to go to school and when I found out, I was thinking, "Oh now I'll never be able to go. Oh now I'll never be able to do this." I thought of all the limitations in my life, now. Like I'll never be able to work, I'll never be able to do this, that, or the other thing. [Mother]

In short, in the months following diagnosis hopes and plans—defining features of any conceptualization of the future—dissolve.

In the months and years following the first annual examination, the absence of a future is replaced with a new view of the future.[33] Parents begin to engage in a process that I refer to as the *Reconceptualization of the Future*. Parents posit a limited future in the face of what at the time of diagnosis seemed to be a situation without a future.

Recall that in the discussion of compartmentalization of information parents of newly diagnosed children see the child as a dying child; they were often afraid of "getting close." After the first annual exam this sense of immediate loss begins to fade and parents begin to think of a future with the child. As one mother described the transition,

> When we brought her home [after she was diagnosed] it was real hard. It was hard for a long time, for me, because I thought that she was just going to die on me. After going through all that I thought, "God, she wasn't going to live that long." And sometimes I felt like I was afraid to love her, because if I got attached and then I lost her, then I'd really be upset. But, it's just normal that you do get attached to them. And, every day that I had her, I thought, "Wow, you know, she was doing much better." And eventually as she got a little older, the coughing stopped. She really doesn't do that much coughing. And then, when she was about a year old [one year after diagnosis], I thought, "Wow, you know, I'm gonna keep her."

---

[33] Charmaz (1991: 75) makes the statement that "illness refocuses one's time perspective. Time seems reduced and reshaped."

The view of the future that is put forward, however, is not the one commonly associated with children in American society, but one that is temporally and qualitatively limited.[34] A future is posited at least as far as high school graduation and maybe even college, job, marriage. At the very least parents see the child as living through adolescence. This is evidenced by the questions that they ask about CF and adolescence. A review of the children's medical charts revealed that by the end of the first year following diagnosis, and certainly by the second, parents ask specific questions about how other parents and children manage treatment when the child reaches adolescence, how the illness affects the child socially and emotionally, and what they can do now, while the child is young, to prepare for adolescence.

In their planning and thinking about the future, many mothers take into account not only their own goals, but also what other responsibilities they might have as the child grows older and perhaps requires more care and treatment.

> I'm always aware that I'm sort of preparing for the future a bit as far as CF goes. And I think with work, for instance, it may be that in the back of my mind I'm thinking if I got very involved in a full-time job or something, I would be less available if something happened. I want to be flexible so that if something happens I'm there. So there may be that in the back of my mind that I want some flexibility and not to be so wrapped up in what I'm doing as far as work that I can't take time off if I want to do something with her or that if she's sick, I'm going to have to spend time dealing with that. It [CF] does affect what plans I make, I think. [Mother]

With the first exacerbation parents feel the future to be closing in once again. In discussing his daughter's first exacerbation requiring hospitalization, eight years after diagnosis, one father remarked,

> I probably think more about the future, now; of what she might have to face in the future. I think the very negative thing: something that is not controlled well by any type of medication or anything, and you just do your best. I guess I feel like it's a very serious situation. I'm more concerned for her future and welfare and everything that's in the future. I am trying to deal with that.

Upon recovery from the first exacerbation parents try to reestablish the view of the future they had before the first exacerbation. They once again posit a future at least as far as high school graduation, and perhaps college, job, marriage. In projecting a life at least through adolescence parents

---

[34] Angst (1992: 90) found that "For many parents . . . their outlook for their child with CF was more narrow than would have otherwise been without the illness." She noted, "Parents were inclined to focus on their child in the present, and were less inclined to entertain thoughts of the distant future" (Angst 1992: 136).

wonder what life will be like when their children reach adolescence and how they will deal with the various issues that emerge at that time.

> I wonder how he's going to react when he gets older and realizes what's going on, and if he's going to be able to talk to us, or if he's just going to hold it in. Because it must be really scary to them when they get sick and have to go in the hospital. And in school and all, people make fun of him and all that. That's a whole new thing we'll have to deal with, when he gets older. [Mother]

With each exacerbation and hospitalization concern mounts, not only about how the child will handle treatments, medication, and relationships with peers, but also with how they will deal with knowledge about the illness and its prognosis, which the majority of parents are fairly certain the child will figure out in due course.

> Eventually he is going to know the statistics of CF. I don't know what it's like to know that you have a fifty percent chance of living to twenty. And I hope he can handle it. And I think he can handle that the best way he can. He has a positive attitude. [Father]

Many parents feel that as the child thinks about his own future he needs to take CF into account. When they speak to the children about their school-work and education they tell them so. One mother recounted,

> He knows that he doesn't have a normal life span. But as far as dying specifically, we never really put a number of years on it as yet. But I know he's aware of the fact. I always did tell him, too, with his cousins. He knew they died, but I always said how sick they were and they didn't take good care of themselves. I said, "You have to get yourself a good education so you can work in a building where they have air conditioning."
>
> Well it's just common sense things. Virgil [a cousin with CF] didn't eat right. He got rebellious, he wouldn't take his pills, he didn't give himself therapy, or they didn't stress therapy. If you put all that together, you get a real negative image and I said, "You cannot afford to do that kind of stuff, you have to take care of yourself." And then a lot of it's risk, too. Chance. But I say all that.

As the child's CF becomes more advanced, parents see the child's future as increasingly limited and diminished by the illness. They speak of the ill child as "needing to adjust career goals to something that will not take so long." One of the hallmarks of the future is independence—supporting oneself, leaving home, and in some cases having children of one's own. As complications develop, parents are concerned about whether or not the child will ever be able to leave home and be financially independent, let alone start a family.

> Let's say she goes to school, moves out, and gets a job and doesn't have hospitalization or enough to pay for all her medical bills. And then she gets sick. What

then? She'll be so in debt that she won't be able to pay her rent. Besides, who will take care of her? [Mother]

They are concerned about the child living long enough and being well enough to raise children. When parents of children who have developed some of the complications of CF talk about the ill child "not being able to have children," at issue is the length and quality of their lives, not simply their reproductive capabilities. Parents know that males with CF are sterile and that were they to have children they would either have to be adopted or the result of donor insemination. They also know that females are fertile, but their conditions often deteriorate more rapidly with pregnancy.[35]

The quality of the child's life, not merely its quantity, concerns parents. The issue emerges not only with regard to what the children will be or do with their lives, but also with how the child is treated by others. Parents of children who needed to be hospitalized for the complications of the disease felt that interns "and other inexperienced people" should not be allowed to start IVs or draw blood. The reason, simply stated by one father:

Since her life may be possibly shortened it should at least be as pleasant as possible.

As the child's condition deteriorates, the future is conceived in an ever more limited way. In the face of marked deterioration, limited activity, and more time spent at home, not in school or in the company of peers, parents focus on the immediate future—rarely beyond a year. Over the course of the illness parents are often told of the need to "take it one day at a time." They would often say, as this mother of a newly diagnosed child did,

Everybody tells you to take it one day at a time, take it day by day. But that's so hard.

Yet many parents felt that they really did not grasp what it meant to "take it one day at a time" until their child's condition began to deteriorate. As the mother of one such child said,

Now I really know what it means to live one day at a time. I have to so that I can go on and give him what he needs.

However "necessary" it may be to "take it one day at a time," it is nonetheless difficult. Some like Mrs. Foster find it impossible,

"I worry ahead." Mrs. Foster giggled nervously. "And I shouldn't. I keep thinking to myself, 'Take it day by day.' But I don't. I'm really ahead all the time."

When it is clear that the child's condition is terminal, the CF team meets with the family to help them to plan for the last days or weeks of the child's

[35] Not surprisingly, then, birth control is an issue for parents of female adolescents with CF.

life. Plans for the future go no farther than what is involved in the care for the child until death and in some cases immediately thereafter (e.g., autopsy, funeral, and burial arrangements). Recall that two days before Casey died Mrs. Bailey "called around to several funeral homes to see if they could handle the viewing and cremation as well as bring Casey's body to the hospital for autopsy."

The future does not extend much beyond the child's death. The furthest into the future the parents will go is the next few days, perhaps the upcoming weekend. Two days after Casey had "come home to die," his mother arranged for an uncle to take him in a van to his grandparents' fortieth wedding anniversary that weekend. His grandfather's birthday was the following week. When I asked her if she was also going to use the van to take Casey to his grandfather's birthday the following weekend, she replied, "No, I can't plan that far in advance right now. Who knows what will be by then?"

For brief and fleeting moments parents think about life without the ill child. "It becomes just a matter of time."

2. STRATEGIES, NORMALCY, AND CONTROL

Recent studies indicate that there is little difference in family functioning between families of children with CF and families of children with other chronic disorders (e.g., asthma) or "healthy controls." In reviewing the literature on families of children with CF, Angst (1992: 11–12) notes that "despite these acknowledged stresses encountered by families of children with cystic fibrosis, more recent studies revealed that overall family functioning in these families was not statistically different from functioning either in families with asthmatic children or healthy controls (Cowen, Mok, Corey, Mac-Millan, Simmons, and Levison 1986; Lewis and Khaw 1982). Eigen, Clark, and Wolle (1987: 1512) in their discussion of knowledge about psychosocial aspects of CF, note that "no differences in emotional problems were found among the CF families studied, when data were compared to those for families in general." Fosson, D'Angelo, Wilson, and Kanga (1991: 309) go so far as to say that "families of children with CF function at least as well, if not better, than typical families and support a model of positive adaptation to chronic illness."

I would suggest that the lack of difference in family functioning between families of children with CF and other families is due in large measure to the strategies that parents adopt to deal with the care the ill child requires and the concerns the child's condition engenders. The strategies described in the previous section allow parents to live, at least for long periods of time, with some modicum of normalcy, some level of control. In this section I show how the strategies that parents adopt contribute to a sense of normalcy and control. I maintain that parents deal with CF by containing for as long as possible the intrusions it makes into their lives. Parents endeavor to preserve as much of their previous normal way of life, as well as their ideas of a normal life, for as long as possible.

It is important to point out, however, that in the early periods of the illness the strategies offer a means to achieve a sense of normalcy in family life and a way to deal with the care the ill child requires and the concerns the illness engenders. As the disease progresses and the perception of the child's condition becomes more bleak some of the strategies are no longer used and others change in such a way that their presence ceases to contribute to a sense of normalcy. They do, however, continue to provide a way to respond to the care the child requires and the concerns the illness engenders.

Period I: Diagnosis Through to the First Annual Examination

The diagnosis of CF places parents in the center of a largely unfamiliar and unknown world—the world of chronic, life-threatening, incurable illness. Parents describe the diagnosis as the "worst," "most devastating," "most painful" experience in their lives. Images are violent and visceral: "torn apart," "ripped apart," "crushed," "run over." They have a sense of everything as "out of control." The diagnosis has wrested any sense of mastery and control over their own lives, their children's lives, their futures. Their lives and the lives of all of their children are not going to be as they had imagined them. Their ill child's life, which they had eagerly anticipated and planned for, is to be cut short. The child will need a great deal of care and attention. Efforts will not be to cure, but rather to stay the inevitable, progressive deterioration for as long as possible. In what parents see as a very limited amount of time they must find a way to give this child all that he/she will need physically, emotionally, and socially and at the same time "go on with their lives"—attending to the mundane tasks of everyday life and balancing the needs of other family members.

Over the course of the first year following diagnosis parents try to regain some of the sense of mastery and control that was lost when their child was diagnosed and to return to what was familiar and "normal." Two areas receive immediate attention: (1) tasks of CF care (2) information about the disease and the child's condition. Parents begin by integrating the tasks of CF care into everyday life. They begin the routinization of CF treatment-related tasks. The emotional charge and concern that comes in the wake of treatment is reduced as the tasks of CF care are added to the list of other chores—just one more item on the "to do list." By making the tasks of CF care into chores equivalent to other daily chores, they are no longer out of the ordinary. The tasks of CF care become familiar, normal, manageable. The chaos of everyday life with all of the additional work that comes with the care of a child with CF is reduced. Life is more like that of other "normal families"—organized, without chaos.

Through routinization CF becomes increasingly manageable. Parents report a growing sense of mastery and control—a sense that, as one father put it, "was stripped away when our child was diagnosed."[36] When one performs the tasks one is no longer passive. The doing of something in the face of the disease, if only to stay its course, renders a sense of power and control. As other researchers have proposed, "parents of children with CF experience a sense of gratification or control from their commitment to the daily CF treatments and responsibilities (Cowen, Corey, Keenan, Simmons, Arndt, and Levison 1985; Gibson 1986)" (Angst 1992: 12).

Many parents also feel that the daily routines of physical therapy are not only useful, but also, in the words of one father,

> A way of saying there is this condition of CF and it's got to be respected and this is what we are going to do to respect it.[37]

Also through the process of routinization of CF-related tasks, the ultimate questions CF raises can go out of awareness.[38] As one father, half jokingly, explained to me,

> The questions are there, like your teeth are there when you floss them. But every time you floss your teeth, you don't think about the fact that if you don't floss your teeth, you may lose them.

It is not surprising then that in tandem with the development of the routinization of CF-related tasks is the development of the compartmentalization of information about CF and the child's condition, for it too provides a way for the ultimate questions that CF raises to go out of awareness. Recall that in the first year following diagnosis parents endeavor to push information about the fatal prognosis to the back of their minds and information about the

---

[36] Brett (1988: 51), in her extensive review of the literature on coping in families of chronically ill children, found that "the ability to master the specific demands imposed by chronic childhood disorders tends to decrease family feelings of anxiety and despair and increase levels of confidence and sense of self-control."

[37] It is important to note that as the disease progresses and the child reaches adolescence, many of these positive feelings about chest physical therapy and the routines around it fade.

[38] Angst (1992: 85) makes a similar observation, illustrated by a similar quote. "For the majority of parents the physical care of cystic fibrosis was not a major issue in itself, and was just an accepted part of life. At times, care was a nuisance, but no more than other aspects of family life. For most parents, care was a routine that was often done without thinking about the actual disease or the significance of therapies. 'It's just something that you do every day. It's like getting up and going to work. You give her the medicine and the treatment, and yet, you're not even thinking about why she has to have it. It's just like telling her to go into the bathroom and brush her teeth and wash her face. . . . It's part of life.'"

potential for cure to the front. When parents spoke to me about how they sorted the information that they received, they talked about how necessary it was not only for "your own sanity," but also for "getting things done." As one father put it,

You just can't dwell on it [the dying] all the time and live and work.

Also, many parents feel that if one focuses on the fatal prognosis, "you will not be able to do therapy and help your child to grow in other ways." The strategies of routinization of CF-related tasks and the compartmentalization of information about CF and the child's condition are mutually reinforcing. They lend a sense of control not only over the disease and over one's daily life, but also over one's thoughts.

Period II: Months and Years Following the First Annual Examination, When the Child Is Relatively Healthy, Through to the First Major Exacerbation Requiring Hospitalization

In the first year following the first annual examination, the strategies of routinization of CF-related tasks and compartmentalization of information are more firmly established. The tasks as well as the thoughts have been assigned a place, and with that assignment comes a sense of mastery and control. The child's relative good health reinforces parents' sense of mastery and control. Parents report "relative calm," "things back to the way they were—almost." Many parents say that they feel "more in control" or "in control again." There is a real desire on the part of parents "to keep things the way they are," "to lead as normal a life as possible."

In the years following the first annual examination, when the child is doing relatively well, parents act to remove or minimize the presence of CF from various aspects of their lives and to contain its intrusion. The ways in which parents deal with the reminders of the disease and its consequences, approach the child and the family's difference from others, establish priorities, and conceptualize the future at the very least mute the presence of CF and contribute to both an appearance and a sense of normalcy and control.

Recall that when the child is doing well parents begin to engage in the avoidance of reminders of CF and its consequences. They avoid, whenever possible, situations where the negative aspects of the illness might have to be confronted. Parents often stop going to parent meetings, reading about the illness, talking to other parents about the overall course of the disease. Those situations where reminders abound, but which cannot be avoided, are carefully managed. For example, some parents do not tell the staff about troublesome symptoms or engage in long discussions about the illness. Talk could disturb the delicate balance. In the words of one father:

When you talk about it, you think about it, and I think that's when you start to center your life around it.

Each time the parent minimizes the child's condition, emphasizes how much the ill child is like other children, or jokes about what may be at the root of apparent difference between the ill child and well children (behaviors associated with the redefinition of normal), then the presence of the disease is muted and the difference between the child with CF and well children is reduced.[39] The atmosphere of normalcy is reaffirmed. Not surprisingly many of these behaviors continue well into Period IV. Recall that even as further complications of the disease began to develop parents were reluctant to attribute changes in the child's activity level to the disease. They emphasized the child's continued participation in extracurricular activities. Again, if the child does what other children do the child is not different, despite the underlying presence of the disease.

The image of the child as like other children is reinforced when the ill child is treated like the other children in the family with the same behavioral expectations and household responsibilities (behaviors associated with the redefinition of normal and the reassessment of priorities). This behavior is unlike that observed in the year following diagnosis when the ill child is given special preference.

The ill child's likeness to other children is enhanced through the presentation of the child as growing up, going on to college, having a career and marriage. With the presentation of a future (behavior associated with the reconceptualization of the future) the parents make a claim for a place for the child with CF within the world of normal healthy children. In so doing, they are also then more like other parents. At the very least, they are talking about the child in the same terms as parents with normal, healthy children. Parents often talk about their children in terms of what they will be and do when they grow up.

With the first major exacerbation requiring hospitalization CF once again makes its presence felt. CF dramatically intrudes into the family's life. Routines are broken as more therapy is required and trips to the hospital become more frequent. Information about the course of the disease, lung deterioration, and the prognosis, which had been carefully tucked away, surges forward. The reminders of the disease and its consequences abound as one goes to the hospital to visit the ill child and talk with the staff. Visiting one's child in the hospital is certainly not within the realm of the normal. It is once again difficult to maintain a balance between the needs of the ill child and those of the well children in the family. The future seems to be closing in again. The barrier has been breached.

---

[39] Robinson (1993: 19), in her study of chronically ill adults, noted that "some adult participants reported making jokes in order to convey the message that they were just like everyone else."

Period III: Recovery from the First Major Exacerbation, When the CF Is Relatively Stable, Through to the Time When Hospitalizations Begin to Increase and Lose Their Predictability

After the first major exacerbation, parents once again act to contain the intrusion that the disease makes into their lives. All of the strategies discussed are again in evidence as parents move to reduce the presence of the illness and reestablish the sense of normalcy and control challenged by the first major exacerbation.

Order is restored, as therapy, which in some cases had slacked off or needs to be increased, is once again integrated into everyday life (behavior associated with the routinization of CF treatment-related tasks). At the same time, by formulating a view of the illness that "they can live with" (behavior associated with the compartmentalization of information about CF and the child's condition), parents feel a renewed sense of control. Granted this view includes some disturbing elements (e.g., chronic character of CF, lung deterioration, course of the illness); but by balancing these elements with thoughts of the potential for cure, the negative aspects of the illness do not dominate one's thinking. Since the negative aspects are easily brought forward, however, avoidance of reminders of the disease continues in much the same way as it had before the first major exacerbation (e.g., not attending parent groups, not seeking new information, not initiating discussion about the course of the illness). Cystic fibrosis, or at the very least the negative aspects of it, can remain in the background.

Emphasis on the way in which the child is like other children is renewed and activities that the child participated in before the exacerbation (behaviors associated with the redefinition of normal) are resumed. Parents minimize the role of CF in the child's condition and limit participation in activities that may show the child to be different (e.g., appearance in telethons). The ill child is again treated like other children in the family (behavior associated with the reassessment of priorities) and future goals (behavior associated with the reconceptualization of the future) are reasserted. All contribute to a reaffirmation of the child as like other children. Once again the presence of CF is muted and with that comes some sense of normalcy and control in daily life.

Each succeeding exacerbation is a potent threat to parents' sense of mastery and control. With each exacerbation the issues that were raised by the first exacerbation return. At this time differences in the way that parents treat their ill and healthy children are attributed to the child "being sick," i.e., symptomatic and hospitalized (behavior associated with the reassessment of priorities). In so doing, even though the parents are treating the child differently from the healthy children, they are still maintaining a sense of the child as like other children; for all children receive special consideration and sometimes treats when sick or hospitalized.

Periodic hospitalization, however, is not commonly associated with childhood. It marks one as different, outside the realm of healthy children. But when parents attribute that hospitalization, as they often do, to something other than CF (e.g., asthma), they are reserving a place for the child in the realm of the normal. In the first instance the child takes that place at all times. In the later instance the child has that place at least as often as when he/she is not sick. The concept of normal is expanded, redefined to include illness of a sort. In that way there is still a major portion of time when the child can appear like other children, and through that appearance parents retain a sense of normalcy and control.

Parents urge their ill children to lay claim to a place in the realm of the normal. They continually stress the importance of remaining active, doing what other children do, and minimizing their differences. They tell their children not to use the illness as an excuse, for to do so sets them apart.

With each recovery parents renew their efforts to define their situation as within normal limits—and to a large extent they can by the way that they handle the situation. The appearance of normalcy comes not so much from the situation itself (as treatment is still given, clinic visits and hospital stays are necessary, more vacations are taken than in like situated families of healthy children), but rather from how the situation is presented. As one mother explained,

> Sure she needs treatments, but we make them so no one else sees them. We schedule clinic visits around school vacations and holidays. That way she's not missing school and no one has to know why she's out. Even hospitalizations, especially "tune-ups," can be managed with the right schedules. And the extras we give her, the vacations, we just explain as the way we do things now.

Seeing families do what "normal" families do and not what one associates with families who have chronically ill members, one is less inclined to perceive them as different. Parents derive a sense of mastery from that perception. Recall how pleased parents were when between hospitalizations others commented on how well, "unsickly," and hence like other children the ill child looked. It is as if their efforts at care as well as the presentation of the child to others has paid off.

Period IV: Development and Increase in Complications Through to the Discussion With the Physician that the Disease Has Advanced

In the face of ever-increasing hospitalizations and the development of complications (e.g., shortness of breath, Burkholderia cepacia, diabetes) family life is more frequently disrupted. There are more trips to the clinic and hospital as the child becomes sick more frequently and with less warning.

Treatment regimens are augmented with additional medications and forms of therapy. Oxygen is sometimes needed. Complications impinge on family members' activities. In short, as complications develop it is far more difficult for parents to contain the intrusion CF makes into their lives. Yet they do try. Some try to deal with the hospitalizations through increased home treatment and home IV therapy. As one mother explained,

> Home IV therapy takes up a lot of time. It's a lot of work too. But it's better than having him in the hospital. At least we can be at home together, have dinner together, like other families. There isn't the running back and forth.

That home IV therapy and all the other chores that go along with it (e.g., increased number of sessions of chest physical therapy, more frequent nebulizer treatments) should be part of the definition of normal seems almost a contradiction in terms. But for many, normal has a great deal to do with control of everyday life. Home IV therapy offers a way to achieve some of that control, not to mention distance from the reminders of CF that come with hospitalization.

In the face of further complications parents continue to strive for control, however elusive. The strategies that have been discussed are a means to that control. However, since the circumstances to which they are directed have changed, their manifestations are somewhat different. The tasks of CF care continue to be a significant part of the daily routine, but the tasks are often scaled back in such a way as to make them a part of everyday life, not life itself. Integrating CF care in this way leads more often to cutting back on treatments.

As parents process and sort information about the disease (part of the compartmentalization of information), hopes for a cure begin to fade. Thoughts focus on control of the disease. And while parents do think about the progression of the disease and the prognosis, they do not dwell on these thoughts. By not dwelling on them, one does not give oneself over to them. There is then a measure of control.

At this time parents also continue to maintain control over the ways in which they handle competing needs and priorities within the family; they are still the decision makers. However, some of the ways in which they handle these competing needs and priorities (behaviors associated with the reassessment of priorities) break down a sense of normalcy within the family. For example, the increase in the number of vacations the family takes can be explained in ways other than the disease, and in fact may even represent to some the demonstration of even greater control over their lives (i.e., we are doing this because the family is more important to us than accumulating material possessions), if not normalcy. But giving the ill child more material goods or privileges than one gives to the healthy child is another matter. It does breach the limits of normalcy when one gives more to one child over another in the family because one "will not grow up." One is then not only stating a difference between the ill child and other children (a hallmark of childhood is growing up), but also doing so in a way that indicates a foreshortened future. While this is the case, a limited future is not what one associates with normal children. The sense of the child as like other children is diminished but not totally obliterated, because when parents speak about the child's future the description includes elements that are like other children's, albeit for different reasons. Recall that as the complications of the disease begin to develop parents still posit a future that includes the same elements as well childrens', namely careers and marriage (behavior associated with the reconceptualization of the future). At this point, however, parents speak of the child as needing to adjust career goals to something that will not take so long to prepare for, and marriage as not necessarily leading to children. These adjustments can still be handled in the realm of normalcy, because well children who are seen as lacking self-discipline are often advised not to pursue careers that will require a great deal of preparation. Similarly, many young adults now choose not to have children when they marry.

Other aspects of the child's future, like the quality of his or her life, cannot be dealt with in the same manner. Parents' sense of control in terms of the quality of the child's remaining life derives in part from the medical staff treating the child as the parents want him or her to be treated. Many parents at this point ask that only experienced clinicians be permitted to start IVs and draw blood gases.

Period V: Increased Deterioration Through to the Conference Where the Physician Tells the Parents that the Child's Condition Is Terminal

As deterioration progresses and the child's condition becomes more severe, the ways in which the parents can contain the intrusion of the disease into their lives are increasingly limited. The realm of normal cannot be extended (part of the redefinition of normal) to accommodate the changes that have now taken place. As parents themselves remark, "What is left that is normal?" "Even the hospital isn't normal anymore." In addition, parents no longer feel that they can maintain distance from the reminders of the disease (part of the avoidance of reminders), for they are everywhere—at home as well as at the hospital. At best a hospitalization can be delayed and from the use of delaying tactics gain some sense of control. Parents are determining when, not if, the child will be hospitalized. The disease dictates the need for more intensive treatment. The parents' sense of control rests in part with determining the time and the place.

With reminders constantly about them, the knowledge of the prognosis is at the forefront of parents' minds (behavior associated with the compartmentalization of information). Yet even at this point parents do not constantly dwell on the terminal aspects of the disease, or at the very least they do not always apply the terminal prognosis to their own child. Parents do not consistently connect the terminal prognosis to their own child until the physician has met with them and told them that the child's condition is terminal and they need to plan accordingly.

With the child's continued deterioration the strategies that remain in evidence have more to do with insuring that what needs to be done gets done than with any sense of normalcy or control. Routines for care are now organized around catheters and oxygen equipment (behavior associated with the routinization of CF-related tasks), less time is given to what were formerly the routines of CF treatment-related care. The ill child's needs come first. There is far less of an attempt to balance the needs of other family members against those of the ill child (behavior associated with the reassessment of priorities). For now the future is limited to months, at best a couple of years, and what the child and family can look forward to has certainly changed (part of the reconceptualization of the future). For the parents there is an increasing emphasis on the present, "one day at a time."[40] Parents are aware that this separates them from other parents, but talking about their child's future in terms of college or marriage would not make sense. As Mrs. Foster pointed out,

> When you talk to other mothers with normal children, they're thinking about the future: college, cheerleading, "I want my daughter to do this." When they talk about the future, it's hard. You don't have anything in common. You're living in a more day-to-day life; where a lot of people aren't.

While the strategies that parents use to manage the tasks of CF care, establish priorities in the family, and conceptualize the future no longer effect an atmosphere of normalcy, they do offer a way to meet the demands of CF care and the concerns the disease engenders. Parents endeavor to do what needs to be done in the face of what has become by this point a losing battle that they continue to fight. As Mrs. Bailey told the members of the CF team,

> When he asked me, "Am I going to die this time?" I told him, "You don't have to, but you need to fight."

Period VI: Terminal Phase of the Illness and Death

After parents meet with the physician and members of the CF team about their plans for terminal care, it becomes in the words of many "just a matter of time." The strategies that parents use to contain the intrusion CF makes

---

[40] Charmaz (1991: 178) finds that amongst chronically ill adults the philosophy of "one day at a time" "confers some sense of control. By concentrating on the present ill people avoid or minimize thinking about further disability and death."

into their lives are no longer in evidence. The ultimate intrusion has come—death. It cannot be contained. Its presence cannot be muted.

The strategies that parents use to meet the challenges of living are replaced by strategies families use to meet the challenges of dying. The previously discussed strategies have served their purpose. As one mother explained,

> What is there left to do? I think he had a normal life, as much as you can have a normal life with CF. Why, right up to the end he was outside there with his brothers—the oxygen in his wagon.

Parents' responses to the care the ill child requires and the concerns the child's condition engenders cannot be separated from the illness experiences. As parents' experiences change, so too do their responses. Responses evident at some points in the natural history of the illness are not evident at others. Linking parents' responses to their experiences with the illness helps us to understand some of what motivates parents' behavior. In addition, looking at particular responses as part of a constellation of strategies parents use to contain the intrusion illness makes into their lives, we begin to comprehend how the sense of normalcy and control that has recently been documented in these families is achieved. We also become acutely aware of just when and how that sense of normalcy and control, so important to parents, is diminished.

It is important to remember that while parents may be able to articulate why they respond as they do, or to discuss the consequences of their actions, it does not mean that the strategies that develop over the course of the illness are premeditated, conscious, or deliberate. The strategies emerge in everyday life in response to the care the disease requires, as well as to the thoughts, feelings, and concerns the child's condition and particular experiences engender.[41]

Parents' responses are not without consequences for themselves as well as for family life. In the following chapters I consider the impact that parents' responses have on well siblings' views of the illness, their place in the family, and their relationships with their parents and ill siblings.

---

[41] Gallimore, Weisner, Kaufman, and Bernheimer (1989: 7), in their study of parents of developmentally delayed children, using a concept similar to strategy—"accommodation"—make the same point. "Accommodative efforts are often unconscious and the forces that drive them may be only dimly perceived by the parents—yet as we will show in the excerpts in this paper, the process is reflected again and again in our informants' accounts."

CHAPTER 12

Well Siblings' Views of Cystic Fibrosis and Their Ill Siblings' Condition

> But I still get worried about Britt. I just know that with CF you could die from it. And you get all skinny. And your lungs fill up with mucus. And you can't breathe. And you die.

This is the way Tyler Foster, age nine, views his ten-year-old sister's disease.[1] For him cystic fibrosis (CF) is a chronic, progressive, life-threatening illness. He did not always think of CF this way. His views of CF, like the views of all well siblings, change over the course of the illness.

The well siblings' views are connected to their experiences. Central among these experiences are their parents' responses to the care the ill child requires and the concerns the child's condition engenders. This is not to say that parents' responses determine the well siblings' views. Their views are part of an interpretative process that involves both the parents' and the ill child's condition and illness-related experiences. In the first part of this chapter I trace the well siblings' views in the context of their parents' responses and their ill sibling's condition and illness-related experiences. The well siblings' views as they appear in the natural history of the illness are summarized in Table 3. In the second part of the chapter I discuss how their views are formed.

1. WELL SIBLINGS' VIEWS

Serious Illness

Children are keen observers (Bluebond-Langner 1978). Well siblings perceive their parents' struggles.[2] They sense the seriousness of their sibling's illness and reveal their awareness in their play and speech. At the time of diagnosis and for several months thereafter some well siblings were observed pretending to feed enzymes to dolls and crying when they spilled. Several gave their dolls chest physical therapy (PT). In this play they placed the

---

[1] The age given is the age at the time the statement was made. Since the study was conducted over a two-year period, more than one age may be given for a particular individual, reflecting the different times of the interviews. See also note 2 of Chapter 11.

[2] Kupst (1986: 174) found this to be the case in the well siblings of children with leukemia. "Even when siblings do not understand what leukemia means or are not informed of the diagnosis they may realize that something is seriously wrong from the reactions of parents."

TABLE 3.
The Well Siblings' Views of CF and Their Ill Siblings' Condition

Periods in the Natural History of the Illness

Siblings' Views	Diagnosis (I)	First Annual Exam (I)	Years Post Annual Exam (II)	Annual Exacerbation (II)	Recovery From First Exacerbation (III)	Increased Hospitalizations (III)	Development, Increase in Complications (IV)	Conference With Dr./Team (IV)	Increased Deterioration (V)	Conference With Dr./Team (V)	Terminal Phase (VI)	Death (VI)
Serious illness	●	▲					⇑		⇑		⇑	
Condition one does things for		●	⇑									
Essentially like other children			●	▲	⇑		■		■			
Not merely a condition				●	⇑		⇑					
Series of discrete episodes of acute sickness and recovery					●[a]	⇑	■		■			
Questions about cure, course of the disease control, and the efficacy of treatment						●	⇑					
Chronic progressive incurable disease that shortens the life span							●		⇑		⇑	
One's own sibling will die from CF									●[b]		⇑	

Key: ● = Begins ▲ = Changes ■ = Ceases ⇑ = Intensifies

[a] If ill sibling has had colds, flus or common childhood illnesses where everyday treatments change, this view can develop earlier.

[b] Well siblings' views may vary in terms of how close to death they perceive ill sibling to be (months, years).

masks used in the inhalation treatments over the dolls' faces and expressed the same frustration they had seen in their parents when the masks fell off and the children began to cry.

Well siblings also express their awareness of the seriousness of CF in the comparisons that they make between their ill siblings and infirm relatives. As one seven-year-old well sister informed me,

> My brother is real sick. He is sicker than even Grandmom.

This seven-year-old, like many of the children between the ages of five and seven, was hesitant to give the name of the disease and had difficulty pronouncing cystic fibrosis. But it was clear from her description that she knew the seriousness of the illness. For example, when I asked this child, "Do you know the name of the disease your brother has?" she answered,

> CHILD: I can't say it, but I know it.
> AUTHOR: Do you want to try it?
> CHILD: Pith (clears throat).
> AUTHOR: That's close.
> CHILD: Fiboscix.
> AUTHOR: That's very close. Cystic Fibrosis. Can you tell me anything about it?
> CHILD: They cough a lot. Take enzymes. And stuff to help him breathe. They [parents] worry about his breathing.

The child's mention of breathing is noteworthy because breathing is an important element in children's definitions of living (Bibace and Walsh 1981). Even very young children associate lungs with breathing (Bibace and Walsh 1981). Many of the well siblings mention the ill child's "lung problems" or "bad lungs" (as some refer to them) as distinguishing features of the illness.

Condition One Does Things For

For well siblings the hectic days of the first year, of running to the hospital, frantic phone calls, and tears pass. What follows are busy days that include ingestion of medication and regular stints of PT. Well siblings know the practices employed to alleviate some of the symptoms of CF. For example, one day in the clinic, a well six-year-old accompanied her three-year-old sister, diagnosed one year earlier, to the bathroom. The well sister commented on the role of enzymes (which she called beads) in the control of rectal prolapse (which she referred to as a flower).

> When Emma used to go to the bathroom a flower used to come out. But not anymore. She takes medicine. She used to take beads in her food.[3] Now she takes capsules. She can swallow them.

[3] For babies and young children the enzymes are often mixed into foods like applesauce.

Recall that thirteen-year-old Liam Sherman expounded on the efficacy of aerosols, breathing exercises, PT (referred to as thumping), and exercises in dealing with the mucus that "gets clogged" and makes it "tougher to breathe."

> Her mucus is thicker and stuff. The aerosol is used to bring up the mucus or at least thin it because it clogs. And it's good for her to have a lot of breathing exercises so it doesn't get quite as thick and stuff, and it gets brought up a lot. Like thumping is to bring it up. And trampolines and swimming now are good.

In the years following the first annual examination, when the child is doing relatively well, the well sibling's view of CF as a serious illness becomes tempered.[4] Now emphasis is placed on the many tasks that must be accomplished to take care of CF. The illness comes to represent a set of procedures and tasks.

> There's a lot she has to do for her CF. But it's like she doesn't have it, except for her therapy and all, which she acts like is a normal routine. [Well brother, age fourteen]

This view of CF comes largely from the routines parents adopt to integrate the tasks of CF care into their daily life. As discussed in Chapter 11, parents put PT on a regular schedule and limit it to those times. Care requirements become chores like any others. Like their parents, well siblings report that more time is spent attending to what needs to be done and less in thinking about CF and its implications.

> Most of the time I forget she has it because the things become quite routine. So, we're having therapy in the morning. It's like, I don't even think about it anymore. It's just sort of normal. I don't look at her as having it at all. I just forget about it. [Liam Sherman, age thirteen]

Granted, when the child is sick, with a cold or other childhood illness, there is more to do than there would be ordinarily, but it is manageable. For example, in describing their brother Cody's care, his sisters noted that when he had a cold he received therapy on a regular basis.[5] Twelve-year-old Holly Farrington pointed out that,

> If he has a cold he has to take his treatment . . . He doesn't do it every day. If he has a cold he'll have to do it every day because he coughs a lot. Other times he gets it once in a while.

---

[4] This is not to say that their sense of CF as a serious illness disappears. It is that, like their parents, they put the gravity of their sibling's condition at the back of their minds, where it is not readily retrieved or discussed (see Chapter 11).

[5] As discussed in Chapter 11, in the second period, when the child is doing relatively well, adherence to PT regimes sometimes slacks off.

Essentially Like Other Children

As long as the ill child's condition remains mild and stable, well siblings continue to see CF as a condition one does things for—sometimes more, sometimes less. This view is buttressed by what the well siblings see when they look at their siblings. At this point the child with CF looks like any other normal, healthy child. There are no outward signs of the disease. The affected child contracts and recovers relatively easily from the same illnesses that afflict otherwise healthy children, and also behaves as they do.

Parents' actions confirm the resemblance between the ill child and healthy children. In the majority of cases there is little observable difference between the way that parents treat well and ill children. Parents report similar expectations for both. They give them equivalent responsibilities. Well siblings take note. Remarks from well siblings like, "We both have to do chores," "She does the same amount," "We get treated the same" are not uncommon. Also recall that when the child is doing relatively well parents minimize the child's condition and emphasize how much the child is like other children. They present all of their children's futures in similar terms. The sense of imminent debilitation and death, notable in their presentations of their child with CF at the time of diagnosis, is absent from their presentations in the years following the first annual examination, when the child is doing relatively well.

Well siblings present their ill sibling's condition in much the same way as their parents. At this time well siblings, like their parents, often openly minimize the differences between the ill child and healthy children. They frequently proclaim that the ill child "isn't really any different." As one well brother, age nine, said of his two sisters, one of whom has CF,

> Helen [the ill sister] is just like June [the well sister]. Helen doesn't look like she has CF. If I didn't know she did, I wouldn't know she has the disease. She looks regular, like a regular girl.

Like their parents, well siblings joke and in other ways make light of differences between other children and the ill child.

> He eats all the time, 'cause he's a pig. [Well sister, age six, of her ill brother]

> It's nothing much other than she has to have therapy and aerosol and take some pills. [Well brother age thirteen]

In many homes, the ill child's enzymes, vitamins, and some antibiotics are kept in the center of the kitchen table or on the counter along with other family members' vitamins. As many of the well siblings point out, the enzymes are taken without comment, and in many cases with little or no direction. In discussing Cody's care Holly Farrington, age twelve, noted that

He takes enzymes too. We always have to remember to give them to him. Sometimes he forgets. Sometimes my mom says, "Holly, get him the enzymes." Or other times he says, "I need my ennies." He calls them that.

Also like their parents, well siblings call attention to the aspects of the ill child's life that are like healthy children's. They frequently mention the ill child's athletic abilities and activities. There is almost a formula to what the well siblings say when describing their ill brother or sister: (*Name of ill child*) is just like ("*anybody else*," "*other kids*"). (*He/She*) plays (*name of sport*). Participation in athletic events is a measure of just how much the child with CF is just like any other normal child.

Cystic fibrosis and the child's condition are no longer frequent topics of conversation between parents or with others who come into the home to talk with parents. Parents' concerns are no longer in public view. Well siblings neither see nor hear their questions and concerns. Discussions at home about CF and their ill sibling's condition are rare. For well siblings, however, no discussion can mean not only no further acquisition of information about the disease, but also no further quest for such information. Well siblings depend on their parents and ill siblings for information. At the time of diagnosis well siblings are told: what medications the child will need to take; when and why enzymes, treatments, and PT are necessary; and that the cough is not contagious. In the main, parents do not discuss the genetic nature of the disease, its course, or prognosis in these early conversations.[6]

If the ill child continues to do well (as is often the case in a subsequent period of relative health following diagnosis) parents tend not to give siblings any more information. By this time well siblings are not only older, but also often ready for more information, yet the parents do not offer it—nor do the well siblings ask.[7] As one well sister, age fourteen, commented,

> Maybe I should ask, learn more, but I don't.

Other opportunities to gather information also diminish at this time. With the parents not reading about CF, less literature is about for the well siblings to pursue. Also, as parents stop attending parent groups and withdraw from CF fund-raising and social activities, there is less contact with other children who have CF—a major source of information. Many of the children indicated that they also learned about CF and their ill siblings' condition from going to the CF center. By the time they are school age, however, they rarely accompany their siblings to outpatient visits, even on school holidays.

> I went to clinic [outpatient visits at CF center] when I was younger. I think maybe it was about the summer; no, not this past summer but the summer

---

[6] Parents' reasons for not telling the well sibling more about CF and their ill sibling's condition are given in Chapter 13.

[7] For further discussion of this point see Chapter 13 and Afterword.

before that. I think I was down. I think I went because I don't think there was anybody else home to baby-sit me. So I think I went down. God, was it busy. Everybody seemed to be rushing around and it was, well, it was different. Because for a kid, for a girl my age, you know, there wasn't too much to do, but it was interesting to just be there and watch people come in and people leave. I thought it was interesting what they did to check Mady over.

I liked that little thing where she blows into the circle and then she sees how high she can get it. I thought that was neat. But when they took blood I had to leave the room because I can stand the sight of blood, except I can't stand the needle. Even to see it happening to her, I'm like, "Oohhhh don't show me that needle." I can't stand needles. It used to take six doctors and maybe a nurse to hold me down when I used to get a shot. I can't stand shots.

I like to see how much she weighs and see if she gained any or lost any. Things like that. [Well sister, age eleven]

In short, when the child is doing relatively well, well siblings have fewer opportunities to learn about CF. Their knowledge of the disease is limited in the absence of further experiences with the illness and remains so for quite some time.

Not Merely a Condition

With the first exacerbation, CF again forcefully intrudes into the family's lives and minds, disturbing their sense of normalcy. Well siblings become concerned about their ill brothers and sisters. As ten-year-old Adam Campbell explained, when he recalled his sister's first hospitalization,

"One time she was sick. She had something wrong with her—I forget what it's called, but she had to come to the hospital for about a couple of weeks. It was frightening, but she came out, so—I was glad. That she doesn't get hurt a lot or anything. Like she might get like sicker and die or something because." Adam stopped for a moment, the word "because" holding his place.

"We were like, 'Where's Zoe?' 'She's at the hospital.' And then my mom and dad went there in the morning. I went to see her one time when she was in the hospital. And it was weird because she wasn't here [home]. When she got back everyone was happy and everything."

The first major exacerbation requiring hospitalization challenges the well siblings' sense of CF as simply "a condition one does things for." With hospitalization CF becomes less benign than a condition that is handled by some pills and some thumping on the chest would imply. CF is not merely a condition. But it is not overwhelming either. The presence of the disease is noted, but bounded. From now until the time when hospitalizations occur with greater frequency, and with little to no warning, the menacing presence of the disease is limited to the exacerbations requiring hospitalizations. One well brother, age ten, explained in terms similar to those of other well siblings,

> My sister was only sick when she had the pneumonia. Otherwise it's just the same.

In the household, as discussed in Chapter 11, after the first exacerbation, parents and siblings alike endeavor to contain the disease's intrusion into their lives. They once again approach the illness as one would a condition one does things for. They reestablish routines for care that emphasize doing things for the condition. They minimize the significance of the hospitalization in the child's life and in CF in general. Parents call attention to the child's extracurricular activities. They do not allow the ill child to participate in activities that would distinguish them from healthy children or call attention to their illness. Family activities resume to the same level as they were before the exacerbation. After the hospitalization, talk about CF is once again limited to what happened at an outpatient visit. The exacerbation takes on the character of an isolated event, not a portent. After all, the ill child looks the same and is involved in the same activities as before the first major exacerbation.

Series of Discrete Episodes of Acute Sickness and Recovery

Well siblings realize that CF does not go away—regardless of what one does for it. As ten-year-old Heather Farrington put it, "It stays your whole life." In the early periods, however, it is not always there out front. It comes out when the child is sick (e.g., at the time of exacerbation or acute illness) and then retreats. It is always there underneath, coming out when the child is sick, but limited to those times. In short, CF manifests itself as a series of discrete episodes of sickness and recovery. Holly Farrington, a twelve-year-old, explained,

> If he doesn't have a cold or anything, it's really like he doesn't have it. But if he gets a cold, it's pretty bad. He coughs a lot.
> Now he has a cold, but I don't think it's real bad. It's just a small cold.
> Mostly it's like he's a normal kid. If he doesn't have a cold or anything, then it's like it's not there.

Well siblings of children who have had episodes of acute sickness before the first major exacerbation requiring hospitalization view CF as a series of discrete episodes of acute sickness and recovery earlier than the well siblings of children whose first exacerbation was the first episode of sickness and recovery. For the latter children the view of CF as a series of discrete episodes of sickness and recovery comes with succeeding exacerbations and acute illnesses. However, in both cases this view of CF changes when the child becomes sick more frequently without warning.

Until the hospitalizations begin to increase and complications develop, well siblings do not list CF as one of their ill sibling's primary characteristics. In their descriptions of their ill brothers and sisters they acknowledge that they have CF, but they do not give it more weight than other characteristics. For example, in describing his brother with CF, one sixteen-year-old said,

He's normal, but he has cystic fibrosis. He's an average bright kid.

Like their parents, at this point siblings tend to see the ways the child with CF is more like other children, rather than the ways that mark him as different. As discussed in Chapter 11, even in the face of "tune-ups" and hospitalizations for exacerbations, parents encourage the child with CF to do what other children do and to minimize the differences between their ill and healthy children.

Questions About Cure, Course of the Disease, Control, and the Efficacy of Treatment

Limits are difficult to maintain when exacerbations increase to the point of requiring intensive therapy and more frequent hospitalizations. The view of CF, as a disease present only when the child with CF is sick, becomes increasingly untenable when the affected child begins to become sick more frequently and, without warning, require unscheduled hospitalizations. CF begins to assume a more ubiquitous quality and talk of it in episodic terms is less in evidence.

With ever-increasing hospitalizations CF becomes a more prominent feature of daily life. Like their parents, well siblings try to routinize episodes of sickness. In describing her brother Jason's condition over the past year Regan Chase, age eleven, reflected on her own reactions.

He's been sick a lot this year. He's been sick a lot, really. But I kind of get used to him being sick. And now I just think of it as, "Well, he's gonna be out a whole week; I might as well stop by the teacher and tell him and get his [Jason's] stuff." So now, I kind of don't really worry a lot, because I am kind of pretty much used to it and stuff.

At this time cure and control of the disease are major issues for the well siblings. While well siblings continue to hope for a cure and to see adherence to therapy and medicine regimens as important for the ill child's well being, they have questions. The questions occur most commonly when the child has an exacerbation or when the well sibling is in contact with other children with CF or in connection with CF fund-raising activities. For example, Louise Chase, age twelve, mentioned that episodes of sickness and bikeathons were the times when she started thinking about CF and her brother's condition. As Louise spoke she wondered aloud about the possibility of cure. That issue raised, her remarks turned to the issue of the prognosis.

> "I think about it at the bikeathon [Cystic Fibrosis Foundation fund-raiser] or when he's sick. I think if they're ever going to find a cure for it or not, 'cause we were raising money to find a cure. And a couple of months ago my mom told me they found what causes it or something about it.
>
> "I heard that they don't live to be . . ." Louise didn't finish that sentence. She started anew. "Like if I live to be a hundred, they'll probably live to be seventy or fifty or something like that. They don't live as long as we do. They get not like real sick. Like he's still talking and bossing me around and I'm just thinking he's a pain.
>
> "Well, I don't think he's gonna die right now or soon or something, but in around forty or thirty. But by the time he gets older, the medicines will be better, so then he'll live longer."

While thoughts and questions about the prognosis emerge at this time, well siblings distance themselves from the eventuality.

> There's a lot of people that put some bad stuff in peoples' heads. They have it that you're going to die and stuff like that. But I'd rather her just think that she's going to be OK all her life. I'd rather think that too—which I know she will be. She'll outlive me. I know that. I don't have no fear because I know she'll pull through anything. She's tough. She's pulled through several times. Now if she would have been a wimpy chick then she would have probably been a lot worse off. I think. I'm serious. She'll stay in the hospital for the least days she has to and she'll make herself better. She's not one to stay in. No way. Neither am I. [Well brother, age twenty-one, referring to his own convalescence after an accident].

Like their parents, well siblings focus on the potential for cure, the possible improvements in treatment, the positive aspects of the ill child's condition. They talk about how much the ill child does and can do to stabilize his/her condition and keep it from deteriorating.[8] As two well siblings from two different families explained,

> It matters how good you take care of it. If he treats himself good, or if he doesn't. Like if he takes his medicines and his PTs [chest physical therapy]. He doesn't have it as severe as other people might. I don't know. Like my mom was

---

[8] As the disease progresses well siblings drop adherence to the treatment regimen as a necessary criterion for longevity.

saying, some people could die at the age of ten or twelve, and he could live to be fifty-five or sixty [well brother, age sixteen].

Every night you [a person with CF] have to get on this machine. And it's because you get all this mucus in your lungs and it's hard to breathe. And when you get sick, you really get sick. And after you get on the machine you have to get clapped [chest physical therapy]. You get that two times a day, in the morning and in the night. And when you're sick you get it three times a day, sometimes four. And he [brother with CF] wheezes. Whenever he wheezes that means he really needs his machine [nebulizer treatment]. And you have to kind of take real good care of yourself. You can't really ever smoke or be around smoke or anything, because then your lungs get real clogged up. And, well, you get allergy shots every, I think, month; it might be every two weeks, I'm not sure. And you take a lot of pills. For every meal you have to take some pills. And in the morning you have to take a lot. And sometimes you die at an early age. But I don't think that will happen to Jason [Regan Chase, age eleven].

It is important to bear in mind that well siblings are trying to work out answers to questions of cure, control, and course of the disease in a context in which parents are trying to present what is happening to the ill child as within the realm of normal. Though they have expanded the realm of normal to include illness of a sort (see Chapter 11), the emphasis in their presentation remains on how much the ill child is like other children. Similarly, the well sibling tries to eschew differences in their presentations, despite their questions. A consideration of the following statement by Louise Chase, age twelve, along with the statement she made above, illustrates the juxtaposition of questions and reiteration of normalcy by well siblings of children who have had a number of exacerbations but no complications.

"If Jason were here [in this room] you could never guess in a million years that he has it, because he is always yelling or something or doing something. If he had something else that's more serious, I would worry about that a lot. But he seems pretty healthy to me.

"Once in a while he'll get real sick, because I mean he gets real sick sometimes, real sick. But I don't worry. Not really.

"Once after I read this book, called. . . . I can't remember what it's called. It was about the Capallettis. They lived near here, but they moved away. When this kid Joey [a child] got real sick [with leukemia], he had chicken pox and he was sick all these five months and he got real sick . . ." Louise didn't finish, she hurried on. "And after I finished reading that book Jason got real sick and I thought, 'Ooh, maybe he could die.' And I said, 'No.' Because I knew he was going to get over it or something like that. He was like over it in a week and back to himself. So I don't worry anymore.

"He's like a regular kid to me. He's like regular. I don't think of him as anything else but a brother. It's normal. And I don't think of him as cystic fibrosis. But I think of him as a brother. I don't know. It's just everyday stuff. Even if he didn't have it, I would think around the same.

"We treat him the same as any other person. But if he was just a regular person, who couldn't run super fast, then we would not let him slide. When we're playing kickball or something like that we know he can't run as fast. He can run fast, but he's not strong. So we let him slide sometimes, because he's cute, smiling."

Chronic, Progressive, Incurable Disease that Shortens the Life Span

As the disease progresses and further complications appear, well siblings notice changes in the ill sibling's condition. Like their parents, they are concerned about the use of oxygen, the development of Burkholderia cepacia (a difficult-to-control infection that is thought by some to be a poor prognostic indicator) as well as the more frequent hospitalizations and complex home care. They notice how hard their parents work to meet their ill sibling's physical and psychological needs. Aaron Woodward, age twelve, discussed how both of his parents tried to help his sister Alyson with her weight and how his mother helped her with her fears about various procedures.

My dad tries to keep her going when she's losing weight. Like, he'll want to have a race. Or he tries to lose weight and she tries to gain weight. And that's what my mom does too. . .

My mom gets all frustrated sometimes when Alyson loses too much weight. She tries to keep a going type attitude at it and tries to keep Alyson happy so she does better. And she talks her through difficult situations and stuff like that.

They are aware not only of their parents' concern, but also of the toll that having an ill child takes on them.

She has no time to herself anyway. She's a twenty-four-hour, seven-day-a-week worker. Constantly working. Everything's on her mind. And then when the girls are in [hospitalized] it gets really hectic. She has to drive down to Philly on Sunday morning or Friday night—it's a four hour drive. The hardest thing's got to be driving to Philly and back and listening to the doctors—what they tell her about how the girls are doing. [Well brother, age nineteen]

Maintaining any sense of a normal life is difficult when parents are running back and forth to the hospital. Well siblings long for uneventful and less hurried times. They want to be like other families. They share their parents' enthusiasm for home IV therapy citing several of the same reasons. As one well sister, age thirteen, explained in terms not unlike her mother's six months later (see Chapter 11),

Home IV therapy is a lot of time and work but it's better than the hospital. There's a lot we have to do for my brother. He can't do everything because of the catheter in his arm. But I'm glad he's here [home] now, not in the hospital, because when he's in the hospital it breaks up the family. And when he's in the hospital Mom's barking orders: "Get this. We have to get to the hospital now." And it's a real mess in the house. I mean that because she is busy running down there and then she has to go over and weed in the garden. And then it's just no one's hardly home. It's horrible when he is in the hospital. We're separate. It's so hard. I don't like it when he's away. And really if he's in the hospital, because he is so far away, lots of times I don't go down there. I go down to see him once in a while, but there's things I have to do here, so I don't get to see him that much. I go down and see him at night, but it's not that much. It just really breaks into family life.

In the midst of these experiences it is increasingly difficult for well siblings to avoid the issue of the prognosis. Well siblings begin to see CF as a chronic, progressive, incurable disease that shortens the life span. As Tyler Foster, age nine, put it,

But I still get worried about Britt. I just know that with CF you could die from it. And you get all skinny. And your lungs fill up with mucus. And you can't breath. And you die.

Acknowledging a shortened life span or a terminal prognosis for persons with CF does not necessarily mean acknowledging that one's own sibling will die at an early age from CF. Well siblings do not necessarily internalize it as an outcome for their own brother or sister, at least not in the near future.

When questions about the prognosis first begin to arise (when the need for hospitalization increases) well siblings also distance themselves and their siblings from the eventuality of death. There is, however, an important difference between the way in which the prognosis is conceptualized when questions first emerge and the way that it is when complications appear. When the well siblings first entertain thoughts about the relationship between cure, course of the disease, control, efficacy of treatment, and prognosis; death is in the far distant future (see previous section). Estimates of the age of death are put well beyond the median age of survival for CF, and in some cases well beyond middle age, almost to a normal life expectancy. In the face of increased complications, however, death, while still nothing like imminent, moves closer.

There is also a subtle, yet important, difference in the way in which the prognosis is discussed when the issue first presents itself and now when complications begin to appear. The tone is far less optimistic. Well siblings' views are sprinkled with conditions and qualifiers, as in this remark by Aaron Woodward, age twelve.

It's one of the deadliest diseases. You are in the hospital a lot. Your chances of surviving are almost zero. That's a lot really scary.

The disease as a despised enemy to be fought, comes through in several of the children's descriptions of the disease. For example when Tyler Foster, age nine, dictated a story he said,

My sister has cystic fibrosis and I hate it. I wish there was a miracle; that they could have a medicine for cystic fibrosis.

In their eyes there is still room to do things. As another well brother, age nine, whose sister required oxygen during hospitalizations said,

There are still things they can do. I'd worry with the oxygen and all, but I know Andrea's a fighter.

Adherence to the prescribed course of chest physical therapy, however, is not necessarily linked to longevity as it was before complications began to develop (see preceding section). Non-adherence to the prescribed regimen does not necessarily mean that one will succumb to the disease in the near future. Many well siblings noted, like the well sister, cited below, that there were "non-compliant patients" that lived longer than "compliant patients" and vice versa.

Somebody could never take their medicine, neglect themselves and live into their thirties, like Toby. She smokes two packs of cigarettes a day, has diabetes. And then other people live by the book and take their treatments three and four times a day, stay out of drafts and everything else, and they die at five. It's highly variable. You try to figure out in your head what the future holds, but you never know. [Well sister, age twenty]

At this point well siblings are well aware of their sibling's difference from healthy peers. They note the trouble that the ill child has keeping up.

All his friends are running around the backyard. He gets so tired and starts coughing. Even when you tell him a joke, he'll sit there and laugh and laugh until he gets to the point where he is choking himself. And you feel so bad. He can't even enjoy a joke without coughing and being uncomfortable and that bothers me. I hate that, when he can't run with his friends. My brother doesn't like to see that he's not keeping up. [Well sister, age eighteen]

Well siblings would rather not see CF as chronic, progressive, incurable disease that significantly shortens the life span; or at the very least not be reminded of the fact. As one well brother, age nineteen, explained,

My mom always asks me how come I never go down to the hospital to see them [his siblings who have CF]. I don't want to go to the hospital. I don't want to go down there and see them in the hospital. Not the fact that I don't want to go see them; it's just that I know what's going to happen. You know it's inevitable. You know the progression of the disease will get worse. That's inevitable.

For well siblings hospitalization is as potent a reminder of the disease and its consequences as it is for the parents.

One's Own Sibling Will Die from Cystic Fibrosis

As the deterioration becomes more marked, with the ill sibling more oxygen-dependent, activities more restricted, and thought given to more invasive procedures (e.g., surgical insertion of intravenous catheters for administration of medication), well siblings find it increasingly difficult to separate the disease and its sequelae from what will happen to "my brother" or "my sister."

> She acts like she's gonna grow old some day, and have a real nice car and stuff. [Pause] It would be nice, but sounds impossible. Everybody never makes it (pause) that far. All of her friends die. She thinks that maybe she'll beat it. I don't, but it's hard to say. Maybe she'll beat it. [Well brother, age eleven].

It is not long before many well siblings come to see CF as a chronic, progressive, incurable disease that will claim their sibling's life in the near future.[9]

In coming to this perspective, a quality of hopelessness begins to permeate the well siblings' statements about CF and their ill sibling's condition. Gone is the subjunctive (e.g., "could die"), and the use of qualifiers (e.g., "chances of surviving are *almost* zero"). Well siblings express their views of CF and the ill sibling's condition in short declarative statements.

> I know they're not going to find a cure. With the lungs filling up you die. [Well brother, age nine]

> She'll never be OK. She's got cystic fibrosis. She'll never be OK. There's no cure for her. [Well brother, age eight]

Acceptance of the imminence of death comes in the terminal phases of the illness. Like their parents, well siblings find that, as death nears, they are unable to think about much of anything else. Several sisters reported crying a great deal. Other siblings spoke of not being able to concentrate at school or at work. Recall that when Casey went home to die his brothers did not want to go to school. When Gavin finally did get to school, his teacher spoke to him about not thinking so much about his brother when he was there.

---

[9] Well siblings' views on just how close to death their ill siblings are may vary from months to years.

2. FORMATION OF WELL SIBLINGS' VIEWS

In this chapter I have presented the well siblings' views of CF and their ill sibling's condition over the course of the illness. I have concentrated on the formation of their views in relation to two significant aspects of their lived experience: (1) their parents' responses to the care the ill child requires and the concerns the child's condition engenders; and (2) their ill sibling's condition and illness-related experiences. Factors such as gender, the family's socioeconomic status, and parents' marital status have not been included in the discussion, since they were not determining factors. Similarly, while I have noted the children's ages, I have not discussed that factor in the presentation of views. In my analysis I did not find age to be a primary factor in well siblings' views of the disease or their own sibling's condition. For example, the statements of the well siblings revealed nine-year-olds who viewed CF as a chronic, progressive, incurable disease that shortens the life span and who were concerned about their sibling's condition; fourteen-year-olds who saw CF as a condition one does things for and saw their sibling as essentially normal; and twenty-four-year-olds who knew that one could die from CF, but did not internalize that their own sibling was dying until hours before the death (see Chapter 13). None of the views presented were unique to any one age group. For example, those who saw CF as series of discrete episodes of acute sickness and recovery ranged in age from nine to seventeen.

Also important is that while the presented model of well siblings' views of CF and the ill child's condition suggests an orderly progression, with each view being gradually replaced or superseded by the next, this is *not* an essential feature of the model. As illustrated by the two cases discussed below, a well sibling does not first have to view CF as a condition one does things for in order to view it later as a chronic, progressive, and incurable disease that shortens the life span. Nor is the well sibling limited to only one view at a time. Other factors (e.g., contact with other children in advanced stages of CF, seeing the movie *Alex*, the death of another sibling, discussions with parents or ill siblings about the disease) can alter the progression.[10] It is noteworthy, however, that while these factors can affect the progression, they do not change how the well sibling's view is formed. The well siblings' views remain bound to their lived experience, not age, developmental level, socioeconomic status, and the like. The lived experience continues to be of paramount importance in the formation of the well sibling's view of CF and their sibling's condition.

Fern Hopkins, age twelve, viewed her sister Ivy more like a well sibling of a child with advanced disease than a well sibling of a child with mild disease and no hospitalizations.

---

[10] For further discussion about parent and sibling communication see Chapter 13.

She's going to die. I know that she has a problem with her lungs and I know that they're filling up with like fluid or something and that maybe in later years (pause). I know that they're not going to find a cure hardly, because I don't think there's any way that they can cure that, with the lungs.

In this particular case, while Ivy had mild disease and had never been hospitalized, she was not looking well and coughed a great deal, even with therapy. Fern noted that,

Usually she's coughing a lot. And she'll cough and then she'll stop and then she'll (makes sound of swallowed cough) and she'll cough some more. But she coughs a lot even when she does have her therapy. It's not like it's continuous coughing, but she will cough through the day and you can hear that there is mucus in there.

Further, Fern's parents' responses were more like those of parents of children with advanced disease than like those of parents with children who were relatively well. For example, unlike the parents of children with mild disease, these parents were heavily involved in CF activities, talked to the well sibling and each other frequently about the ill child's condition and the fatal prognosis—responses usually seen only in parents of children with more advanced disease. In addition, because of the father's occupation, this well sibling was often confronted with the terminal outcome of CF.

Tad Campbell, age sixteen, was three years old when his eighteen-month-old sister, Ariel, died of CF. Another sister, Zoe, born several years later, also has CF. I interviewed Tad three years after Zoe's one and only post-diagnosis hospitalization. Her condition was quite good and the parents did almost no therapy. As you will recall from the account in Chapter 5, Mr. and Mrs. Campbell encouraged active participation in athletic activities. While they had had contact with other parents of children with CF when Zoe was diagnosed, they no longer did. They did not talk about Zoe's condition. Their behavior was like that of other parents of children who had had only one major exacerbation requiring hospitalization. Nothing that would raise the specter of CF's progression or the prognosis was discussed. They did not talk about the deceased child's death. In fact, the only person that Tad had spoken to about Ariel's death had been his grandmother.

Tad had two views of CF and Zoe's condition. One was like that of well siblings with a brother or sister who has had at most one exacerbation and is doing well.

It doesn't show, the disease, so it's nothing really. It's not a part of her. We wouldn't think of it. I don't think of it when I think of her. She's really normal.

His other view was like that of well siblings of children who already have suffered some of the complications of CF and are reluctant to apply their knowledge of it to their own sibling.

"I just think of it," the smile fading from Tad's face, "as a condition that some-times gets too out of hand, and it drains the body. Because one of the people I knew in Alabama [where the family was living when Zoe was diagnosed] was very thin, and that's only because not much of the food got to the body itself. I know that some people have lived until thirty-five. They're really healthy. And, I don't really think about Zoe dying early. But she says, 'I'm going to be this when I grow up.' And I always think about it. Just for an instant, though. I don't give it. I thought about when she would die. I don't want to think about it. It's not what I plan to do either.

"I think about maybe pancrease and that the kids can grow up—some can, some can't—and that my sister has it."

While Tad had thought about the possibility of Zoe's dying, he was reluctant to incorporate that eventuality into his view of her. Like other well siblings with such a view, he qualified his statements about the prognosis, refrained from generalizing to all children with CF, especially to his own sister. And when his thoughts did turn to her, he quickly refocused to what could be done.

The well siblings' views of CF and their ill siblings' condition play a signifi-cant role in their relationships with their parents and well siblings. In Chap-ter 13 I consider the role of their views in the ways in which they deal with their parents and ill siblings on issues of central concern to all of them.

CHAPTER 13

Well Siblings' Relationships with Parents and Ill Siblings

When a child is diagnosed with cystic fibrosis (CF) a new element is introduced into family relationships. In this chapter I look at the place of CF in the well sibling–parent relationship and in the well sibling–ill sibling relationship. Two issues dominate discussions of well sibling–parent and well sibling–ill sibling relationships: (1) the allocation of material and non-material resources; and (2) communication about CF and the ill child's condition. I selected these two issues because of their centrality to both relationships. I found that the most common topic when parents spoke about their relationships with their well children, and when well children spoke about their relationships with their parents, was the allocation of resources, particularly the resource of time in the form of attention.[1] Moreover, running through discussions about the allocation of resources was the issue of the course of the disease and the ill child's condition. In describing their relationships with their ill sibling, well siblings often noted the presence or absence of differences in how their parents treated each of them—what each received in time, attention, goods, and services—and whether these differences were related to the ill child's condition. At such times they often revealed how they felt about their ill sibling, the concerns that they had about their condition, and how much of this they shared with their sibling, and their ill sibling with them.

The ways in which the well siblings handle the issues of the allocation of resources and communication about CF and the ill child's condition reflect a keen awareness of the place of the illness in family life. Specifically, well siblings understand what they can expect from their parents and siblings, as well as what they must do, given the circumstances in which they find themselves. In the first section I discuss the issues of the allocation of resources and communication about CF and the ill sibling's condition over the course of the illness. I show how well siblings' approaches are linked to their parents' responses to the care the ill child requires and to the concerns the child's condition engenders (discussed in Chapter 11) and to their own

---

[1] Many researchers and clinicians have mentioned the prevalence of the themes of differential treatment and lack of attention in their interviews with well siblings of children with cystic fibrosis and other chronic life-threatening illnesses (cf. Chesler, Allswede, and Barbarin 1991: 238).

views of CF and their ill siblings' condition (discussed in Chapter 12). In the second section I consider what the well siblings' behavior (as presented and observed) suggests about their position in the family and their feelings about their position. I also discuss well siblings' rights, privileges, duties, and responsibilities from their own viewpoint and from that of others.

1. RESOURCES AND COMMUNICATION

Period I: Diagnosis Through to the First Annual Examination

The issues of the distribution of resources and communication about CF and the ill child's condition are present in bold relief as soon as the diagnosis is made. Parents immediately turn their full attention to the ill child, who becomes the focus of their time and energy. For many well siblings this is the first time that their needs and desires are second to anyone's, let alone to a child who, in their parents' minds at this point, is dying (see Chapter 11). Their parents' attention is elsewhere and continues to be, even after the child comes home from the hospital. One mother commented,

> I remember with my two girls [well daughters], you're so concerned with the sick one you forget about the others.

And yet as Kupst (1986: 174) found in her study of well siblings of children with cancer, "this is the time when they [well siblings] are fearful and their needs for attention are high."

The majority of children with CF are hospitalized at the time of diagnosis, leaving well siblings separated from their mothers, often for the first time in their lives. Many are cared for by relatives and friends, some in their own homes, others outside the home. They may see their mothers only briefly, if at all, during the sibling's initial hospitalization. Several weeks can elapse before the well sibling(s) see their sibling, who often is a newborn diagnosed shortly after birth and transferred directly to a CF center. As one mother described her six-year-old well daughter's reaction to her brother's initial hospitalization,

> When Devin was in the hospital, my mom couldn't find Sylvie. And here she was in our bedroom, and, like, our bed was here and the crib was there. And Sylvie was sitting on our bed, holding Devin's blanket, and crying. And my mom said, "Well, what's wrong?" And she said, "I just want my Mommy and my brother to come home." And then she asked why Devin couldn't come home. So she has had a rough time, but she was aware of everything that was going on.

Some well siblings (those five years or older at the time of diagnosis) recalled the experience. Said one ten-year-old well brother, five years old when his sister was diagnosed,

I didn't get to see her much [when she was diagnosed]; only about once a week I would see her, because we weren't allowed in there [in her room in the hospital] much.

And then we waited. I was sitting there doing nothing. I would stay out in this waiting room and the nurses would make me hot chocolate. And I would have a Popsicle they would give me. Or I would bring my cars to race. When other kids came I would play with them and my cars.

And then when I did have a chance to see her, I was happy to see her.

Well siblings are concerned about their newly diagnosed brothers and sisters, as is evident in this father's account of his experience telling his five-year-old well son about his sister's illness.[2]

When it got to telling him, we had got this little comic book from St. Christopher's Hospital.[3] He was just starting to read. Now he couldn't put any of those words together, but he sounds his words out. He's very slow about reading, but he's positive. And I sat down with him while his mother was up to the hospital with Abby [child with CF] after I brought that home.

Now we brought a pack of them [comic books] home to take to school to the kids and explain to them that Abby is not going to kill them if she comes back to school. But anyway we went through the book and I read it. Of course he likes comic books and he thought it would be fun with that.

And I told him how serious it was and explained to him everything that was explained in there, in the little comics.

And that's when it really hit him that she was not going to get better right away. He didn't think she was ever going to come home at the time. And until she did come home, he didn't think she would ever come home.

Some well siblings express their concern quite directly, others more indirectly.[4] But whether it is through constant questioning about when the child will come home, or by a look, or a gesture, or through tears, parents grasp the well siblings' concerns.

When we didn't come home with her; he [Darrell] cried, and that just struck me. I didn't think he really understood what was going on but I guess he did. And he really cried.

---

[2] This conversation took place while the child's sister was in the hospital, where she had remained since her diagnosis. While the parents had told their son the diagnosis, this was the first in-depth conversation either parent had had with the child. The age given is the age at the time the statement was made. Since the study was conducted over a two-year period, more than one age may be given for a particular individual, reflecting the different times of the interviews.

[3] The comic book focuses on care and treatment. There is no mention of death, or suggestion of a progressive course.

[4] Chesler, Allswede, and Barbarin (1991: 19) found "constant worry about their ill brother or sister" to be a "major theme" in their study of the well siblings of children with cancer.

You can tell there is emotion there. He gets very upset. I often wonder what they think of when I'm doing the treatments. Darrell has never asked us. We've tried to explain to him as we do it. [Mrs. Daley]

Some well siblings try to comfort their ill sibling in the hospital. One two-year-old well sister, whose parents thought "she didn't understand what was going on," brought her cherished bear, "the one she could not sleep without," to the hospital when she came to see her brother, Jan. She left it with him after the visit. Her mother described the scene,

> Funny thing about Diedre is that she brought her brown bear. Her two favorite toys are Cookie Monster and Popple [the brown bear]. Well at the time she used to sleep with that bear. Cookie Monster and Popple were Christmas presents. So this was in October, and the bear was her favorite toy. And like I said, I didn't come home [from the hospital], just once in a while. I would stay up there, and he [husband] would bring the kids [well sisters] up on weekends.
>
> Anyway, when she left, she left the bear with Jan. And I said, "No, Diedre. Take him home." Because I thought for sure that she would pitch a fit once she got home. Well she didn't. She wanted her bear to stay with him.
>
> I just think that was her way giving something to him that was special.

Well siblings are also concerned about their parents, and often try to comfort them as well.

> Even when he was only two, when Carl was diagnosed, we told Stuart, because he needed to know. Well, all I could do was cry. I would say for the first two weeks that's all I did. And Stuart kept telling me, "I'm sorry Mommy." [Mrs. Reynolds]

Well siblings observe much, with little to no comment from adults. As discussed in Chapter 12, at the time of diagnosis and for several months thereafter well siblings view CF as a serious illness. It is a view formed more through observation of others' behavior, especially that of their parents, than from direct communication, of which there is little.

Recall, when the child is diagnosed parents give well siblings only the most rudimentary information about the disease and their ill sibling's condition. Notably absent is any mention of the genetic component of the disease, its course and prognosis. Parents give a variety of reasons for their decision. Most commonly cited is the well sibling's age. Parents feel that the well sibling is too young to understand much more than the basic facts (e.g., the cough is not contagious, there are treatment and medication requirements). They vow to tell more when the children are older.[5] One mother, speaking of her three-year-old well daughter, said,

---

[5] Some keep this vow only to find, by their account, that the children seem to have forgotten what they had been told. One father said, "They forget everything when you tell them. It's like teaching them about sex. You lay the whole thing out and a few months later, the same questions come up again. It's like anything that doesn't make itself clear and the experience is such, they just have questions about it again."

We told her he has CF, but she doesn't know what that is. We don't tell her he is sick; just that he has something he has to live with and that's why Daddy goes out to smoke. She reminds him not to smoke around him. And she reminds us about his enzymes. And sometimes she pats him and says, "PT [chest physical therapy], Mommy." We will tell her more when she gets older.

In addition to age, many parents feel that there is no need to tell well siblings much beyond the requirements for care as their sibling is "not sick" (i.e., acutely ill, coughing, in pain). As one father explained,

I could see [telling more] if he [child with CF] was going in the hospital a lot, stuff like that. But he's not. He doesn't cough. And he gets these things that are almost everyday things, everyday things for her, so she [well sister, age seven] doesn't think he's being sick.

For still other parents it is not simply the well children's ages or even the ill sibling's relatively good condition that limits what they tell them. The child just does not ask, and hence they see no reason to discuss the illness in any general or particular way (e.g., care or treatment requirements).,

Maya [well sister, age six] doesn't ask. All she knows is we tell her to ask every night in her prayers to make her brother well. [Mother]

For the child who asks, information is given. As one father comparing his two daughters, ages two and six, explained,

One time I was in the car and Avrie asked me, "Why does Devin take enzymes?" And I told her that he takes them because he has a prob— [father did not complete the word]. It helps him get his food.

And she said, "Why?"

I said because Devin has a problem and this helps him get his food so he can get strong.

She said, "Well, why?"

And I said, "Well he has something that will make him—" I don't know exactly how I put it, but "he'll get weak and he can get sick if we don't take care of him."

And then she said, "Well did I have to do that when I was a baby?"

And I said, "No. It's that Devin has this problem that you didn't have."

Then she just went, "Oh." And it was the end of it. But it's hard, especially with a two-year-old, to really explain to them at their level of understanding.

Now I think with Sylvie I could have even said the name of the disease by now and explained it a little bit more thoroughly and she would understand, but she hasn't asked, so why say?

In some cases, parents claim that they limit what they tell well siblings for fear the child might misunderstand or tell other people, who might then treat the child with CF differently from other children. One mother speaking of her well daughter, age seven, explained,

I was afraid to give her the name of the disease, because if she went to school or even to the kids in the neighborhood and said it, and have them say, "Oh No! Tara's brother has cystic fibrosis." And then maybe that kid would overhear her parents talking to someone else and say, "Oh, you know there's no cure for that." And that kid will come back and say to my daughter, "Your brother's going to die," or whatever.

I just worry about that. And that's why I really didn't want to give her the name.

And then if they saw *Alex* they might tell her things. And Dusty is not that sick.

In still other cases it may be, as Meyerowitz and Kaplan (1967: 260) have suggested in their study of parents whose children have cancer, that parents limit what they say because they find it stressful to have the sibling know, to have it out there in no uncertain terms.

In the months following diagnosis parents find allocating their time amongst all of their children particularly vexing. As one mother reported, three months after her infant's diagnosis,

I'm feeling manipulated by Eli [infant] and not as close with Philip [well son, age nine]. I don't have the time with him anymore. And yet he is very understanding of Eli's need for extra attention.

Another mother spoke of "not going out with" her two daughters, ages five and eight. Her statement of "I used to go out and be on the go all the time" was echoed by many parents. There is just so much to think about, so much to do (see Chapter 11).

Parents worry about the time that they will need to spend with the ill child, often to the exclusion of the healthy child. Several parents of newly diagnosed children felt that not being able to give the well sibling as much attention as they needed might be the cause of many of the problems they had heard or read that many well siblings have. Several parents whose children with CF were now experiencing some of the complications of CF traced their well children's difficulties in school back to the time of diagnosis when the well child was, as many said, "lost in the shuffle," "ignored," "slid aside," or "overlooked."

Parents felt that, regardless of whether or not the well children show it, they must feel "left out."

The girls [well sisters, ages four and six when brother diagnosed] were pretty young. I guess it kind of upset them, because we were so busy with him; trying to get him organized, and worrying about him. So they probably felt left out. They had to feel left out during that time. [Mother]

Parents pointed out the various ways that the well children would try to get their attention: from feigning illness and asking for medication, to interrupting physiotherapy, to engaging in generally disruptive behavior. Parents handled these bids for attention in various ways. One mother, whose three-year-old well daughter asked her for medicine, gave the child fluoride; another gave her five-year-old well daughter vitamins; and another took her three-year-old well son, who complained of headaches, to the clinic "to see what his brother went through." Interruptions during therapy were handled directly and in much the same way as Mr. and Mrs. Reynolds had done. Recall,

> If Stuart got demanding while Carl was getting his therapy I just said, "Whoa, you can't do this. You'll have your time when we're done."

Thinking that disruptive behavior was rooted in jealousy over the time spent in care of the ill child, several parents tried to involve the well child in the care. As one mother explained,

> When Hilary came home from the hospital [after she was diagnosed] I think it went to a jealousy kind of thing. They [Hilary, age nine, and Rudy, well brother, age six] went through a jealous period, because we were spending four hours a day just on therapy. Every time she eats a piece of fruit or even takes a candy bar you're asking, "Did you take your pills? Do you need pills?" It seemed like every turn you made was headed in Hilary's direction.
>
> So then we had some trouble, so to speak, with Rudy. He became impish. He got into things. And I think we realized that he needed some attention. So that's when we started to involve him in PT. We'd say, "Rudy, go start Hilary's PT for her, while I'm doing dinner." He saw it as not something that we were giving him, an order or more attention, but as he was just involved on his own.
>
> And we were surprised that he knew how. But evidently from watching he knew.
>
> And of course we had a time. "Well don't do that." Or, "Don't slap too hard." Or "Watch the cupping." Then it was like a shared kind of thing.

Some parents even hoped that involving the well children in therapy might not only stave off jealousy, but also bring the siblings closer than might otherwise be expected. At this time the majority of well siblings are too young to be able to do much more than just watch the chest physical therapy and the administration of enzymes and various oral and inhaled medications.[6]

---

[6] Interestingly, while the parents in this study often raised the issue of jealousy, the parents in Burton's (1974: 199) study in Ireland did not. She found that "very few [parents] regarded the well child's jealousy as a real problem to them," at any point in the illness. In contrast, I found that parents raised the issue at the time of diagnosis and continued to over the course of the illness. At the time of diagnosis, parents commented on whether or not they thought it would

Very few of the well siblings recalled feeling jealous. Perhaps this was because they were too young at the time of diagnosis to recall much of what happened in any specific way. Or it could be that now, given their ill siblings' condition, it would be difficult for them to voice these feelings.[7]

Some parents tried to handle the well siblings' bids for attention by finding time when they could give the well children their undivided attention. One mother would have her husband look after the ill child when he came home from work, leaving her free to play with the well child. Another took her well son out one afternoon a week during the two months her other child was hospitalized. Others asked grandparents and other relatives and friends to look after the ill child during naptime so that they could go out with the well children.

Even with these efforts parents did not feel terribly sanguine about what they were doing. Recall Mrs. Foster's comments about how she treated her son Tyler, only a baby himself when his sister, Britt, was diagnosed.

> I gypped him of a lot of holding, handling, holding, loving. And I really feel bad about that now. All I can remember him as a baby is I would just stick the bottle in his mouth. I wouldn't even hold him to feed him. And I wonder if that somehow didn't affect him."

Parents see more than simply the limitations of time and attention as making their well children's lives difficult.[8] Some are concerned about the impact that their own preoccupation with the ill child might have on the well sibling. Recall in Chapter 11, as parents begin the process of the compartmentalization of information they are at first focused on the prognosis and the course of the disease. Not until well into the first year following the diagnosis do they push this information to the back of their minds. Parents describe themselves as feeling "tense," "pressured," "anxious," and then as several put it, "losing it" with their well children. One mother explained,

> Milt [husband] and I get anxious about Felicia. Something happens with Felicia and it all falls apart. Like yesterday when Felicia threw up all over Milt. We just lost it with the kids [well children].

Several parents reported that it "did not take much to set them off." Their feelings are close to the surface.

> The thing is, like in the morning when I know I have to do the treatments, I can feel myself get, not nasty with the kids, but impatient, like "No Genna, I can't

---

develop, considered how they would handle it if it arose, and asked professionals and other parents whether in fact it could be avoided or alleviated given the circumstances.

[7] The well siblings' reluctance to speak of being jealous or wanting more attention is discussed later in this chapter.

[8] Also noted by Angst (1992: 91) in her study of parents of children with cystic fibrosis.

read you a book right now." You know, where I used to say [before son was diagnosed], "All right, I'll read it to you in half an hour." I can feel myself like that. [Mother]

Several parents also expressed concern about the responsibilities that the well siblings would incur as a result of having a sibling with a chronic, life-threatening illness; responsibilities that children without an ill sibling just would not have. They wondered if these added responsibilities would not make life harder for them than it is for children without such siblings. As Mr. and Mrs. Daley, point out,

> "I think both of them are going to have to make an adjustment. I mean they're going to be in a different situation from most kids, knowing they have a sister with a chronic illness."
>
> "Yeah," agreed Mrs. Daley. "Sticking up for their sister if anybody ever teases her or something."
>
> "Well I guess that's the way. I mean, once they begin to understand she has a serious illness. I guess there's got to be a social adjustment there."

Additionally, unlike other children the well siblings will have to witness things that are difficult for anyone to witness. Parents are concerned about what it will be like for their well children when their child with CF becomes ill, is hospitalized, or undergoes daily chest physical therapy and nebulizer treatments.

> "But taking enzymes all the time and getting sick, getting this treatment done and their sister getting clapped, getting PT. I think that should be hard to see." [Mr. Daley]

Some parents feel the need to keep the children separated, afraid that the child will "catch something, a cold, and get sick," and are concerned about the impact that their decision to keep them separated will have on the siblings' relationship, as well as on the siblings themselves.

Despite the distance created for fear of contagion, the added responsibilities and the loss of attention, parents are convinced that the well siblings care very deeply about their ill sibling. Parents speak of the spontaneous kisses and pats the well siblings give to their ill sibling, the proclamations of love, and even the ways in which the well siblings yield to the ill in disputes. One father in describing the way in which two well sisters, ages seven and three, and their younger brother with CF get along noted,

> Carla's really good with him. Her and Nora sometimes get into little battles. But when it comes to Derrick she always seems to just kind of back down and let him have his way. Nora does too. Nora sticks up for herself. And if anybody

ever wants anything, forget it. It's mine and it's tough. But when it comes to him, she's pretty good too.

The actions that the parents described were observed at home as well as at clinic. For example, several well siblings would let the physician examine them first (e.g., listen to lungs, look down their throats and into their ears and nose) if the ill child was at all hesitant. One mother commented to the doctor,

> Polly [well sister] used to swallow empty capsules for Hannah [child with CF] so she could see how to do it.

Well siblings expressed their desire to help care for their siblings through reminders to their parents to give the enzymes, by mixing the enzymes in applesauce and feeding them to their siblings, as well as by their willingness to entertain their siblings during physical therapy, or at the very least not interfere or bother their parents at this time. One six-year-old well sister described such an occasion, which her parents later said occurred "rather often."

> Last night I went over and fed him some of his enzymes. I was sitting next to Mommy. Mommy was going to go do something and she asked me if I wanted to feed Colby, and I did. I picked up the spoon and got him out as much applesauce [mixed with enzymes] as I could get on there. And then I fed him. If some fell I did what Mommy did. I scooped it up and put it back in.

Period II: Months and Years Following the First Annual Examination, When the Child Is Relatively Healthy, Through to the First Major Exacerbation Requiring Hospitalization

During this period well siblings continue to demonstrate their care and concern about their ill siblings. If ill siblings are old enough to take the enzymes on their own, well siblings will sometimes remind them to do it. If the ill child is not old enough to take them without assistance, well siblings will often remind the parents. Many well siblings continue to keep ill siblings occupied during therapy. Recall ten-year-old Heather Farrington's statement,

> He doesn't like the machine because he doesn't have anything to do. But now me and my sister play with him when he's on the machine. We play cards with him.
>
> We just go there and play with him. We made that up so that Cody won't scream and holler. He would scream and holler. He just doesn't like it [the machine with the mask]. He was bored when he had it on. He was just sitting there watching TV so we started playing with him.

At the very least, over the years as the child continues to do relatively well, well siblings no longer interrupt these sessions. Eventually therapy ceases to be a time when well siblings try to enlist their parents' attention. Well siblings recognize that the time parents take for therapy is not time taken away from them, but rather time that must be given to the ill sibling out of necessity.

> We're treated the same, except Pru has to have more time for her therapy and things like that. Otherwise we both get the same amount of time with our parents. [Well sister, age twelve]

Interestingly, some well siblings see therapy as, in part, what draws the mother and ill sibling "closer" to one another than to other members of the family. One well sister, age twelve, in describing who in the family she was closest to, said,

> Probably my sister [sibling with CF]. We're close. We're best friends. And I know that if I'd ever, if something would happen in school that I would never have a friend who I could really trust; I know I could always trust Serena.
>
> But Serena's closest to my mom because she and my mom do therapy together. And she's usually, well she gets home from school before I do. I don't know what they do before I get home, but I think maybe they do a lot of things together. But I think [in terms of who Serena feels closest to] it would maybe be between Mom and me.

While well siblings no longer make their bids for attention during daily at-home therapy sessions, they still sometimes do on clinic days and at the clinic. For example, one eight-year-old well sister interrupted her mother's conversation with the doctor in the waiting room with plaints of, "Look at my arm," pointing to a scratch. Her mother turned to her and said, "Honey, let me talk, this is important. I know your elbow's important too, but I'll deal with it later."

With each succeeding month of relative good health the illness moves further into the background of everyday life. Recall thirteen-year-old Liam Sherman's remarks,

> Most of the time I forget she has it because the things become quite routine. So, we're having therapy in the morning. It's like, I don't even think about it anymore. It's just sort of normal. I don't look at her as having it at all. I just forget about it.

The illness is not forgotten, but it is not the focus either. As discussed in Chapter 11, when the child is doing relatively well parents act to mute and contain the intrusion. They want "to keep things the way they are." Talk could disturb that delicate balance. For the parents discussing the illness among themselves or with the well sibling raises issues that they would prefer not to think about (see Chapter 11). Hence, talk at home is minimal.[9]

Well siblings report few conversations with their parents about the illness, beyond what treatments and medications are required. "We don't talk about it much," was a common refrain. The few illness-related discussions well siblings (and in some cases parents) did recall dealt with reminders not to be around children with colds or flus, and certainly not to bring anyone home to play who might be ill or harboring an infection (an admonition that continues throughout the course of the illness).

They do not report talking to their parents about what it is like to have a brother or sister with cystic fibrosis. As one ten-year-old well brother described the parameters of discussion,

> I ask them about the lungs and all, her treatments, what she has to do, because I have to know about it. But I don't tell them what I think about it, the sad feelings. She has it. It's not good to have.

When asked, "Who do you talk to about CF and your sister's condition?" he responded,

> Myself. I think about it in my head. I don't talk to nobody about it.

Even though well siblings may want to engage in further conversation they are reluctant to do so. Some sense their parents' unwillingness to pursue discussion.[10] Not uncommon are remarks like "I don't think they [the parents of this nine-year-old well brother] want to talk about it."

Some parents feel, however, that it is the well siblings' silence that thwarts discussion. They point out that the well siblings do not "say much or ask much about it." Believing that if the well siblings wanted to know they would ask, parents do not open conversation. Recall Mr. and Mrs. Sherman's remarks,

> "Liam likes to be cool about it. He doesn't want you to tell him things about it. He doesn't want to know. Most of the time he really doesn't need to know anything bad about it, but he might after her future."
>
> Mr. Sherman agreed. "He's quite quiet about it. I think he'd probably just as soon have it all go away. I don't mean just for jealousy, but because it is a painful thing for him. So I think, judging from the way he deals with some other things, he's working out of a 'if you don't talk about it, it'll go away' kind of concept."

Parents also continue to cite the well sibling's age and the ill sibling's good health as reasons for not telling the well sibling more about CF and their

---

[9] Kupst (1986: 181), in her study of families of children with cancer, found that "the longer the remission progressed the more families tended to think and talk less about leukemia."

[10] Other reasons for the well siblings' reluctance to discuss the illness and their siblings' condition with their parents are suggested in the second section of this chapter.

siblings' condition. Echoing many, one mother of a fourteen-year-old well child and a twelve-year-old child with CF, said,

> We don't discuss it much. She hasn't been that sick, so there is no sense in telling her [the well sibling] much at this point.

And still other parents introduce the notion of undue worry for the well sibling and fear that their questions will not end.

> I think when the time comes, when he's [well brother, age seven] eight or nine and he can understand more and reasonings why, and also be able to see that there's hope in the future, and so forth and so on, he'll understand it and accept it a little better and I'll tell him more. Right now, if I said, "Haley [age four] has cystic fibrosis and he's probably going to die," Cliffie would be flipped out. He would, he would go into, he would question me about it all the time then. "But why is he going to die?" "But Mommy—. . ." you know.
>
> I tried explaining the other night why we wanted them to hit a home run so that everybody had to pay five dollars to Cystic Fibrosis [Foundation] and he couldn't understand. "But why do we want to give them money?" I said, "Well, if we give them money then the doctors can find a way to make Haley better." And he just didn't quite, didn't quite fathom that.
>
> He [Cliffie] understands he [Haley] has mucus and that if he has a cold he can't go near Haley because we don't want Haley to get the cold. 'Cause Haley can get more, you know, sick than he can. And then Haley would have to go in the hospital and get special medicine. But other than that—see, Haley's been so healthy—.
>
> And there hasn't really been a need to answer too many questions. And there's only so much that they're going to understand 'cause they're so little. [Mother]

Several parents were also concerned that talk about the illness could lead to problems in the siblings' relationships with one another. Recall Mrs. Sherman's discussion of her reluctance to talk to her thirteen-year-old son about his sister's condition,

> I don't want CF to be something big between them. Because he doesn't need to be worrying about her or feeling sorry for her. He has to be what he would be anyway for her.

As a reason for not telling the well sibling very much beyond the requirements for care, a few parents raised the issue of the well sibling giving the ill sibling information that they would rather the child not have.

> I would never tell Ross [well brother, age eight] and not Jordan [child with CF, age five], because Ross would relay it to Jordan, I'm sure. And then you get a lot lost in the translation and it would be worse. [Mother]

While parents may not discuss the illness, they feel that the well sibling will learn about it. They continue to be concerned about how the well sibling might find out, and they vow to tell eventually.

> Eventually they're going to read it, or they're going to . . . Their curiosity. There's libraries, there's TV programs. And they're going to eventually find out, and I don't want them to come to me and say "Mommy, why didn't you tell me?" They're going to hear it from somebody else—a kid at school's—"Oh, I had a cousin that died of that." You never know.
>
> When I think when the time is right and they're old enough to understand, I'll tell them. [Mother of son with CF, age four, and well son, age seven]

Well siblings do not report talking about CF, their ill sibling's condition, or their feelings about it with their ill siblings either. And the ill siblings do not report talking to the well. While at this point lack of discussion about the illness has no impact on their relationship, it does in later periods of the illness [see discussion in Period IV and the second section of this chapter].

At the same time that conversation about the illness declines, so too does differential treatment among the children. After the first annual examination, when the child is doing relatively well, parents also strive to redress the balance between the attention that the well child and the child with CF receive. As discussed in Chapter 11, they try to respond to the needs and desires of the ill child and the healthy ones equally. Recall that in the main the parents report treating their children in the same way, except when the child with CF is sick or has a clinic appointment. They act on the ill child's difference from other children only in those settings where the difference cannot be overlooked. In the daily course of events, without acute illness or visits to the clinic, parents treat the child with CF as they would their other well children, and they present the child as such. They emphasize the activities that the child with CF participates in that are like other children's. They talk about all of their children in terms of a future that includes career, job, perhaps college, and marriage.

Like their parents, the well siblings treat and talk about their ill sibling as if he or she is like any other child (see Chapter 12). The well siblings do not give in on fights, as they had at the time of diagnosis. As one well brother, age sixteen, put it,

> She's just like everybody else, except she takes some pills when she eats.

Well siblings feel that parents should require the same of their sibling with CF as they do of them and are not, as their parents note, shy about telling them so.

> The other evening, she [well sibling, age thirteen] says, "I'm carrying out all the garbage bags for my allowance, and Nita's [child with CF, age eleven] not carrying them. You should make her for her allowance." I said, "Well Camy, the bags

are larger than Nita." So then we try to find something for Nita to do like clearing the table or something that's a little easier [for Nita to do for her allowance]. [Mother]

Parents often report that the well siblings admonish them if they feel that the ill child is getting something more or his or her needs are being placed before theirs. One mother recalled how, once the child with CF started to do well, his older brother, then nine, would say things like,

Since he's come along, it's like we don't even exist.

This mother added that such phrases "never crossed his lips when Vene was diagnosed."

Although the potential for jealousy and resentment between the siblings is a concern for parents at the time of diagnosis (and, as we will see again, later in the illness), it is not a concern when the child is doing relatively well. Parents do not see the illness or the way in which they deal with the siblings as an issue in the sibling relationship. And the well siblings do not report it as such either.[11]

Well siblings describe their relationships with their ill siblings as "friendly," "fun," "close." They speak of "playing together," "going places together," "doing stuff together." The easy give and take in the sibling relationship is reflected in the remarks of this seven-year-old well sister.

I tease her, she teases me. I jump on her, she jumps on me. I pull her hair, she pulls my hair. We race. We play hide and go seek. We wrestle. And I sleep in her room sometimes. Sometimes we get in trouble with our dad for that.

Their descriptions of their relationship sounds like those of many siblings who do not have ill siblings. As one twelve-year-old well sister noted,

We are close. I mean we have an occasional fight once in a while, but it's nothing like we go around saying, "I hate you," and things like that. And, you know, we might make jokes about each other. We may call each other a name every now and then, but we're usually real nice to each other. We're usually on the friendly side.

The ill siblings corroborate these reports. As the ten-year-old sister of the twelve-year-old quoted above put it,

Sometimes we fight, but not a whole lot. We play together and sometimes we do homework together. And then sometimes we sleep together.

Parents' descriptions of the siblings' relationships for the most part matched the siblings' descriptions, with one notable exception. Several par-

---

[11] Possible explanations for the well siblings' omission of direct statements of jealousy are discussed in Section 2.

ents added to their descriptions of the siblings' relationships a comment on how "protective" the well sibling is of the ill sibling. For example, in describing the relationship between her nine-year-old well daughter, and her seven-year-old child with CF, one mother noted,

> She [well daughter] treats her [child with CF] very normal. She doesn't feel sorry for her or anything. But she's protective of her. If they're out in the neighborhood if anyone would get rough with Emmy, Madeline would jump right in and say, "Don't bother her." She doesn't want anybody hitting her or anything like that.

Some parents attributed this protective quality directly to the illness. One mother said of her five-year-old well son's actions towards his ill eight-year-old brother,

> I think he protects his big brother a little bit. And I think that will come out more and more over the years; as he realizes what he's doing. Ira [well brother] just thinks the world of Neal. And he knows something, because I think he knows something's different. I mean you can't help it what with the therapy [chest physical therapy] and all.

Other parents simply commented on the protective quality without reference to the illness. One mother said, in describing the relationship between her well son, age five, and her child with CF, age three,

> They're *very* close. They always want to sleep together, every night.
> Luke's very protective of Trevor [child with CF]. And I don't know if that's because he's his younger brother or what.
> He finds a lot of humor in Trevor. I'll hear Luke laughing hysterically and he'll say "Mom, come see what Trevor's doing!"
> Trevor likes to follow after Luke and pretend exactly what Luke's doing. He gets frustrated when he can't keep up or he can't do something the same. "But I want to do what Luke's doing!" "I want to go to school like Luke!"
> But yet Luke will. Luke lets him. Luke taught him how to make friends in the neighborhood and what not. He's a good teacher.

Many parents see the well siblings' protection of their ill sibling, coupled with the ways in which they deal with the requirements of care (discussed in the beginning of this subsection), as evidence of the well siblings' continued concern for their ill sibling, concern that at the time of diagnosis was demonstrated by kisses, pats, proclamations of love, and yielding in disputes.

> He's [well brother, age eight] so concerned about her. Like last night. It was really nice yesterday afternoon, and then just before dark, we had had dinner, it got cold out. And they [well brother and older sister with CF, age twelve] went out and sat on top an old junk car out here and the wind came up. And I could see it was blowing in her face. Well I knew she wasn't going to be able to get her

breath if she didn't soon come in, so I called out for her first time and then her mother did. She went to the door and called out for her. And Orin said, "Ava, we better go in."

He knows now that we know when she's had enough and she needs to come in. And I've seen him stop her in the summer jumping rope here on the back step. She'll jump rope just to prove to us how many jumps she can make before she's completely out of wind. [Father]

While the well siblings may not mention "protection" in their descriptions of their relationships with their ill siblings, they often voice protective sentiments in their discussions of the care and treatment their sibling requires.

But I know that if anybody else is ever sick I'm not allowed to go around that person because I don't want to bring it home. And if I get it, I know she'll probably get it, and I don't want to have that. I don't want to take that chance. [Well sister, age twelve]

As the child with CF continues to do well there is little reason for well siblings to change their views or approach. The well siblings receive no information that would lead them to think or act in any way other than as having a sibling who has a condition that can be managed. There are no notable changes in their parents' behavior or their siblings' condition. Their parents treat them evenhandedly. Their ill sibling does what other children do—extracurricular activities, sports programs, etc. Well siblings see little difference between themselves and their siblings with CF, "except a few pills when they eat, and some therapy in the morning." As the well siblings tell it, CF is not a factor in how they conduct their relationships with their ill siblings. Recall Liam Sherman's [age thirteen] depiction of life with a sister with CF,

Having a sister with CF is just normal. I think I just act about normally, like anybody that has a sister who's a brat. But that's the way it is with all sisters. I made sure. I talked with my friends. They all have brat sisters. She's OK. She's fine. I don't look at her any differently. I don't think anybody does. No. Not at all. Except for that hour she has to have therapy and stuff and aerosol. It's nothing more than that and taking pills.

The first exacerbation poses a threat to the well siblings' approach to the conduct of their relationships with their parents and the ill sibling. During the first hospitalization well siblings become concerned about their sibling as well as about family life. Some even worry if they might be the cause of the problem necessitating hospitalization.[12] In retelling what it was like when his

---

[12] Burton (1975: 195) in her study of families of children with CF noted that well siblings' "feelings of responsibility and worry escalated when the child [with CF] was unwell or hospitalized."

sister Zoe was hospitalized for her first and only exacerbation, ten-year-old
Jeremy Campbell remarked,

> She was in the hospital for pneumonia. She had pneumonia. I gave it to her. I
> knew it because I had it before she did and she just got it. Sometimes I think it's
> my fault and it bothers me.

They vividly remember their first visit to the hospital. One nine-year-old
well brother said two years after his sister's first hospitalization,

> I remember I came in the room and she was in this bed and she had all these
> cards around her from school and everything. The class made cards for her. She
> got lots of cards.

During the first hospitalization daily life as they had come to know it over
the months and years of relative health ceases. The daily order, as discussed
in Chapter 11, is disturbed. They note the link between the change in their
sibling's condition and family life. As Adam Campbell [age ten] explained
when he recalled his sister's first hospitalization,

> "One time she was sick. She had something wrong with her—I forget what
> it's called, but she had to come to the hospital for about a couple of weeks. It
> was frightening, but she came out, so—I was glad. That she doesn't get hurt a
> lot or anything. Like she might get like sicker and die or something because."
> Adam stopped for a moment, the word "because" holding his place.
> "We were like, 'Where's Zoe?' 'She's at the hospital.' And then my mom and
> dad went there in the morning. I went to see her one time when she was in the
> hospital. And it was weird because she wasn't here [home]. When she got back
> everyone was happy and everything."

Period III: Recovery from the First Major Exacerbation, When the CF Is Relatively Stable, Through to the Time When Hospitalizations Begin to Increase and Lose Their Predictability

The well siblings do not discuss with their parents or ill sibling their feelings
about the exacerbation or the illness at the time of the first exacerbation or in
the period of recovery and relative good health that follows. The pattern of
communication remains the same as it was during the period of relative
health, following the first annual examination. There is little conversation
about CF-related matters beyond necessary care and treatment.

Parents attribute the lack of dialogue to the same factors that they had
before the first exacerbation. They still report that the well siblings do not
probe about CF and pledge to tell them more when they get older. The fear
of being asked "millions of questions" is reiterated. As the time without inci-

dent increases, parents again cite the child's relative health as a reason not to pursue further discussion.

The ill siblings do not recall speaking to their well siblings about CF or their condition. They think that the well siblings may speak to their parents.

As discussed in Chapter 11, after the recovery from the first exacerbation parents again act to contain the intrusion CF makes into their lives. They want things to be as they were before the exacerbation. There is a real desire to "hold on to what you've got." Parents again try to define the situation as within the realm of normal.

With recovery from the first exacerbation there is renewed emphasis on the ways in which the child with CF is like other children. Parents continue to claim that they make the same demands of all of their children, making exceptions for the child with CF only when he or she is sick, much as any parent would, whether they had a well child or a child with a chronic illness. "All parents make exceptions when their children are ill."

The well siblings' behavior reflects this principle. They only yield in disputes when their sibling is sick. Recall ten-year-old Heather Farrington's remark,

> When he gets sick I don't yell at him. I don't get mad at him. If he does something I get mad, but I don't say anything to him.

This is not so different from the parent who makes exceptions when the child is ill; otherwise, the ill child is treated in the same way as the well child.

Ill siblings agree. They claim to see no differences in the way that their parents and their well siblings treat them that could be attributed to the illness. Such differences as do occur are related to factors that arise in families that have only healthy children—gender and age, for example.

> My mom treats me a little different, but I'm a girl and they [well siblings] are boys. [Girl with CF, age eleven]

In short, life at home returns to what it was before the first exacerbation. Well siblings have the same expectations of their sibling, and once again conduct their relationships with their ill siblings as they had before the first major exacerbation. As in the period before the exacerbation parents' descriptions continue to contain the elements of protection (whatever the reason—illness, age, or gender) and concern. As the mother of three children, two well older daughters, ages nine and eleven, and one son with CF, age six, put it,

> Oh, they get along good. They take care of Buddy. Like if I'm not here they give him his enzymes and stuff. They're close. And they get along good.
>
> I guess I'd say that Doreen's closer to Buddy, but Tina and Buddy play together better. I guess because they are closer in age. But Doreen takes good care

of him. If I'm not here or something she gives him his enzymes and dresses him. And when he was little, littler, she used to give him a bath, stuff like that; like a big sister. That's why I'd say they were closer. But him and Tina, they can play together better because they're closer in age.

Well siblings do not change the way that they relate to their parents, either. Well siblings clearly voice their demands for the same degree of attention and special privileges the ill child receives. Recall the scene in the clinic waiting room when Zoe's brothers wanted something to eat.

> "I'm hungry," Jeremy announced.
> "Me too," echoed Adam.
> "Can we get something to eat? Please?" pleaded Jeremy.
> "Not right now," their mother replied.
> "When then?" the boys asked in chorus.
> "When Zoe's finished."
> "When will that be?"
> "When she's been examined."
> "But that's a long time.
> "It won't be long, she's in getting weighed."
> "Please can we go?" Adam begged.
> "No. We'll wait 'til Zoe's been examined."
> "Can we go by ourselves?" Jeremy offered.
> "We'll come right back," Adam assured.
> "No!"
> "If Zoe wanted something to eat you'd get it for her right away."
> "Yeah. You'd let her eat."

Mrs. Campbell did not respond. She continued to look straight ahead, her expression unchanged, while the boys pouted in their chairs and waited for Zoe to return.

According to parents, if the well siblings feel that there is a difference in the way that they and their ill sibling are being treated they say so. Recall Mrs. Farrington's discussion of her well daughters Holly and Heather's behavior in this regard,

> "But the girls, they don't say that we spoil Cody [age seven] because of the CF. They say it's because he's the youngest. That's what they say. I don't know. Maybe the older one [age thirteen] might think that it's because of the CF. I don't think the younger one [age ten] thinks that. She's still young yet.
> "Holly just thinks we let him get away with too much. She'll say, 'You can't just let him get away with everything because he's sick.' And then I'll say, 'Well that's easy for you to say.' And she says she understands, 'but you can't have the kid turn into a monster.'" Mrs. Farrington laughed.
> "I tell her something could happen to him," explained Mrs. Farrington, her

voice becoming increasingly somber. "And she knows that." Mrs. Farrington nodded. "And then I just say something could happen to him and we would feel bad or something.

"The youngest one doesn't ever say anything like the older one. It's just the older one that says, 'Well, you can't let him get away with everything because he's sick.' I just ignore her. It doesn't make me not do it anymore. I still do it.

"Holly says those things when she gets mad. See if we tell him 'No,' not to do something, and if he goes ahead, if he keeps doing it, we don't just stand there and yell at him, and say, 'Don't, don't, don't!' And she doesn't like that. But I think that even in a normal family, the youngest one is likely to be spoiled. But with Cody it's just even tougher."

While well siblings may feel that the differential treatment the ill sibling receives is related to the disease, in most instances they try to attribute it to something other than the disease, to something that would differentiate children in a family with no ill children. To explain differences the well sibling might say of the child with CF, "He's the youngest," or "She's the only girl," attributes that are within the realm of the normal and ordinary. Well siblings raise the issue of CF only as a last resort, when they feel that there is no other way to get what they want.

Both parents and well siblings present the illness as a series of discrete episodes of acute sickness and recovery. After each exacerbation or tune-up attempts are again made to return to everyday life as it was before the first exacerbation, or at least to where it was before the last exacerbation. One area in which this becomes increasingly difficult for parents is around the issue of attention and differential treatment. With more hospitalizations there are more occasions when the needs of the ill child are placed before those of the well, when the children are treated differently. This is especially the case during hospitalizations themselves. One mother pointing to the scar on her older well son's neck said,

> That's another thing I feel guilty about. When Edmund was in the hospital Judd got lymphitis. His stepfather was not responsible about getting him to a good doctor, and I wasn't paying attention. It got bad and required surgery that led to this scar. It's one of those things, Edmund became the focus.

As parents themselves point out, the child with CF is the center not only of their own attention, but also other family members'. Recall Mrs. Reynolds's comments about Carl's episode of acute sickness and hospitalizations,

> Because times when Carl's sick, all the phone calls are, "How's Carl?" Everybody who sees Stuart, "How's your brother doing?" And all the presents. Carl gets all the presents. It has to have some kind of effect on him [Stuart]. Like the last time Carl was in the hospital, my mother-in-law dropped off a box of toys, presents to bring down to Carl.

Balancing the needs of the well and ill children during periods of acute sickness and hospitalizations is difficult, but parents do try.

About five years ago the disease got a better hold. They [daughters with CF, then ages eleven and thirteen] started to be hospitalized more often. The boys [her well children, ages ten and fourteen] got shipped to my mother's. And then as they got older, left alone. I went down [to the hospital] on my one free day, on Sundays, to the girls. They needed me at that point for encouragement to get better. And yet realizing that the boys were suffering because even though they weren't home, even though the kids went out to play, or like now there's softball games or something like that; I wasn't there. I was with the sisters. [Mother]

In the face of increasing hospitalizations and more frequent episodes of acute sickness concern about the impact that the illness will have on the well children returns. Parents begin to entertain the possibility that while the well child does not say anything directly, the attention the ill child receives during this time (in and out of hospital) bothers them. Recall Mr. and Mrs. Reynolds's comments,

"So I think because we're so aware and in tune with what Carl's things are like," Mrs. Reynolds continued, "Stuart feels, 'Nobody cares what my poop looks like.' Or these other important things."
"He never talks about it, but the way he acts, you can tell it bothers him. You can tell something eats at him.

One area that is of particular concern to parents, even when the child is not sick or hospitalized, is the ill child's special dietary needs. Children with cystic fibrosis often have difficulty gaining and maintaining their weight. Nutritionists often recommend dietary supplements (e.g., Sustecal) and special food preparations (e.g., adding Polycose to cooking) to increase caloric intake. Parents try to explain these "special needs" to their well children.

I worry that Lucky [age sixteen] resents my buying yogurt for Jay [age twelve], but as I've told him, there's just not enough money for him to have it too. And Jay needs to keep weight on. [Mother]

While some well siblings claim not to notice any differences in the way that their parents treat them and their ill siblings, others do, but say that they "understand" and "do not mind." Recall the various comments Regan and Louise Chase [ages eleven and twelve] made about the difference between the ways in which their parents treated them and Jason, their nine-year-old brother with CF.

"My mom would usually take his side on some things because he's a little younger. But if she saw the real [what happened] if she really knew it was not my fault, if she was there, or even if she wasn't there, but she couldn't figure out how it would be my fault and she would see that it was my brother's; then she would treat us kind of both the same.

"I really don't mind. I used to mind when I was little, not really little but like in third grade. My brother would come home and eat all the stuff. I'd say, 'How come he gets to eat more then I do?' Because he gets to eat all this good stuff, like pudding and stuff. And I'd say, 'I want some.' But now I don't. I don't really mind."

Louise would say of her brother's extra eating and special food, "My brother always has to eat more then usual. He can't go without dinner. He has to eat a lot. My mom always buys him these special puddings or something and he has to eat them He has to gain weight a lot. . . .

"Sometimes my parents have to spend more money on him, because I remember something. When I asked for a raise in my allowance or for clothing or something my mom said that once they would have had a lot more money, if my brother didn't have it [CF]. If my brother didn't have it, we would have a lot more money. But I don't care, because I have a lot of stuff.

Yet during hospitalizations as well as in clinic some well siblings (including several who claimed not to notice any difference in the way that their parents treated them as well as some who claimed not to be bothered by the difference in treatment) would often open conversation about their own physical ills—an action many might interpret as a bid for attention (Lask and Fosson 1989). For example, immediately after Wade (nine-year-old with CF) was examined and found to have nasal polyps which bore watching, his five-year-old well brother, Siggy, jumped up on the examining table and declared, "I'm sick like Wade. Look at my nose." His mother responded, "You're not sick. Get down off there." The doctor continued the physical examination. After listening to Wade's chest she said, "I hear some crackles I haven't heard before." As Wade and Siggy's mother got up to listen, Siggy said to the doctor, "I'm like Wade." The doctor replied, "When's your birthday?" Wade whispered into his brother Siggy's ear. Siggy said, "June seventh. Can you look in my ears?" The doctor replied, "I think we have a lot of people here today." "But I'm the sickest of them all," Siggy retorted. Siggy continued in this same vein in the pulmonary function lab with the laboratory technician. "Could you try me on the little one [pulmonary function machine] today." "No not today," said the technician. "Maybe next time," Wade and Siggy's mother added. "Well I have crud in my nose," Siggy pleaded. "Yeah, you have crud in your nose," his mother repeated sarcastically. Siggy murmured to the technician, "Are we allowed to take this [nose clip] home?" "Sure."

Parents interpret the well sibling's expression of physical illness as a means to get attention. Recall Mrs. Reynolds's description of her seven-year-old well son Stuart's behavior,

And when Stuart is sick, when he has a cold, maybe he needs to do the mist, maybe he needs the vaporizer. He stresses for some attention when he just has a little cold. So I try to make a bigger thing out of a little cold for him. I maybe let him stay home an extra day, if he acts like he has a cold.

Sometimes he likes to create sickness and hurts—"Oh my leg hurts"—because he gets attention for that. He's already walked with crutches. People would say, "Oh Stuart what happened to you?" Or he'd wrap his leg with an ace bandage because then people would say, "What happened to your leg?" And that was real important to him.

Parents feel that the well siblings' desire to be sick is an indication of how the differences in the way they are treated bother them. As Mrs. Chase said of her own well daughters, quoted above,

> "Whatever the girls may say," Mrs. Chase would remark, "I think they think he gets special things or that he's treated more special. They just think of him as being more special. They'll say things like, 'Oh he's lucky, I wish I had CF.' I'm there, 'Oh no you don't.' But people say things like. . . ." Mrs. Chase didn't finish. She picked up with a specific example. "Louise had this thing last year where she said she wanted to break her arm or leg so that she could stay out of school, and then she would get lots of presents.

Yet not one well sibling ever made an outright statement stating that he/she was "jealous".[13] And only one child with CF stated outright that he thought his well siblings were "jealous of the attention" he got.

As among the well siblings, some ill siblings did not report any differences between the way in which they and their well sibling were treated and some did. As one adolescent with CF who did not perceive a difference, at least in terms of everyday life, when not sick, put it,

> Not really. Sometimes, maybe when I'm sick and stuff, but otherwise she [mother] bitches at me just like she bitches with them [well siblings]. I don't listen, either. I bitch back at her.

One nine-year-old with CF who did perceive a difference said,

> My mom does treat me a little bit more special, but she still loves them [well siblings] the same way she loves me. It's just that she gives me more things that would help me. Like she gives me more food. She gives me more hugs and lets me do more things. Sometimes I don't think it's fair to my little brother [age five] that I get more food than he does or I get more attention then he does. But he does get a lot of attention. Anytime my Mom tickles me, he goes "Nobody can tickle me. Nobody can tickle me." And then my mom goes over and tickles him.

Whatever their perceptions of the ways in which their parents treated them, this was not an issue that the siblings discussed with one another. In fact, only one well sibling, Louise Chase [age twelve], recalled the subject even coming up between herself and her brother with CF [age nine]. She recounted,

---

[13] This is not to say of course that the well siblings did not feel jealous.

"Once in a while we'll be standing there and say, 'I'm special.' And Jason goes, 'Nah uh. I'm more specialer.' I go, 'Why?' And he goes because I have . . .' He goes, 'You're not special.' And I go, 'Yes I am.' He goes, 'I'm a special kid.' I go, 'You are not.' He goes, 'Yes I am.' I said, 'Why?' He goes, 'Because I have CF.'

"He thinks it's some kind of. . ." Louise didn't finish. "I don't know. He knows about it and he doesn't take it too seriously. And he thinks he's special.

Even in the face of further exacerbations talk about the disease and the child's condition continues to be infrequent. And this is the time, as discussed in Chapter 12, when the well sibling begins to have questions about the course of the disease as well as about the efficacy of treatment and cure. For answers they are left largely to their own devices. Some read, others rely on observations of their siblings and other children with CF. For the most part they receive little information from conversations with parents and ill siblings. Parents report that talk is, at best, infrequent. The difficult issues are not addressed. Recall Mrs. Reynolds's account of the conversation she had with her well son Stuart [age seven] when he asked if his brother with CF, Carl [age five], was going to die,

> One time Stuart asked me if Carl was going to die. One time, I'm trying to remember if it was when he was in the hospital one time or, I just don't remember. And I told him, "Yeah, someday." And I said, "So are you someday." So, we didn't discuss it. We didn't drum on it anymore because we don't dwell on that. You know it's reality, but we don't talk about it. So for Stuart it's just Carl has a disease that he takes enzymes for, and sometimes he gets sick, and sometimes he has to be in the hospital, but that's as far as it goes.

Mr and Mrs. Reynolds, like many parents at this time, do not think that the well sibling, to use their words, "understands that you can die from CF." More often than not, they base their conclusion on the well sibling's age, not what they have or have not told him, or on what the child may have picked up by himself. Statements like Mr. Reynolds's, "I think that at his age that's [referring to requirements for care and treatment] all he can understand," are not uncommon.

Despite whatever sense they have that the well sibling has questions and concerns, parents do not bring up the subject of the prognosis themselves. One mother noted that her well children, ages thirteen and fourteen, would often ask her about a young woman with CF whom they had met when their brother had been hospitalized. "I told them things, but I never told them that she died, though."

There are times when the answers to difficult questions cannot be so easily avoided, when a child puts forth concrete evidence of death from CF (e.g., news of another child's death, the movie *Alex*). At these times parents answer the question a bit more directly than the child's more general hypothetical,

"Can you die from CF?" or "What happens to people who have CF?" Parents, however, are quick to point out to the well sibling the differences between their own sibling's situation and the child who has died. Recall the way in which Mrs. Reynolds handled Stuart's questions about death and CF after he had heard children at school talking about the movie *Alex*, which he had not been permitted to see.

> "But," Mrs. Reynolds rejoined, "since the movie [*Alex*], Stuart has asked me if Carl is going to die. And from kids at school, I think some kids at school had watched the movie and then asked him. I don't know what he told them. He didn't tell me, and I only found out from the teacher because the teacher asked me if he watched it. I sent a note to her the day after the movie to say, 'He didn't watch it. Please don't talk about it.' And so she didn't, but she asked me then because she knew these other kids were talking about it.
>
> "I told him that people do die from having CF, but that Carl has been really healthy so far and that with all the new research and all the new medicines and everything that we just didn't think about that. But that yes, it is a possibility, and that's why sometimes he doesn't understand why I say, 'No, Carl can't go out to play in the mud puddles because it's raining.' And different things like that; because of catching colds and that sort of thing.
>
> "I try to use those times to explain to him why I make the choices that I make sometimes. And he seemed to accept that answer and he's never brought it up again.

Well siblings do not take their questions to their ill siblings, either. They "just don't talk about it." Some well siblings claim that their ill siblings do not want to talk about the illness with them. For example, to the question "Do you ever talk to your brother about CF?" one eleven-year-old well sister replied,

> No. I don't ask my brother. He'd yell at me. He'd go, "No stupid. I don't want to tell you, stupid." He goes on like that if he doesn't want to tell me something. He'll say, "Why should I tell you?" or "I don't feel like talking about it."

The ill siblings' reports are not any different from their well siblings'. They, too, claim that their well siblings do not speak to them about the illness beyond what they should do to take care of themselves. Some ill siblings add that they prefer it that way. A seventeen-year-old who was quite explicit in her views on the matter said of her well sister,

> She reads a lot of stuff and then she always asks me all kinds of questions. "Did you take your machine today?" "Did you take your pills today?" I don't like that. I just walk away and say, "Leave me alone."
>
> I don't want people nagging me about it, really. Because then it makes me not do it if they keep nagging me.
>
> She tells me if I don't do my stuff I'll get real sick and stuff like that. Then I just walk away from it because I don't want to hear it.

To this twenty-four-year-old well sister, however, her "nagging" is evidence of her concern,

> I wouldn't bring it up if I didn't care. Yeah I guess I nag her sometimes. But I get worried when she's not doing what she's supposed to.

Her twenty-one-year-old well brother feels the same, and is far more direct than I heard any other well sibling at this point in the illness,

> If she doesn't do something the doctors tell her [to do] I tell her; I say, "You're going to do it. If not, you're going to mess up your life. And you ain't going to mess up your life 'cause then you're going to mess up mine."
>
> I put it plain, blunt out. You do the machine and take your medicine and stuff.
>
> And she's just, "I don't want to hear it. I don't want to hear it," and walks away. But I said it.

Embedded in the well siblings' directives as well as in their questions is a real concern about the ill sibling. They demonstrate that concern in other ways as well. Seven-year-old Stuart Reynolds knew it was important for his brother to rest after meals and complied with his parents' request that he help by sitting with his brother after dinner, and not run around. As he himself said,

> After dinner Carl's supposed to sit down and rest a little. So I sit down with him and rest and in twenty minutes we're allowed to go play.

Some well siblings continue to be willing to keep the ill child occupied during chest physical therapy (PT), but requests to learn how to do it or to assist with it are far less frequent. The few who had tried it found it extremely difficult to do and did not want to go any further. Only one well brother (age sixteen) in the entire sample did therapy on any regular basis. The ill sibling had been hospitalized several times but had, as yet, shown no complications. His mother was divorced and worked long hours. He also gave his brother his night-time dose of antibiotics. He was responsible for one of the two therapies a day his brother received.

Well siblings also demonstrate their concern in a variety of ways during hospitalizations. Many made regular phone calls to the hospital. A nineteen-year-old well brother commented when describing his sister's most recent hospitalization,

> Every day I'd call her. I ran up a four-hundred-dollar phone bill. Ask her.[14] See, she was doing bad. And for a while she was in the hospital all the time. I just wanted to encourage her not to be afraid.

---

[14] I did ask his mother. She replied, "Oh, yes he did, indeed. I still owe [the phone company] a hundred fifty-seven dollars."

They also try to do things for the ill sibling. For example, Regan Chase (age eleven) made sure to get her brother Jason's homework when he was ill.

Ill siblings appreciate these gestures. As one eleven-year-old with CF said of her thirteen-year-old well brother,

> When I get sick he's very nice to me. Like when I was in the hospital, I said, "Niles, will you send mommy up with this book?" He goes, "Oh sure." He gives it to my mom, and sends up three more, instead of one. He treats me nice.

Despite more frequent hospitalizations and episodes of acute sickness, well siblings continue to consider their ill siblings as "regular playmates" and companions. They do not alter the way in which they deal with them, except as mentioned earlier, when they are ill. The second oldest in a family of four boys, the third of whom had CF, put it,

> I treat him [brother with CF] like a normal kid. (Pause) It gets passed down the line. I got smacked around and he's gonna get smacked around. And pretty soon our little brother's gonna get smacked around.

Ill siblings would agree. They do not think that their well siblings treat them any differently because of their CF. One ten-year-old with CF characterized the way her twelve-year-old brother treated her,

> He's like, this is just my sister. He doesn't treat me any different than if I had or didn't have it.

They, like their well siblings, report the rounds of bickering and arguing about household chores continue. One thirteen-year-old with CF said in describing his relationship with his seventeen-year-old well sister, with whom he shares a room,

> We fight about little things; like who is going to clean up and who is going to do the room. She says I'm messier, but I just tell her she is. And then I always dry and she always fights because she wants to dry, except when my mom dries and washes, sometimes.

They, too, continue to name their well sibling as a "regular playmate." In short, the well and ill siblings share a similar perspective on the well siblings' approach to their relationship.

Parents also continue to describe the well siblings as they had before the first major exacerbation and immediately thereafter. Again, to their descriptions of how they are like any other sibling pair, "usual number of fights, disagreements, disputes" they add "how protective the well siblings are." Recall Mrs. Reynolds's comments on the way that Stuart deals with Carl,

> Stuart's pretty protective of him. Different people have said that when they're out some place that he's protective as far as, "Did you take your enzymes, Carl?"

And when Carl coughs, Stuart sometimes kind of guards him and doesn't fuss over him and doesn't make any kind of explanation, but he's there.

Period IV: Development and Increase in Complications Through to the Discussion With the Physician that the Disease Has Advanced

As the disease progresses, many well siblings not only become more protective of the ill sibling, but also verbalize it.[15] Feelings of responsibility run quite deep; as remarks like twelve-year-old Aaron Woodward's indicate,

> It's like you are responsible for a lot of stuff. Like yelling at her or getting mad at her gets her real mad and makes her do worse. You wish you didn't do that.

Well siblings see protection of their ill sibling from the insults of others as one of their responsibilities. One eleven-year-old well sister explained,

> I know I have to watch out for my sister, especially at school. She gets teased about her cough. I tell kids they can't catch it.

Many well siblings keep a watchful eye on their sibling's daily activities. Many share their parents' concern about their sibling's weight. Recall how nine-year-old Tyler Foster regularly admonished his sister to eat, and how Aaron Woodward tried to think of ways to get his sister to eat.

> My mom usually comes up with the stuff to help gain weight and I add on to it. Like if I drink a Sustecal shake, she will. And stuff like that.

"Looking out for," "being responsible" or "protective" does not mean pitying. Well siblings caution against pity.

> I don't think they want pity at all. In fact, I think that they want the opposite. They don't go around telling anybody about their CF and stuff. [Well sister, age fifteen]

Ill siblings confirm their well siblings' appraisal. As one adolescent with CF said during hospitalization,

> I don't want them [well siblings] down here. No way. I'd say, "Go home." Not being mean; it's just like I don't like them seeing me sick. It's like then they give me all this pity, all the pity in the world. And I hate getting pity. I hate it more than anything. I hate it. It's like, "Don't pity me, whatever you do." I couldn't take that. I don't want to be pitied. I hate getting pity. I like to do stuff myself. Like when I'm here [in the hospital], it's like, "You want me to go get your coat? Want me to get your shoes?" "No. Chill out. Sit down."

---

[15] Kupst (1986: 174), in a study of well siblings of children with cancer, found that "some siblings channel their worry into a kind of protectiveness of the ill child, taking on a nursing role which gives them a sense of mastery in being able to do something for the patient."

At the same time, they know and openly state that their siblings "care about" them. One nine-year-old with CF said,

> He [eight-year-old well brother] knows that I'm sick sometimes and need special care.

Furthermore, they feel that their well siblings are aware of their limitations and are, in the words of several, "helpful."

This is not to say that the siblings do not have their share of arguments and fights. Interspersed with adjectives like "generous," "helpful," "caring," are comments like, "and sometimes we fight."

Well siblings claim that they make the same demands of their ill siblings that they would of any sibling and that they expect those demands to be met. One well sibling (age seventeen) jokingly said in comparing the way in which he treats his sister with CF (age sixteen) and his well brother (age fourteen),

> I treat her just like Arlin. We'll fight. We'll argue when we have to. No different. No leniency at all.
>
> And Beth and I have gotten into some really bad ones. I mean fisticuffs. We really hit each other. She lays a good punch too. She can hit hard.

Well siblings realize that this is not the case for the parents, whom they feel hold the ill sibling to a different standard because of the illness. One fifteen-year-old well brother said of his fourteen-year-old sister with CF,

> Everybody sorta like babies her. Whatever she wants she gets like that. I gotta wait a while.

They frequently remark on how their ill sibling uses CF to get out of school, or chores, or church. A thirteen-year-old well sister spoke about how her eleven-year-old brother would be able to miss church through protestations of not feeling well.

> Sometimes when Lester doesn't feel like doing something, he uses his disease. He uses it to get something from my mother. For a while he didn't feel like going to church on Sundays and he would come up with an excuse, "I don't feel well." That made Mom think that this might have something to do with Lester being sick, and so he wouldn't have to go to church. Finally Mom got smart and said, "Well I think you should go." But sometimes Lester uses his disease to an advantage, you know, and I kind of feel left out. I don't have one.

Some well siblings feel that the differences in treatment, attention, and privileges have led to the child with CF being spoiled and at times bad-tempered; as these two well siblings, ages twenty and twenty-four, suggest.

ALMA: Phoebe [age sixteen] is a spoiled—I'm serious now—she is spoiled, and she's got an attitude problem. But she's got a sense of humor, she does. You can joke with her. If she's not in a good mood, I mean forget it. Watch out.
ESTELLE: She's very moody.
ALMA: Yes, she is, oh my god. But when she's in a good mood, like we happened to catch her on a good night, she's all right. She's good, I mean sometimes she's really a brat.

Along with such criticism is also praise. Many of these siblings, like the two well sisters, ages fourteen and twelve, from two different families, quoted below, are quite specific. They extol their ill siblings' virtues with concrete examples,

Mom and Dad spend a lot of time with him. He's a super brother, and he's always sharing things with me. He never thinks of himself only [crying, she continues]. Like the other day Mom got him these pizzas. There's two pizzas that come in a box. And she told him I'm supposed to make both of them for him. He's supposed to eat a lot, you know. And he said, "You know, Trish, I can eat both of them, but I want to share them with you." I really don't think you can ask for a better brother.

Well, I wonder, you know, what's going to happen after my parents die, and then when my other family dies, and then Celia dies. I'll probably miss my parents and Celia most of my whole life, because Celia sort of, she brings my spirits up. Like if we're ever playing a game and we get mad at each other and we walk off, she'll come over to my room and she'll knock on my door and she'll say, "Natalie, I'm sorry," and give me a hug and it makes me feel good.

As discussed in Chapter 12, as complications begin to increase well siblings come to see CF as a chronic, progressive, incurable disease that shortens the life span. While at this point well siblings do not internalize the prognosis for their own sibling, each additional illness or exacerbation brings a renewed sense of fear and concern.

I get worried when she gets sick. Like when she had chicken pox, I was really worried about her. And I was. I sort of prayed every night that, you know, nothing happened and (pause). I get worried. And she is just sort of there, and you can tell that there's really something wrong. [Well sister, age twelve]

Well siblings do not readily enter into conversations with their parents about their concerns about their ill siblings' condition. One well eighteen-year-old brother summarized the feelings of many when he said with regard to not wanting to talk to his mother about his sister's condition:

We don't talk about it. I try to stay away from it, because I don't like to hear it. I already know for a fact what's going on. I know as much as I need to know. I don't care to hear any more about it. If they come up with a cure, that's great.

Then I won't have to worry about it all. But they haven't, so we don't talk about it.

Parents concur. Even when the child with CF is hospitalized conversations are limited to brief exchanges of the form "How is ———— doing?" In the main, details are not requested, and when they are, parents are surprised. About the only subject that sparks a more protracted conversation is discussion about news of advances in CF research and treatment.

> We talk more about the things that you hear on the news; technology breakthroughs, things like that. Those kinds of things come right up. [Well brother, age seventeen]

No more than well siblings tell their parents of their feelings about their ill siblings' condition do they discuss with them what they perceive to be a real difference between the way in which they and their ill sibling is treated. Unlike in times past they do not initiate conversations about the differences.

Parents, however, are as aware now as they were then. Recall the scene in the waiting room when Mrs. Foster expressed concern about the amount of attention nine-year-old Tyler received.

> Standing in the waiting room she said, "I want to give Tyler more attention. He needs it. He wants to show it, but he can't. He should. It's hard."
>
> Tyler, who had been playing nearby interrupted her conversation and asked, "It's hard for me, what? I should do what?"
>
> "You feel like more," Mrs. Foster called back. "You want some of the attention.
>
> "No. I don't want most of— I know Britt has CF and she needs all the attention."

Parents put forward several possible explanations for the well siblings' reluctance to speak with them about the issues related to the illness that concern them. This mother's comments encompassed the entire range of possible explanations parents presented,

> Maybe it's me; could be. I could seem not open and not realize it. I think the children feel as if, "Well, she goes to work and she's such a crab when she gets home; who wants to sit down and really talk to her?"
>
> Or maybe it's just something very private to them. Or maybe they don't want to sound out because it'll hurt me. Or maybe they don't want to face it. Or maybe they figure I can't face it.

While on one level well siblings do accept the situation, the acceptance is not without disappointment and conflict; as indicated by this ten-year-old well sister's remarks,

When he gets more I understand, but it still hurts. I get extra gifts too, but the gifts don't make up for the hurts and other things inside of me. You know, you may smile on the outside, but inside it hurts.[16]

Attributing differences in attention to the disease rather than to birth order or gender, as they did earlier in the disease process, does not necessarily make things easier for the well siblings. In fact, attributing differences in parental attention to the illness may lie at the root of the indirect and more destructive attention-getting behaviors that several researchers and clinicians have observed in some well siblings at this time (see Chapter 1). Unable, perhaps, to express demands directly because of what they know of the ill child's needs, they show their desire for attention in other ways. At this point in the illness some well brothers acted up in school, and a few others gained weight.[17]

Parents often recognize these behaviors as bids for attention. With ever-increasing hospitalizations and complications the issue of attention becomes more burdensome for parents. Recall Mrs. Foster's remarks concerning Tyler's grades,

And then I was so worried about her failing in school I brought her books every time I came to the hospital and studied with her. Report cards came out and she got all 90s. And Tyler, who usually does better than Britt, had an F. I just wasn't paying enough attention.

During hospitalizations they find it especially difficult to meet the needs of both the well and ill child, but they do try. One mother explained,

When he has to be hospitalized she [well sister, age fourteen] kind of gets put on the back burner. People are calling to ask about Owen [age twelve]. Everybody is Owen this and Owen that. And people are busy bringing things for him.

And she gets very jealous of the fact. So we found that we have to arrange for somebody else to go spend time with Owen so that I'd have an afternoon with her. We go for a bike ride or something, and it was just for that she was an important person too.

But she also had to accept the fact that Owen needed this attention more at the time because where he was at wasn't very pleasant; having to be away from home.

---

[16] Lindsay and MacCarthy (1974: 192) noted that "even older children may understand, but still feel the parents' concern for the sick child as a rejection of themselves. They may be resentful and angry that their needs are not being met and at the same time feeling guilty about having these needs and therefore deny their existence."

[17] Kupst (1986: 174) found that the well siblings "appear quite self-centered and uncaring, immersing themselves in their own interests and activities." She attributes this to "jealousy over attention, anger over the disruption in their lives and anxiety that they cannot dispel."

Some parents report that it is difficult to be sympathetic with their well children when they are sick. One mother said in the course of describing a conversation she had had with her ill daughter about her condition,

I once asked her [eleven-year-old with CF] when was the last time she didn't have any pains. She said, "I think one day last summer." She never has a day without some pain; what they go through.

Then when he's [twelve-year-old well brother] sick, I have no patience. I say to him, "What's your pain? Nothing. Now your sister, she has pain. How can you complain?"

I know I shouldn't say that, but I can't help it. I was talking to Mimi Reardon, Ethan's mother and she says the same thing. She doesn't have patience for normal kids.

And for some the differences in their sympathies and affinities come through in nonverbal gestures.

When we are watching TV I find myself going over to Glenna [nine-year-old with CF], sitting down next to her, and rubbing her back. And then I make up my mind that next time I'll go over and sit with Zane [eight-year-old well child], but I don't. I'm with Glenna again. [Mother]

Many well siblings recognize their parents' bind and know its source, even if it is not mentioned. As discussed in Chapter 12, at this point in the illness, well siblings see CF as a chronic, progressive, incurable disease that shortens the life span.

The girls [sisters who have CF] are angels, you know, as far as my mom's concerned. And, I'm always spiteful at them. I mean, "Aw, come on. How come they get so much and we [well brothers] . . ." You know, like they're going to the shore and stuff. But I'm only saying that because, you know, in a joking manner. You know, I realize what the situation is. How, you know, the disease works and everything. So, I know, she's [mother] just trying to spend as much time with them as she can to make them happy, to keep it out of their minds, you know. It doesn't bother me that much. Every once in a while it will build up and be a big explosion. [Well brother, age nineteen]

With the development of more complications and more frequent hospitalizations family life changes. It is now far more difficult to contain the intrusion the disease makes into their lives. As discussed in Chapter 11 the disease and reminders of it are not so easily pushed aside. Home IV therapy, while offering some measure of control and fewer trips away from home, puts the disease in the center of the living room. It is in the words of one fifteen-year-old well sibling,

Always there. You can never forget that there is cystic fibrosis in the house. It changes everybody's life, I think. Just, it's in your thoughts all the time.

The well sibling is keenly aware of the changes in family life, not to mention the toll that it has taken on their parents. Two well sisters, ages sixteen and twenty, summarize the observations and interpretations of many when they explain,

> SELMA: I think that if everybody in our house was healthy, it would be a lot different there.
> HARRIET: Yeah, there would be a lot less tension, and all of us afraid, you know, of being afraid and everything . . .
> SELMA: I think Mom carries a lot of guilt around. I think in a way she blames herself. When they [ill siblings] are in the hospital, she feels so guilty that they have to go through that that she puts herself kind of through it. She'll stay down there. She'll come home five o'clock in the morning, go to work, make dinner, do whatever she has to do, go right back down there. And my father, too, gets up four o'clock in the morning, drives down to pick her up.
> HARRIET: Yeah. It's true
> SELMA: And you get depressed sometimes just because of it. You feel bad for them. You feel bad for your parents having to go through it. You get aggravated at having to drive down there all the time and you just—it's just always there.

Although well siblings generally share few of these feelings with their parents, they note that when their parents are feeling especially bad, or "depressed," or "worried," they will sometimes discuss their feelings with them.

> When Bianca [age fourteen] was in the hospital for the long period of time and my mom was so worried that she needed to talk to somebody and it happened that I was home one night and she told me how she felt, and was going on down to Philly [Philadelphia] if she thought the doctors weren't doing the right thing.
> But other than that one time when she wanted to get something out of her system, I don't think we ever talked about it. [Well brother, age seventeen]

Parents recognize their well siblings' support in word and in deed. Recall Mrs. Foster's comment about nine-year-old Tyler,

> He knows I worry about her. When I explain things to him he pats me on the back and tells me not to worry.

Talk with ill siblings is not any richer. While the ill and well siblings talks with one another run the gamut from absolutely no real dialogue even about CF care and treatment, to discussions of weight gain and loss, to what happened during a particular hospitalization, to news of other peers with CF, they stop short of their own sibling's course and prognosis. As one well brother, age nineteen (three years older than his ill sister), put it,

I've never had any in-depth conversations with my sister about it.

Ill siblings agree. They, too, report that they talk about day-to-day treatment, weight gain, what happens during hospitalizations, and other children with CF, but not about their own trajectory and prognosis. One adolescent put it quite emphatically when asked if she discussed the course of her illness or prognosis with her well siblings,

No, never. Never ever ever.

Parents seem to be aware of just how circumspect the dialogue is among the siblings.

They [well and ill siblings] talk about school and friends mostly.

They [children with CF] talk about what happens at the hospital, but mostly about the funny things. They might mention offhand someone died, but not necessarily someone with CF. But they'd talk about kids like Roxanne [who does not have CF] that was in their room. Hadley [well brother] met her and he laughed about that. Or they'll talk about some of the fun things they do. Because they do have fun down there [at the hospital]; come home with funny stories. They tend to tell the funnier ones more than the morbid ones.

CF's not something they bring up. I don't think they actually sit down and talk about it the way they do friends and all. [Mother]

The lack of conversation among the siblings does not mean that the well siblings are unaware of their ill siblings' concerns. Recall twelve-year-old Aaron Woodward's rather lengthy discussion of his sister's concerns,

My sister gets scared when she is losing weight or when she has to get her blood gas. She's scared of it sometimes—when she's doing bad and she has to take a test, like the pulmonary function, and she knows she's hasn't been doing good. She gets scared of that. She's scared of getting the tube through your arm that goes to your heart, the Hardy line. She gets scared of that when you miss sometimes. And it's just frustrating . . .

And she got upset when she found out she had that pseudomonas [Pseudomonas cepacia, now known as Burkholderia cepacia]. She got that not too long ago. It's the worst one [bacterial infection]. She got worried because all the people she knows that have died had it. That got her scared.

His eleven-year-old sister Alyson's remarks would confirm her brothers' perception,

It's pretty scary when other kids die from CF, especially my friends. You're like, "Oh no! Are you next?" Because there are so many: Dara, Troy, Leana Linder, Pepper Lyons, Wayne. I know Skip Schmidt, not Skip Lachman, Sonia, Toby. That's all I know, I think. And Nell. There's more, though. A lot. I don't know them all.

Well siblings draw their conclusions on the basis of their own observations of their ill siblings as well as on conversations that they have overheard between their parents, between their parents and staff, and between their ill siblings and their peers.

With all of their knowledge of one another, if at this point siblings do not share information, a distance is created in the relationship that can last until the ill child's death.[18] As one twenty-four-year-old well sister explained after her brother's death,

> We [the ill child and speaker] didn't talk. We weren't that close. My sister [another well sister in the family] did talk to Max—they were close.

For some the reluctance to enter into dialogue about the ill sibling's condition is born of prior experience. Efforts to engage in conversation have been rebuffed.

> Ava carries her own cross totally. Like if I ask her how she's doing she gets annoyed. She just doesn't want to talk about it or anything. [Well sister, age eighteen]

They also are concerned about their own and their sibling's reaction to a discussion of the disease. One well sister, age eleven, said,

> I don't think I'd be able to talk about it. I might say something that would get her mad or upset. I'm really scared about what her reactions will be. Maybe something would come up that my parents don't want her to know.

Or in the words of another well sister, age twelve,

> I don't want to tell [what I know] because I don't know what is going to happen. I don't know how she is going to react, I don't know if she's just going to say, "Well, when it happens," or if she's going to start crying or something like that.

Siblings' reluctance to speak often occurs with full recognition that the ill sibling not only knows the prognosis, but also knows that people are not willing to talk about it.

> I think she sort of feels out in the cold about that we know more about it than what we're telling her. I think she knows, from the people that we have known who have had CF and died. We haven't said that kid had cystic fibrosis, or anything like that. We sort of say it's a shame and leave it at that. We don't really tell her. But she knew one [who died] and that he had treatments like her. [Well sister, age twelve]

[18] Delisi (1986: 75) found in his study of the well siblings of children with cystic fibrosis "a lack of closeness between the siblings and their chronically ill brothers and sisters." He labeled this "an unexpected finding." Yet, if closeness is related to communication (as is suggested here) and the siblings are not talking about their feelings about the illness, Delisi's finding becomes less puzzling.

Like well siblings, ill siblings also worry about the impact that a conversation about the course of their illness and the prognosis might have on their well sibling. Recall, in explaining why she did not talk to her nine-year-old well brother about her condition, ten-year-old Britt remarked,

> "He worries a lot . . . He worries about me mostly. I don't know why . . . Sometimes he talks to me about what he worries about. Sometimes, I wouldn't say much, because he doesn't want me to know. He just, well, I can hear it on the phone that he is.

Others refrain from conversation because they feel that their well siblings "wouldn't understand." One sixteen-year-old with CF put it,

> I don't think they'd [well siblings] understand exactly what I'd be trying to say, or exactly what I meant.

Several children with CF also reported that they found it difficult to engage in such discussions and at the same time to continue to adhere to the prescribed therapeutic regimen, to plan for the future, and to work toward fulfilling those goals. A fifteen-year-old with CF explained,

> It's hard to talk about, to even think about Nell and the others who have died, and still keep doing what you have to. And then if you did as much as they wanted you to do you wouldn't have a life in the outside world, which they want you to do too.

Talking about another's deterioration or death, not to mention one's own, especially when one is beginning to experience some of the complications of the disease, brings the prognosis, of which they are well aware, to the forefront of their minds, where they would rather not have it.

Period V: Increased Deterioration Through to the Conference Where the Physician Tells the Parents that the Child's Condition Is Terminal

For the majority of siblings talk about the course of the illness and the ill siblings' prognosis does not increase in the face of increased deterioration. As one thirteen-year-old with CF put it, when asked, "Do you talk to your sister about CF?"

> Not really. It's just not one of the topics we talk about. She doesn't talk about it either, except when she has a friend over and has to explain things—like when I was getting IVs at home. I have them down in the basement, all the needles and stuff. Our basement's real nice. It's not like some basements. It's where we watch TV.
>
> We have pipes and my mom hangs the IVs and stuff on them. They're over the couch. And my sister's friend was sitting on the couch and looked up. So my sister had to explain everything that I had to do and everything.

Her friend doesn't like needles and there were needles all over. So she just explained what it was for and why I have to do it.

Well siblings would agree. They report that what little conversation there is between them centers around care and treatment (see comments below). Their reluctance to enter into conversations about their siblings' prognosis continues. When topics emerge that raise the specter of the prognosis (now seen as closer and more certain—see Chapter 12), they are not necessarily dealt with in a more forthright manner. For example, one well sister and her brother with CF had planned to move out of their parents' home and share an apartment together. But when her brother's condition became severe and he became oxygen-dependent, they had to abandon the plan. Rather than discuss the change in plans in terms of the changes in his condition, they talked about how difficult it would be to rent an apartment without his income.

> I don't think his dying was as hard on me as before he died. He had to quit work. He started to paint. We'd talk about selling his paintings so we could still buy an apartment.
>
> See, we were supposed to get an apartment together. We were actually looking. He really wanted to get out on his own for a while. Experiencing life on his own. And that just wasn't going to be.
>
> I guess I kind of knew then we were never going to get the apartment. He was too sick, but we didn't say that. We said it was the money.
>
> But that was harder for me than death was itself. And I think it was for him too.

No more than well siblings initiate conversations with their ill siblings about the course of their illness and prognosis do they initiate such conversations with their parents. Parents report that the well siblings "really don't say too much." The subject does come up, however, in the context of other discussions, most frequently those revolving around the issue of attention and special privileges. A father described one such encounter,

> Willa [well sister, age thirteen] felt that Daphney [age ten] was getting all the attention. I said, "Your mother and I don't always get the time together we want. We share it with you and we share it with Daphney. But Daphney's going to take more time. She's not always going to be around; so we want to give her what we can. And she has to have it."
>
> Every once in a while I say to Willa, "You give her PT [chest physical therapy] and see if it's fun." And she'll give her one part of it, then she'll say, "I don't want to, Dad."
>
> But I say, "We're not finished yet." "And how would you like to do this every morning?" I go, "How would you like to take enzymes every time you eat? It's really not that much fun."

She looked at me and, well, you know, that was the end of it.

With increased deterioration the ill sibling becomes the primary focus of parents' attention, a fact of which the well child is well aware. Parents report that the well sibling will often tell them "don't worry about me." Parents feel that at the same time that the well siblings are telling them not to worry about them, they themselves are upset and concerned about their own needs not being met.

> The last time in the hospital when we took her [daughter with CF] up [to the hospital], he's going, "Well, where am I going to go? How am I going to get to school?" He was a little worried, concerned about "Don't leave me here." (Laughs) "Where am I going to stay?"
> It doesn't show too much. It comes out in his school work. He's not with it, or it comes out in those things. [Mother]

As discussed in Chapter 11, parents find balancing the needs of the well and ill children ever more difficult. Home IV therapy continues to represent a useful alternative to hospitalization. At the very least the well child's everyday life is not disrupted to the extent that it would be during hospitalization. Parents "if not available" are present. Recall Mr. Foster's discussion of the advantages of home IV therapy,

> I think it's hard for him to concentrate when Britt's in the hospital. And the fact that sometimes he gets trucked all over the place at those particular times, that doesn't help things either. I think that is a problem too. We've talked about this ourselves. And when she's in the hospital we have to still maintain this house for him and not put him at her mom's or my mom's or somebody else's house. I think, that's not good for him when she's away. And I think he still needs the stability of this house. So that's why we kind of thought really good about it when Britt was home on the IV. I think that helped. That seemed to be a one hundred percent better situation. Even though it was a lot of work. Well not a lot. It was our inexperience more than anything.

Whatever parents' efforts, well siblings become increasingly concerned, not only about their place in the family, but also about what will happen to their family. While they may not share these concerns with their ill siblings or parents, they do, on occasion, share them with others. Nine-year-old Evan Bailey wrote in school,

> I used to think that nobody cared about me, but now I can see why Casey is getting all the attention. It's not because he is better than me. It's just because he needs more of the attention than my brother and me. My parents are doing their very best for us all. I know our family will make it through the good times and the bad, if we just stick together.

As the child's condition begins to deteriorate family life changes. Chores, errands, ferrying well siblings to activities and social engagements, and in some cases even one's job, must be worked around the ill child's care. The ill child's needs come first.

As discussed in Chapter 11, parents' sense of normalcy and control is rapidly diminishing. At best, parents determine the time and place of treatment, certainly not if there will be treatment. If there is care to be done it becomes the focus of family life, if for no other reason than it is now far more time-consuming (e.g., care of oxygen equipment, intravenous catheters).

Parents admit to holding the ill child to a different standard, and some think that the well children do too.[19] Recall Mr. and Mrs. Foster's discussion of differences in expectations for nine-year-old Tyler and ten-year-old Britt, as well as their sense that Tyler also has different expectations,

> "And we let her get away with things. Tyler, we usually don't. And, we're not the only ones that let her get away with things, because Tyler also says he lets her get away with things."
> Mr. Foster nodded in agreement.
> "It's like three of us. And she, I think she . . .
> "She's aware of that."
> "She is."
> "She's very aware of how to get her way, sometimes."
> "And like I said, Tyler will go and get her things. She'll ask him, 'Do this for me. Do that . . .'

This sense is based more often than not on observations of the well siblings' behavior, especially what happens now in a dispute. As Mrs. Foster points out, despite what Tyler may feel, he yields.

> Tyler seems to let Britt go with a lot of it. Sometimes he gets to the point where he will just scream right back at her. But in a sense he lets her get away with things. He'll fight a little bit, but he'll always, he's the first one to give. For an example, one time they were fighting over a sleeping bag. She wanted it, she really wanted it. And it was his turn to use it. And she just kept going on and on and on. I don't know what her reasons were, but it was his turn. They had one sleeping bag and I had said that they had to take turns with it. Well he let her. He gave in.
> And if we tell Britt to clean this or pick up the books or something, put it

[19] Johanna Green, a research assistant responsible for conducting observational studies in the clinic waiting room, found that "the children incorporate a lot of pushing and shoving into their interaction. In families where children are sicker if anyone was reprimanded it was almost always the well sibling. Interestingly the well siblings accepted the scolding and did not try to shift the blame" (Green 1985: 11–12).

away; she'll be moaning, "Oh, I don't feel good. I don't feel like doing it." And he'll end up getting up himself and he'll do it for her.

This was not the case in earlier periods of the illness (see discussion of disputes in Period II). The easy give and take that characterized the period of relative health and even the times between episodes of acute illness are not as much in evidence.

The "protective quality," the sense of responsibility (that parents speak of earlier in the illness, and that well siblings begin to verbalize as complications develop), however, is very much in evidence. Both ill siblings and parents note how the well sibling looks after the ill child. One twelve-year-old with CF responded when asked "How do you think your having CF has affected your sister?"

> She doesn't push me to do something if I don't feel like it; like running or playing or something. She won't push it. Some people keep begging and begging. She doesn't push it that much.

They continue to try to motivate their ill siblings to eat and to do therapy. As Mrs. Foster noted,

> Tyler's always saying, "Why don't you go down and get your treatment already? Do you want to die? Go down and get your treatment." And she'll argue back about the treatment or something, and he'll go, "Go already. Do you want to die?" And then she's all huffy.

While all are not as dramatic in their urgings as Tyler, his remarks reflect not only the concern that well siblings have about their ill siblings' condition, but also the place that the prognosis has now taken in the well siblings' mind. As discussed in Chapter 12, at this the point well siblings' notion of shortened life span is far less academic or theoretical. The future is no longer distant, it is near; how near varies.

Period VI: Terminal Phase of the Illness and Death

Whether voiced or not, well siblings' concerns about the fragility of their ill sibling's life, about the tenuous quality of their condition, does not diminish in the terminal phase of the illness. They are indeed worried about their ill sibling, and in a few cases will even say as much. Recall Gavin's conversation with his mother in the kitchen, on his way out to do his paper route,

> "Mom," he asked, "if Casey rolled over on his oxygen could he be killed?"
> "No! It's the disease that's killing me, not the oxygen," Casey bellowed from the living room.
> Gavin moved closer to his mom and lowered his voice. "What will happen when Casey won't eat anymore?"

"We'll give him Sustecal and Polyviocase?"

"And then when he won't take that?"

"Well, as long as he takes fluids he'll be OK. Now you go do your paper route," said Mrs. Bailey, steering Gavin toward the door.

Note that even at this point [Mr. and Mrs. Bailey had been informed that Casey's condition was terminal and they had decided to bring him home to die] Mrs. Bailey does not say that death will come. The issue remains open-ended, with Gavin needing to pose the next "What if?" Even in the last days when she told Gavin that she and his father knew "what to look for" in order to determine if Casey was near death, she does not tell Gavin what those signs are. Mrs. Bailey is not unique in limiting what she reveals about the child's impending death. Some parents would not even tell as much as she did. One twenty-one-year-old well sister said of her father,

> Like if I went to him and said, "How's Reggie?" He would have told me, "Oh great." He'd want to protect me from feeling hurt over Reggie. He's very protective. He doesn't want anything to happen to his kids if he could take it on himself.

Once the parents have been informed that their child is in the terminal phases of the illness, and that they need to think about how they want to proceed, the atmosphere at home becomes pregnant with death. As discussed in Chapter 11, the strategies that parents use to contain the intrusion of the illness into their lives are no longer in evidence.

Not all well siblings are as aware as others of the immediacy of death. As discussed in Chapter 12 perceptions of the closeness of death (days, weeks, months) varies. According to several well siblings, the imminence of death for them is a function of "how close" they were, and/or "how much we talked." As two adult well sisters commented,

> FAITH: Right up until the end, even with the morphine, I didn't quite get it together that he was really going to die then. Sally and the others [other family members] could, even before, but not me. But then I wasn't as close to him as Sally was.
>
> SALLY: I knew he was dying probably before anyone else; probably even before my mother, because I talked to him about it.

Without speaking they could maintain distance from the imminence of death. As Faith continued,

> I was afraid to talk to him because I didn't want him to tell me that he was dying. I didn't want to talk to him because of that. So I would go in and he'd be in his room, on oxygen, and I would talk to him, but I would never; you know I didn't want it to get to the point where he would start telling me, "You know, it's going to be over soon."

Many well siblings would like their ill siblings to die at home. Some promise to do more around the house, to be generally more cooperative if it will allow the sibling to be at home to die. They do not want to be a stumbling block. As Mrs. Bailey noted,

> Gavin says he wants to learn how to do the IV. I told him that if he wanted to help he'd have to go to school and then he could help later. And they both offered to do jobs if Casey could come home.

Well siblings know that their parents' attention is elsewhere. While not making any requests for attention directly, parents interpret (as they do earlier in the illness) the well siblings' physical complaints as an indication of their desire for attention. When one mother went into the kitchen to get Pepto-Bismol for her son with CF, I heard her say to one of her well sons,

> You don't have a stomachache. You're just saying that because I'm giving Bruce Pepto-Bismol.

Some well siblings try to get close to their dying sibling, only to find their efforts rebuffed. For some time after Casey died, Gavin, age eleven, found he could not forget the way in which his brother rejected his efforts to comfort him,

> He [Casey] kept calling, "Rub me! Rub me!" I tried going over to him to rub him, and he told me to go away. He like pushed me away.

Casey agreed. He said that he did not want his brothers around or to play with his toys. When they did he would yell from his place on the bed in the living room, to stop and go away. His mother tried to intervene.

> He wouldn't let his brothers do anything. Finally I said to him, "Look at the couch. See your brothers, crying. They want to help too. Let them." He said he was sorry, and Gavin and Evan got up and sat on the bed.

But it was not until two days before his death that he allowed his brothers to be near him, to do anything for him. As his mother recalled,

> Friday he let Gavin rub him, which was good. And he called Evan over and asked him to give him juice.

Other siblings cannot seem to face their dying sibling. One mother said of her eighteen-year-old son,

> Marshall couldn't bring himself to come in the room. So finally, he came in the room. And Woody was kind of in a coma at this point. And he said, he said to me, "Could I talk to Woody?" And I said, "Yes, come on over here." Even though Woody wasn't, you know, wasn't talking, he was in a coma. He said, "Alone." So everybody left the room, we left him in there. To this day I have no

idea what he said. And when he was at the undertaker's that night, the under-taker said he put a note in his [Woody's] pocket. Even though the two never got along, you know what I mean? Marshall resented all the things Woody got, the attention, the special privileges, but what else could I do?

Woody, in contrast to Casey, wanted his siblings around. He requested that they be called and asked to come to the hospital.

The terminal phases of the illness are a time of tremendous turmoil for well siblings. As Evan Bailey said to his teacher,

> Do you think I'm cold-blooded? I just couldn't stand him that way,—just laying there with his oxygen in his nose yelling, "Rub me! Rub me!"

Well siblings find it increasingly difficult to go on with their activities, to go to school, let alone concentrate on their school work. Recall Mrs. Bailey's response to Gavin's reluctance to go to school,

> I just told him, "If something were going to happen, do you think I'd go to school? And I'm going."

They also question what they should say and do, as this conversation be-tween two well sisters illustrates. The sisters are recalling their brother's deci-sion to take the morphine that had been offered to ease his pain, even though this could affect his breathing and perhaps hasten his death:

> SALLY: Just like right before he took it [the morphine], he asked us. He said, um . . . It was just you [Faith] and I there. And he said, "Do you think I'm a real asshole for doing this [taking the morphine]?" You wanted to say, "Yeah, don't do it." But that would have been for us.
>
> FAITH: And the kid couldn't breathe, as it was. [He had been on oxygen for quite some time.]
>
> SALLY: And I could see you [Faith] were just about to tell him not to do it.
>
> FAITH: Oh God, it was on the tip of my tongue, "No! No! No!" But I was . . .
>
> SALLY: That was hard.
>
> FAITH: Yeah, that was hard. He didn't want us to think he was copping out, like he wasn't a survivor. He couldn't breathe. I mean he was saying good-bye to us, and he couldn't even breathe. (Pause.) It was the hardest thing. He didn't want us to think that he was giving up.
>
> SALLY: We knew that he had to do it. And we were all there with him. And we all did get to say good-bye. How many of us will get to say good-bye to every-body before we go?

Neither the dying nor the death is easy to accept. A mother recalled after her son's death,

> Even when he died, he [well brother, age eleven] knelt by the bed and said, "He isn't dead." He knelt by the bed and said, "See, he's still here."

He would come home every day after school and say how much better he looked. He'd go, "See how much better he is." I had to shake him and say, "He isn't going to get better."

But he knew that. His teacher told me he knew.

2. THE WELL SIBLINGS' POSITION IN THE FAMILY

The ways well siblings handle the allocation of resources and communication about CF and the ill child's condition with their parents and ill siblings reflect a keen awareness of the place of the illness in family life, as well as what they can and must do, given their own circumstances.

At the time of diagnosis and for some time thereafter well siblings are adrift. They are outside their parents' sphere of attention, seeing little of them or of their ill sibling, and receiving little information about that which will soon become a defining feature of family life. Not lost on their parents are the ways in which well siblings try to find their way back into the purview of their parents' attention. Techniques that have worked in the past, including "acting out" and statements of physical pain and discomfort, are in evidence as well as newer approaches that reflect the new element of family life. Well siblings evince interest, and in some cases even participate, in the newest feature of family life—the tasks of caring for an ill sibling. This is the domain of family life where the presence of the disease is most prominent and where their parents are spending much of their time and energy.

While for the most part their responses parallel their parents' efforts, there are occasions in the first year following diagnosis when chest physical therapy sessions become the scene of negative behavior. This is not surprising, given the place that these sessions occupy in family life.

As the child with CF continues to do well, the visibility of CF in everyday life decreases. Well siblings' attempts to gain attention in ways that would call attention to its presence or reintroduce it into the center of family life also decreases. Well siblings not only do not talk about the illness with their parents or ill siblings, but in those situations where the subject could or does come up they minimize the ill child's condition, especially those aspects related to CF. They focus on just how much their ill sibling is like other children. With their parents they emphasize how important it is for them to treat their ill sibling like any other child—a precept that well siblings follow in their own dealings with their ill sibling.

With the child who has CF perceived and responded to as if he/she is like any other child, the well sibling can remain on relatively equal footing with the ill child. The well sibling is then justified not only in expecting and maintaining a reciprocal relationship with the ill sibling, but also in making the same demands of parents, for attention and privileges, that the ill child receives—a right the well sibling did not have when their sibling was diagnosed or acutely sick. In short, by fitting their line of action to that of their parents (e.g., not talking about the illness, emphasizing the ways in which the child is like other children) well siblings gain a place for themselves in the sphere of their parents' attention, as well as a means to make demands of them and their ill siblings that they would not have were the illness in the forefront of their lives.

Like their parents, well siblings continue to contain the intrusion that the illness makes into their lives for as long as possible. Episodes of acute sickness, exacerbations and hospitalizations bring the illness into the center of family life and make the approaches of the period of relative health less feasible. Like their parents, well siblings place boundaries around these experiences and try to return to the behaviors that they had engaged in before such episodes occurred (e.g., not talking about the illness, treating the ill child in the same way that they had before the exacerbation). In this way well siblings can continue to operate as they had when the child was doing relatively well, with all the rights and privileges that accrue from such a position including expecting and receiving from their parents and ill siblings what any child would.

This approach, however, is not without problems. While well siblings have questions about the efficacy of treatment, cure, course, and control of the disease, they do not ask them. For to put them forward would raise the specter of the illness, move it out of its carefully constructed boundaries where it could threaten the normal life each is trying to maintain. It would then be far more difficult to demand of their parents and ill siblings that the ill sibling share in household chores as well as in wins and losses at play. Instead, behaviors like expressions of a desire to be ill reappear. This signals to parents, at least, where well siblings perceive their parents' attention—on the one who is ill. Being sick is an acceptable reason for claiming extra attention and special privileges. The well siblings have seen it. They have applied similar reasoning themselves in their relationships with their ill siblings. And now they use it for themselves.

When complications begin to develop and increase there is in some cases a return to even more of these "attention getting-behaviors," as some well brothers begin to act out in school and others gain weight. For these children as well as for those who do not exhibit such behavior there is still a reluctance to share concerns about CF and the ill child's condition with their parents and ill sibling. And neither the parents nor the ill siblings encourage such discussion; for to do so would place what lies ahead for the ill child before each of them, in no uncertain terms. For the well sibling this would then mean that distance from the ultimate outcome would not be possible. Also since the well sibling does not face disability or death, having the ill child's condition discussed would make criticism of their parents' behavior vis-à-vis the ill child (e.g., giving the child "more" in the way of material goods or special privileges) or even the ill child's behavior (e.g., using the illness to avoid school, church, or household tasks) less legitimate.

With the illness in the foreground "normal" social relationships with parents and ill siblings become increasingly difficult. While well siblings look out for their ill siblings, yield to their demands, "cut 'em some slack" because of the illness, they also want from them what one would expect from any sibling—mutual aid and reciprocity. They understand why they "should not ask for more attention," but they still would like to have what the ill child receives, or at least that there not be such a disparity—what to their way of thinking would be the case if their sibling did not have CF.

With further deterioration of their siblings' condition, well siblings feel increasingly left out and unable to do anything about it. As neither caretaker, nor ill person, well siblings are outside the major focus of family life.[20] With oxygen use more regular, home IV therapy more frequent, and the ill child's activities more restricted; CF is literally more visible in the center of family life. It is in every room of the house as the ill child spends more time in the living room or family room, equipment by his/her side. There is so much to do. Parents and increasingly well siblings yield to the demands of the ill child.

As death approaches there is little that well siblings can ask of their parents or ill sibling. There are no culturally approved ways now for the well sibling to gain or even expect to gain equal attention from parents, not to mention reciprocity with siblings. The well have a future, the dying none; and what little time the dying have is further diminished by pain and suffering. As Bank and Kahn (1982: 79–80) point out,

> The parents [of a dying child] essentially must put "first things first" and with time running out feel about the well child, "I'll take care of you later."
> Thus the well sibling must put aside his or her own needs and assume a greater caring role with the victim sibling and the emotionally taxed parents.

Well siblings are losing a sibling and in a sense their parents as well. Their relationships with their siblings are not necessarily fulfilling and the means open to make them such are now in large measure in the hands of the ill children—some of whom reach out and some of whom do not.

In sum, through an examination of the ways in which well siblings deal with the issues of the allocation of resources and communication about CF and the ill child's condition we gain insight into the well siblings' sense of their

[20] Kramer (1981: 158) characterizes the position of the well siblings of children with cancer in a similar way, using the term "outsider."

position in the family, their perceptions of their rights, privileges, duties, and responsibilities as well as the feelings their position engenders. As in the discussion of the parents' responses described in Chapter 11, well siblings' approaches are not necessarily conscious or deliberate. They emerge in everyday life in response to the situations in which they find themselves.

In the next chapter I consider the implications, for clinical practice, of the well siblings' behavior, their views and responses, as well as the context in which they emerge.

Afterword

Meeting the Needs of the Well Sibling

WELL SIBLINGS of children with cystic fibrosis (CF) struggle with thoughts and feelings that are not easily managed. Despite the tremendous challenges these children face, the majority of them (and other well siblings who have recently been studied) are not appreciably different from children in families with only well children (e.g., Gayton, Friedman, Tavormina, and Tucker 1977; Drotar and Crawford 1985; Tritt and Esses 1988; O'Brien 1987; Binks 1982; Switzer 1984; Breslau, Weitzman, and Messenger 1981; Cadman, Boyle, and Offord 1988; Harder and Bowditch 1982; Kupst 1986).[1] I attribute this lack of difference in large measure to the strategies that well siblings and their parents use to contain the intrusion that CF makes into their lives.

The strategies that I have described in this book allow well siblings and their families to live with some modicum of normalcy, some sense of control for long periods of time. At no time, however, do their approaches remove the conflicts or the pain that comes from living with a child who has a chronic, progressive, and ultimately fatal illness like CF. Well siblings face a number of problems, some stemming from the strategies themselves, that can benefit from the kinds of special support skilled clinicians can offer. In this chapter I consider some of the ways that clinicians might help well siblings. In the first section I discuss some general guidelines for working with well siblings. The guidelines proceed from a perspective that assumes neither increased well being nor pathology as a result of growing up with a sibling who has a chronic, life-threatening illness (see Chapter 1). These guidelines can be useful in dealing with a wide range of responses and issues, including those where, owing to other factors, there are indications of risk for social and emotional difficulties. In the second section I look at a particular issue that concerns both clinicians and family members—communication about the illness and the ill child's condition. I suggest an approach to intervention, one that I refer to as "shuttle diplomacy."

---

[1] As discussed in Chapter 1, for the small number of children who did experience behavioral problems there was more to their problems than having a chronically ill sibling. The illness was, as others have suggested, one factor among many (Drotar and Crawford 1985; Lobato, Faust, and Spirito 1988; Leonard 1983; Delisi 1986).

1. GENERAL GUIDELINES FOR CLINICAL INTERVENTION

At the outset of this book I raised the question, "How does chronic illness affect well siblings?" I stated that in order to answer that question one must become familiar with the well siblings' experiences over the course of the illness, information that my work would attempt to provide. I suggested that we begin by looking at the well sibling in the context of the family. I argued that examination of how well siblings understood and made sense of their experience, how they dealt with the situation in which they found themselves, would provide insight into what impact chronic, life-threatening illness has on well siblings. Indeed, with this approach we not only can see how the well siblings interpret their experiences over the course of the illness (Chapters 12 and 13), but also we can begin to posit an explanation for what shapes their views and responses so as to make sense of their experience (Chapters 11 and 13).

My approach to clinical intervention proceeds from the same premise that guided the research: namely, that we begin by considering the situation in which well siblings find themselves. Understanding the experience allows one to see, not only what is open for change, but also what may be un-changeable or unavoidable. I say unchangeable or unavoidable because all too often when faced with psychosocial problems in practice, clinicians think that they are amenable to change. They feel it is simply a matter of how to effect the change. Given the meaning and nature of chronic illness, its place in the life of the individual and in the family, the kinds of changes that we may want to see in an individual's behavior or emotional state may not be possible. No more than all physical illnesses can be cured or prevented, can all social and psychological problems be prevented or remedied. For exam-ple, all of the explanations and justifications parents offer to well siblings about the changes in family lifestyle, priorities, responsibilities, and attention will not, and perhaps cannot, alleviate the feelings of loneliness and anxiety that accompany living with a sibling who has a life-threatening illness (Chesler, Allswede, and Barbarin 1991: 36). Much of what the well sibling feels in the way of lack of attention, disruption of family lifestyle, concern for the ill child, and fear of the illness's consequences may be not only unavoid-able, but also appropriate (Kupst 1986: 187).

Beginning at the macro level of the experience, one must never lose sight of the fact that well siblings and their families live in a society where chronic illness and disability are stigmatized, and normalcy, control, and order are valued. It is a society where parents are charged with the responsibility of providing for the well being of all of their children. Yet in these families if parents do for one child it is often at the expense of the other. And that "other child" is more often the well sibling, who must master the tasks of childhood, adolescence, and adulthood despite whatever difficulties may come as a result of growing up with a child who needs so much care and attention from parents.

At the micro level one needs to assess: (1) ill child's condition and experiences with the illness, (2) the well siblings' interpretation of the ill child's condition and experience, (3) the parents' responses to the care the ill child requires and the concerns the ill child's condition engenders, and (4) the well siblings' interpretations of those responses. More specifically, one needs to focus on how well siblings and parents: (1) deal with the tasks of care, (2) handle information about the disease and the child's condition, (3) deal with reminders of the disease and its consequences, (4) approach the ill child's difference from other children, (5) assess needs and establish priorities within the family, and (6) conceptualize the ill child's future. Their approaches are not without consequences for their own thoughts, feelings, and relationships with others.

While age and stage of development cannot and should not be overlooked, they alone should not be used to determine what well siblings know or are concerned about, let alone how they are best approached. As is evident from the material presented in Part III we would do well to begin by considering the well siblings' experiences.

2. COMMUNICATION IN THE FAMILY: THE CASE FOR "SHUTTLE DIPLOMACY"

From the material presented in Chapter 13 we know that well siblings are reluctant to discuss openly CF and the ill child's condition with their parents and ill siblings, and vice versa. Well siblings' comments indicate that they find it difficult to engage in open communication and at the same time make the "normal" demands for parental attention that other children do. Maintaining "normal" relationships with the ill sibling in the face of open communication is also seen as problematic. Moreover, well siblings are concerned that open communication with their parents and ill siblings might upset them, and they want to protect them from such pain and discomfort (Chesler, Allswede, and Barbarin 1991: 32; Carpenter and Sahler 1991: 204).

From the perspective of the well siblings as well as from that of other family members, there is good reason not to communicate openly (see Chapter 13). Open communication is fraught with risk, risk to what they see as essential for the conduct of everyday life and family relationships. Discussion of CF and the ill child's condition, especially the course of the disease and the prognosis, would put CF where they do not want it, in the center of family life and in forefront of their lives, making it difficult for them to accomplish the tasks before them.

We also know from the material presented in Chapter 13 and from the work of other researchers and clinicians (see Chapter 1) that the absence of discussion about CF and the ill siblings' condition can lead to misinformation and misunderstanding. Without discussion distance can develop in relationships that is, to say the least, difficult to deal with. All of this is still to say nothing of what we know is the sense of isolation that comes from holding inside what one fears cannot be revealed to another. As Chesler, Allswede, and Barbarin, from their studies of the well siblings of children with cancer, suggest,

> Acting "normal" and keeping one's thoughts and feelings to oneself may be common and may reduce the pressure of the immediate situation, but this behavior may also increase stress by intensifying feelings of isolation. It may cover up important issues that need to be discussed (Chesler, Allswede, and Barbarin 1991: 31).

What is a clinician to do when he or she feels that a family member (in this case a well sibling) needs or wants to discuss an issue with other family members and that individual or the others do not want to enter into such discussion?[2]

The best position to take may be one that has always been available, the one that one customarily takes, consciously or unconsciously, "shuttle diplomacy." How do we manage this approach that we associate with the larger global sociopolitical arena (e.g., Henry Kissinger, Jimmy Carter, and Warren Christopher dealing with issues in the Middle East) in the smaller psychosocial arena of clinical care? Below is a suggested course of action.

1. Consider what you or the family member, in this case the well sibling, need or want to discuss (e.g., course of the illness, allocation of resources, treatment alternatives). Family members may wish to be open with one another on some topics, but not on others. For example, parents and well siblings may be willing to discuss openly with each other the care and treatment the disease requires, the progress in medical research, even the course of the disease, but not the ill child's prognosis.

2. Try to determine why the particular issue is being raised. Is the purpose to disseminate (in the case of the clinician) or to gather (in the case of the well sibling) more medical information on a given topic (e.g., alternative modes of chest physiotherapy, the techniques of chest physical therapy, or procedures and efficacy of heart–lung transplantation)? Or is the purpose in raising a particular topic to explore some of the psychosocial aspects of the issue (e.g., the attention the ill child receives because of the required chest physical therapy, or concern

---

[2] For purposes of this discussion the issues are presented and discussed in terms of the well sibling; however, the model could be applied to any family member or any number of issues.

that their sibling might die during the heart–lung transplantation, or the question of who will take care of them during the long hospitalization)?

3. Consider who is raising the question and with whom the individual wants to discuss the issue. Family members find that the extent to which they can be open on any given topic depends to a degree on whom they are speaking with. Well siblings have different concerns about discussing the issues of fertility, reproduction, carrier status, and CF with their parents than they do with their ill siblings. To discuss the issues with their ill brothers, for example, raises the issue of sterility, a condition they do not share.

4. Assess where the family is in the natural history of the illness. We know that well siblings' views, like those of other family members', vary over the course of the illness. Changes in responses are linked to pivotal experiences or events in the illness trajectory (see Chapters 11, 12, 13). A family member may be willing to discuss a particular topic at one point in the illness but not at another. Recall how not only the parents' and well siblings' willingness to discuss the course of the illness, but also the reasons that they gave for speaking or not speaking were different when the child was doing well than when complications began to develop.

5. In short, before embarking on a particular course of action review the situation (see Section 1) and assess what the advantages and disadvantages are to open discussion of that particular issue, among those individuals, at that particular time. In other words, do a kind of cost-benefit analysis. One may decide to stop right there and go no further at that point. Or one may decide to proceed further, in which case I would suggest the following.

6. Ask every family member to be involved in the discussion what concerns they would have if the particular topic to be addressed came up in a conversation in which that family member (A) was present. Perhaps begin with the question, "What is the worst that could happen if subject X were to come up in conversation with A?" Then go on to elicit other concerns that may not have been expressed, by listing concerns that others whom you have worked with or read about have mentioned, and asking if they share these concerns.

7. Discuss with each individual how he or she would want concerns to be addressed. Perhaps the individual would like you to arrange a meeting with A and/or others present; in which case you might want to discuss the possible consequences of such a meeting—positive, negative, and otherwise. Or perhaps the individual would like you to pursue the issue with A and/or the other family member(s), but leave him or her out. In this case, you would return to the individual (from whom you or a colleague heard or sensed the need for an open discussion) and discuss with that person the fact that "some people do not like to talk about X, because Y (insert individual's worst-case scenario for what would happen if X came up)," and continue what needs to be discussed without the other(s) present. This may well be the result when family members want or need an outlet for their feelings, but feel that doing so would make it difficult to maintain "normal" social relationships or to carry on with the business of every-day life.

8. If one or the other of the parties does not wish to proceed with open discussion with other family members, do not persist. It is better to avoid statements like, "It would be better if you all spoke openly to each other about this issue." To do so is to suggest that their approach to life with a chronic, life-threatening illness is flawed, a notion that would be difficult for them to accept given their perception and presentation of their experience, and it may present other difficulties in your relationship with them. Besides, some of what you have wanted to accomplish has been, through your dialogues with the individual. As Kleinman (1988: xii) points out, "witnessing and helping to organize experience can be of therapeutic value."

Shuttle diplomacy is a time-consuming process; however, given what is gained through the process, not to mention what is not lost or damaged, it is time well spent. Through the process of shuttle diplomacy all parties are to a degree unburdened. Each has an opportunity to discuss concerns without risking what they see as essential for the conduct of everyday life and relationships. The foundation is laid for further communication. In addition, two of the greatest consequences of closed communication are averted. Misinformation and misunderstandings are corrected. Not insignificantly, the participants are not alone with their fears. They have shared them with one another, however directly or indirectly. And finally, because of what is accomplished through shuttle diplomacy, the clinician can enjoy a sense of accomplishment instead of the failure and frustration that often attends the goal of getting family members to be "open with one another."

Ratjen (1989: 19–20), citing the work of Chodoff, Friedman, and Hamburg (1964: 744), defines coping as "consisting of two aspects, an externally directed one, judged for its effectiveness in social terms . . . and an internal or defensive aspect which serves to protect the individual from disruptive degrees of anxiety and which is judged for adequacy by the degree of comfort resulting." Shuttle diplomacy emphasizes preserving what family members see as essential for the maintenance of everyday life and relationships, while giving both permission and venue for discussion of feelings necessary for a sense of well being; it facilitates coping in every sense of the word at every level. Shuttle diplomacy allows the clinician to meet the needs of family members at both the social and intrapsychic level.

With advances in CF care and research, children with CF, their parents, and their well siblings will be able to enjoy relatively normal lives for much longer periods of time. Even now, as in so many other chronic and life-threatening illnesses, it is not unusual to find well siblings growing up and leaving home before the disease begins to take its toll. For them, growing up with a brother or sister who has CF will have a far different impact than it did on those who grew up with a brother or sister who became severely ill and died in the developmental years. The challenge to clinicians, however, will remain relatively the same: that is, to design and implement intervention programs that take into account the entire multifaceted and dynamic context in which any given response is situated—the social, psychological, and temporal dimensions of the experience.

Glossary

Here are explained the significance of unfamiliar terms that occur in the personal accounts and other places in the book where individuals are quoted. In compiling this glossary I have used information from publications of the Cystic Fibrosis Foundation (1994, 1995) as well as a booklet prepared by Cunningham and Taussig (1991) and *Taber's Cyclopedic Medical Dictionary*.

annual — yearly outpatient examination.

antibiotics — used in treatment of bacterial infection (e.g., ticarcillin, ceftazidime, tobramycin)

beating — see chest physical therapy

blood gas — a test whereby blood taken from an artery is measured for oxygen saturation, pH, and carbon dioxide levels

bronchodilator — medication that opens bronchial tubes to allow freer breathing

Broviac — see central line

Burkholderia cepacia — see Pseudomonas cepacia

carrier detection test — a test that detects the presence of the cystic fibrosis (CF) gene

central intravenous catheter — see central line

central line — intravenous catheter that is placed into a major vessel, such as the subclavian vein, for the delivery of medication (e.g., Broviac)

chest physical therapy — percussing the lobes of the lungs by thumping or pounding on the chest and back, thereby dislodging mucus; attention is paid to body position to make removal of mucus easier

chest physiotherapy — see chest physical therapy

clapping — see chest physical therapy

clinic — see cystic fibrosis center

clubbing — a manifestation of CF, related to oxygen deficiency, in which the tips of the fingers and toes become rounded and enlarged

Cotazym — a proprietary pancreatic enzyme-replacement preparation

CPT — see chest physical therapy

cystic fibrosis center — a designation bestowed by the Cystic Fibrosis Foundation to major teaching and community hospitals that provide comprehensive diagnosis and specialized treatment for people with CF and their families. Families in this study refer to the facility as "the clinic" when visiting on an outpatient basis, and as "the hospital" when they are inpatients. The center at St. Christopher's Hospital for Children, where this study was conducted, is one of the largest CF centers in North America

Ensure — a high-calorie dietary supplement

enzymes — see pancreatic enzymes

exacerbation — the result of excessive bacterial growth in the lung and increased mucus production, leading to a further compromised airflow; signs include increased coughing and production of thick sputum, fever, weight loss, and decreased lung function; treatments include increased chest therapy, intravenous antibiotic therapy, and hospitalization

fat malabsorption — inadequate removal and uptake of fat during digestion, leading to foul-smelling stools

gastrostomy feeding — feeding through a surgically created opening in the abdominal wall

InspirEase — a portable drug-delivery system or metered-dose inhaler that helps deliver medication to the lungs

mask — see nebulizer

meconium ileus — an obstruction of the intestines of a newborn infant with abnormally thick meconium (first stool); it is the earliest symptom of CF, occurring in 7 to 10 percent of patients

mist — see nebulizer

mist machine — see nebulizer

nasogastric feeding — feeding directly into the stomach through a tube inserted through the nose and down the esophagus

nebulizer — a device used to deliver bronchodilators and anti-inflammatory agents (e.g., albuteral sulfate, cromolyn sodium) and/or antibiotics (e.g., tobramycin, colimycin, gentamycin). The mist is inhaled via a mask that fits over the nose and mouth

Pancrease — a proprietary pancreatic enzyme-replacement preparation. The term is sometimes used by family members and patients in this study as a generic reference to any pancreatic enzyme-replacement preparation

pancreatic enzyme — a substance produced by the pancreas, which aids and accelerates the chemical processes in digestion. Persons with CF often need enzyme replacements (see Pancrease, Cotazym)

PDs — see chest physical therapy

PFT — pulmonary function test

postural drainage therapy — see chest physical therapy

pounding — see chest physical therapy

Pseudomonas cepacia — a bacterial infection found in persons with CF; considered a poor prognostic indicator. Now called Burkholderia cepacia

PT — see chest physical therapy

pulmonary function test — a battery of tests that measure lung capacity and efficiency

rectal prolapse — a protrusion of the rectum occurring in children with CF because of their digestive complications

slapping — see chest physical therapy

Sustecal — a high-calorie dietary supplement

sweat test — the diagnostic test for CF done by measuring the amount of sweat chloride; in CF the amount present is high

the machine — see nebulizer

therapy — see chest physical therapy

thumping — see chest physical therapy

treatments — see chest physical therapy

tune-up — scheduled, periodic hospitalization during which persons with CF receive more aggressive PT and intravenous antibiotics.

Works Cited

Works listed here are those cited in the text and footnotes, as well as in research proposals, presentations, and publications related to my studies of well siblings, parents, and individuals with cystic fibrosis.

Abrams, Sandra J.
  1986   *The Self-Concept of Sickle Cell Children and Their Siblings and Related Maternal Attitudes*. PhD Thesis. Columbia University.
Abramson, H. A., and Peshkin, M. Murray
  1960   Psychosomatic Group Therapy with Parents of Children with Intractable Asthma: Sibling Rivalry and Sibling Support. *Annals of Allergy*, 18:87–91. May/June.
Adams, David
  1979   *Childhood Malignancy: The Psychological Care of the Child and His Family*. Springfield, Ill.: Charles C. Thomas.
Allan, J. L.; Townley, R. W.; and Phelan, P. D.
  1974   Family Response to Cystic Fibrosis. *Australian Pediatric Journal*, 10 (3):136–46.
Allen, Hugh D., and Lemen, Richard J.
  1984   Cardiovascular Manifestations: Cor Pulmonale. In *Cystic Fibrosis*. Edited by Lynn M. Taussig. New York: Thieme-Stratton.
Ames, L. B.
  1982   *He Hit Me First: When Brothers and Sisters Fight*. New York: Dembner Books.
Andersen, D. H.
  1938   Cystic Fibrosis of the Pancreas and Its Relation to Celiac Disease: Clinical and Pathological Study. *American Journal of Diseases of Children*, 56:344–95.
  1959   Cystic Fibrosis of the Pancreas. *Journal of Chronic Diseases*, 7:58.
  1960   Cystic Fibrosis and Family Stress. *Children*, 7:1. Jan./Feb.
Anderson, C. M., and Freeman, M.
  1960   "Sweat Test" Results in Normal Persons of Different Ages Compared with Families with Fibrositis Disease of the Pancreas. *Archives of Disease in Childhood*, 35:581–89.
Anderson, J. M.
  1981   The Social Construction of Illness Experience: Families with a Critically Ill Child. *Advanced Nursing*, 6 (6):427–34.
Anglim, Mary Ann
  1976   Reintegration of One Family After the Death of a Child. In *Home Care for the Dying Child*. Edited by Ida Martinson. New York: Appleton-Century Crofts.
Angst, Denise
  1992   *Defining and Managing CF: The Experience of School Age Children and Families*. PhD Thesis. Rush University. Illinois.

Balk, David E.
   1981   *Sibling Death During Adolescence: Self-Concept and Bereavement Reactions.* PhD
           Thesis. University of Illinois at Urbana-Champaign.
   1983   Adolescents' Grief Reactions and Self-Concept Perceptions Following Sibling
           Death: A Study of 33 Teenagers. *Journal of Youth and Adolescence,* 12 (2):137–60.
Bank, Stephen, and Kahn, Michael
   1975   Sisterhood-Brotherhood: Sibling-Subsystems and Family Therapy. *Family
           Process,* 14 (3):311–37.
   1982   *The Sibling Bond.* New York: Basic Books.
Bearison, David
   1991   *"They Never Want to Tell You": Children Talk About Cancer.* Cambridge, Mass.:
           Harvard University Press.
Bearison, David J., and Pacifici, Caesar
   1984   Psychological Studies of Children Who Have Cancer. *Journal of Applied De-
           velopmental Psychology,* 5:263–80.
   1989   Children's Event Knowledge of Cancer Treatment. *Journal of Applied Develop-
           mental Psychology,* 10:469–86.
Becker, Marshall H.
   1976   Role of the Patient: Social and Psychological Factors in Noncompliance. In
           Patient Compliance. Edited by Louis Lasagna. Mt. Kisco: Futura Publishing.
Bedell, J. R.
   1977   Life Stress and the Psychological and Medical Adjustment of Chronically Ill
           Children. *Journal of Psychosomatic Research,* 21 (3):237–42.
Bellisari, Anna W.
   1984   *Beating CF: Patient Compliance with Chest Physiotherapy in Cystic Fibrosis.* PhD
           Thesis. Ohio State University.
   1987   Owning Cystic Fibrosis: Adaptive Noncompliance with Chest Physiotherapy
           in Cystic Fibrosis. In *Encounters with Biomedicine.* Edited by Hans A. Baer.
           New York: Gordon and Breach Science Publishers.
Bendor, Susan J.
   1986   *New Approaches to the Supportive Treatment of Siblings of Pediatric Cancer Pa-
           tients.* PhD Thesis. City University of New York.
Berger, Peter, and Luckman, Thomas
   1966   *The Social Construction of Reality: A Treatise in One Sociology of Knowledge.*
           Garden City, N.Y.: Doubleday.
Bergmann, Thesi, and Wolfe, Sidney
   1971   Observations of the Reactions of Healthy Children to Their Chronically Ill
           Siblings. *Bulletin of the Philadelphia Association for Psychoanalysis,* 21:145–61.
Beuf, Ann H.
   1989   *Biting Off the Bracelet: A Study of Children in Hospitals.* Philadelphia: Univer-
           sity of Pennsylvania Press.
Bibace, Roger, and Walsh, Mary E.
   1980   Development of Children's Conception of Illness. *Pediatrics,* 66 (6):912–
           17.
   1981   *Children's Conceptions of Health, Illness, and Bodily Functions.* San Francisco:
           Jossey-Bass.

Binger, C.
1973   Childhood Leukemia—Emotional Impact on Siblings. In *The Child and His Family: The Impact of Death and Disease*. Edited by E. J. Anthony and C. Koupernik. New York: John Wiley.

Binks, Elizabeth Tate
1982   *Impact of Cystic Fibrosis on Children's Emotions: Behavior and Concept of Death as Seen by Parents*. PhD Thesis. Adelphi University.

Bluebond-Langner, Myra
1978   *The Private Worlds of Dying Children*. Princeton: Princeton University Press.
1983   *Illness in the Child's Social World*. Grant proposal to the National Science Foundation, Washington, D.C.
1985   *Preliminary Findings from Study of the Well Siblings of Children with Cystic Fibrosis*. Paper presented at the Regional Cystic Fibrosis Retreat, Philadelphia, Pennsylvania.
1985   Field Notes, Field Journals, Transcripts of Interviews. Unpublished.
1986   Field Notes, Field Journals, Transcripts of Interviews. Unpublished.
1991   Living with Cystic Fibrosis: A Family Affair. In *Young People and Death*. Edited by Jack Morgan. Philadelphia: Charles Press.
1991   Living with Cystic Fibrosis: The Well Sibling's Perspective. In *Medical Anthropology Quarterly*, 5 (2):133–52.
1994   *Chronic Illness and Society: Implications for Clinical Practice*. Paper presented at the annual meeting of the Cystic Fibrosis Foundation. Orlando, Florida.
1995   *"How Did You Do It?": Approaches to Data Collection, Analysis, Writing and Presentation Used in the Construction of a Book on Well Siblings and Parents of Children with Cystic Fibrosis*. Paper presented in a seminar on Methods and Techniques in Social Research. Rutgers University, New Jersey.

Bluebond-Langner, Myra; Perkel, Dale; and Goertzel, Ted
1991   Pediatric Cancer Patients' Peer Relationships: Impact of an Oncology Camp Experience. In *Journal of Psychosocial Oncology*, 9 (2):67–79.

Bluebond-Langner, Myra; Perkel, Dale; Goertzel, Ted; Nelson, Kathryn; and McGeary, Joan
1990   Children's Knowledge of Cancer and Its Treatment: Impact of an Oncology Camp Experience. In *Journal of Pediatrics*, 116 (2):207–213.

Blumenthal, M. D.
1969   Experiences of Parents of Retardates and Children with Cystic Fibrosis. *Archives of General Psychiatry*, 21 (2):160–71. August.

Bonchek, Rita
1983   *A Study of the Effects of Sibling Death on the Surviving Child: A Developmental and Family Perspective*. PhD Thesis. University of Wisconsin-Milwaukee.

Bosk, Charles
1992   *All God's Mistakes: Genetic Counseling in a Pediatric Hospital*. Chicago: University of Chicago Press.

Bossert, E.; Holaday, B.; Harkins, A.; and Turner-Henson, A.
1990   Strategies of Normalization Used by Parents of Chronically Ill School Age Children. In *The Journal of Child and Adolescent Psychiatric Mental Health Nursing*, 3 (2):57–61.

Bowlby, John
1980 *Attachment and Loss.* Volume III: *Loss.* New York: Basic Books.
Boyle, Ivy R.; Sack, Sallyann; Millican, Francis; di Sant'Agnese, Paul A.; Kulczcki, Agnes; and Lucas, L.
1976 Emotional Adjustment of Adolescents and Young Adults with Cystic Fibrosis. *The Journal of Pediatrics,* 88 (2):318–26. February.
Breslau, Naomi
1982 Siblings of Disabled Children: Birth Order and Age-Spacing Effects. *Journal of Abnormal Child Psychology,* 10 (1):85–96.
1983 The Psychological Study of Chronically Ill Children: Are Healthy Siblings Appropriate Controls? *Journal of Abnormal Child Psychology,* 11 (3):379–91.
Breslau, N.; Weitzman, M.; and Messenger, K.
1981 Psychological Functioning of Siblings of Disabled Children. *Pediatrics,* 67 (3):344–53.
Brett, K.
1988 Sibling Response to Chronic Childhood Disorder: Research Perspectives and Practice Implications. In *Issues in Comprehensive Pediatric Nursing,* 11 (1):43–57.
Brodie, B.
1974 Views of Healthy Children toward Illness. *American Journal of Public Health,* 64 (12):1156–59. December.
Bronheim, S. P.
1978 Pulmonary Disorders: Asthma and Cystic Fibrosis. In *Psychological Management of Pediatric Problems.* Volume I. Edited by P. R. Magrab. Baltimore: University Park Press.
Bryant, Brenda K.
1982 Sibling Relationships in Middle Childhood. In *Sibling Relationships: Their Nature and Significance Across the Life Span.* Edited by M. Lamb and B. Sutton-Smith. Hillsdale, N.J.: Lawrence Erlbaum.
Burhmann, M. V.
1970 Death:Its Psychological Significance in the Lives of Children. *South African Medical Journal,* 44:586–589. May.
Burns, W. J., and Zweig, A. R.
1980 Self-Concepts of Chronically Ill Children. *Journal of Genetic Psychology,* 137 (2):179–190.
Burr, Carolyn Keith
1985 Impact on the Family of a Chronically Ill Child. In *Issues in the Care of Children with Chronic Illness.* Edited by N. Hobbs and J. M. Perrin. San Francisco: Jossey-Bass.
Burton, Lindy
1974 *Care of the Child Facing Death.* Edited by Lindy Burton. London: Routledge and Kegan Paul.
1975 *The Family Life of Sick Children.* London: Routledge and Kegan Paul.
Bury, Michael R., and Wood, Phillip H.
1979 Problems of Communication in Chronic Illness. *International Rehabilitative Medicine,* 1 (3):130–34.

Bush, Andrew
 Forthcoming   Cystic Fibrosis: The Disease and Its Treatment. In *Psychosocial Aspects of Cystic Fibrosis*. Edited by Bryan Lask, Myra Bluebond-Langner, and Denise Angst. London: Chapman and Hall.
Bywater, E.
 1981   Adolescents with Cystic Fibrosis: Psychological Adjustment. *Archives of Disease in Children*, 56 (7):538–43.
Cadman, D.; Boyle, M. H.; and Offord, D. R.
 1988   The Ontario Child Health Study: Social Adjustment and Mental Health of Siblings of Children with Chronic Health Problems. *Journal of Developmental and Behavioral Pediatrics*, 9(3):117–21.
Cain, Albert C., and Cain, Barbara S.
 1964   On Replacing a Child. *Journal of the American Academy of Child Psychiatry*, 3 (3):443–56.
Cairns, N. U.; Clark, G. M.; Smith, S. D.; and Lansky, S. B.
 1979   Adaptations of Siblings to Childhood Malignancy. *Journal of Pediatrics*, 95 (3):484–87.
Caldwell, S. M.
 1985   Systems Theory Applied to Families with a Diabetic Child. *Family Systems in Medicine*, 3 (1):34–44.
Carandang, M. L.
 1979   The Role of Cognitive Level and Sibling Illness in Children's Conceptualization of Illness. *American Journal of Orthopsychiatry*, 49 (3):474–81. July.
Carpenter, P. J., and Sahler, O. J.
 1991   Sibling Perception and Adaptation to Childhood Cancer: Conceptional and Methodological Considerations. In *Advances in Child Health psychology* Edited by J. H. Johnson and S. B. Johnson. Gainesville, Fla.: University Press of Florida.
Carr-Gregg, M., and White, L.
 1987   Siblings of Pediatric Cancer Patients: A Population at Risk. In *Medical and Pediatric Oncology*, 15:62–68.
Cassady, Lucinda
 1982   *The Forgotten Children: A Study of the Interpersonal Perceptions of Healthy Siblings of Children with a Life-Threatening or Chronic Illness*. PhD Thesis. California School of Professional Psychology. San Diego
Charmaz, Kathy
 1991   *Good Days, Bad Days: The Self in Chronic Illness and Time*. New Brunswick, N.J.: Rutgers University Press.
Chesler, Mark; Allswede, Jennifer; and Barbarin, Caesar
 1991   Voices from the Margin of the Family: Siblings of Children with Cancer. In *The Journal of Psychosocial Oncology*, 9 (4):19–42.
Cohen, D. S.
 1985   Pediatric Cancer: Predicting Sibling Adjustment. In *Dissertation Abstracts International*, 46:637. University Microfilms, No. ADG 85-08044, 8505.
Cicirelli, V. G.
 1977   Children's School Grades and Sibling Structure. *Psychological Reports*, 41:1055–58.

1982   Sibling Influence Throughout the Life Span. In *Sibling Relationships: Their Nature and Significance across the Life Span.* Edited by M. Lamb and B. Sutton-Smith. Hillsdale, N.J.: Lawrence Erlbaum.

Cimini, Maria D.
1986   *An Examination of Behavioral Problems in the Siblings of Pediatric Cancer Patients and an Evaluation of an Information/Support Group.* PhD Thesis. State University of New York at Albany.

Clifford, James, and Marcus, George
1986   *Writing Culture: The Poetics and Politics of Ethnography.* Edited by C. L. James. Berkeley, Calif.: University of California Press.

Cohen, Harriett, and Rosen, Helen
1980   *Children's Reactions to Sibling Loss.* Unpublished manuscript. Rutgers University.

Cook, Sarah Sheets
1973   Children's Perceptions of Death. In *Children and Dying.* Edited by Roberta Halporn. New York: Health Sciences Publishing Corp.

Coopersmith, Stanley
1959   A Method for Determining Types of Self-Esteem. *Journal of Abnormal and Social Psychology,* 59:87–94.

Cowen, Leslie; Corey, Mary; Keenan, N.; Simmons, R.; Arndt, E.; and Levison, N.
1985   Family Adaptation and Psychosocial Adjustment to Cystic Fibrosis in the Preschool Child. *Social Science and Medicine,* 20 (6):553–60.

Cowen, Leslie; Mok, J.; Corey, M.; MacMillan, H.; Simmons, R.; and Levison, H.
1986   Psychological Adjustment of the Family with a Member Who Has Cystic Fibrosis. *Pediatrics,* 77 (5):745–53.

Craft, M. J.; Wyatt, N.; and Sandell, B.
1985   Behavior and Feeling Changes in Siblings of Hospitalized Children. *Clinical Pediatrics,* 24 (7):374–78.

Crain, A. J.; Sussman, M.; and Weil, W. B.
1966   Family Interaction, Diabetes, and Sibling Relationships. *International Journal of Sociological Psychiatry,* 12 (1):35–43.

Crider, Cathleen
1981   Children's Conceptions of the Body Interior. In *Children's Conceptions of Health, Illness and Bodily Functions.* Edited by R. Bibace and M. Walsh. San Francisco: Jossey-Bass.

Crocker, A. C.
1983   Sisters and Brothers. In *Parent-Professional Partnerships in Developmental Disability Services.* Edited by J. A. Mulick. Cambridge, Mass.: Academic Guild.

Cunningham, James, and Taussig, Lynn
1991   *An Introduction to Cystic Fibrosis for Patients and Families.* Bethesda, Md.: Cystic Fibrosis Foundation.

Cystic Fibrosis Foundation
1995   *Foundation Facts.* Bethesda, Maryland: Cystic Fibrosis Foundation.
1995   *A Teacher's Guide to Cystic Fibrosis.* Bethesda, Md.: Cystic Fibrosis Foundation.

Czajkowski, D. R., and Koocher, G. P.
1986   Predicting Medical Compliance among Adolescents with Cystic Fibrosis. *Health Psychology,* 5:297–305.

D'Angelo, S.; Wilson, J.; Fosson, A.; and Kanga, J.
1990   *The Relationship of Family Environment to the Psychological Adjustment of Children with Cystic Fibrosis and Their Parents.* Paper presented at the Cystic Fibrosis Foundation meetings. Arlington, Va.

Darling, R. B.
1979   *Families Against Society: A Study of Reactions to Children with Birth Defects.* Beverly Hills, Calif.: Sage.

Davies, Elizabeth Mary
1983   *Behavioral Responses of Children to the Death of a Sibling.* PhD Thesis. University of Washington.

Davis, Fred
1963   *Passage Through Crisis: Polio Victims and Their Families.* New York: Bobbs-Merrill.

Davis, Pamela B.
1984   Cystic Fibrosis in Adults. In *Cystic Fibrosis.* Edited by Lynn M. Taussig. New York: Thieme-Stratton.
1994   Evaluation of Therapy for Cystic Fibrosis. *New England Journal of Medicine,* 331 (10):672–73.

Deford, Frank
1983   *Alex: The Life of a Child.* New York: Viking Press.

Delisi, Stephen
1986   *Adjustment, Developmental, and Relationship Issues in Siblings of Children with Chronic Illness.* PhD Thesis. Miami University.

Denning, Carolyn R., and Gluckson, Muriel M.
1984   Psychosocial Aspects of Cystic Fibrosis. In *Cystic Fibrosis.* Edited by Lynn M. Taussig. New York: Thieme-Stratton.

Denning, C. R.; Gluckson, M.; and Muhr, I.
1976   Psychosocial and Social Aspects of Cystic Fibrosis. In *Cystic Fibrosis: Projections into the Future.* New York: Thieme-Stratton.

di Sant'Agnese, Paul A.; Darling, Robert; Perera, George A.; and Shea, Ethel
1953   Abnormal Electrolyte Composition of Sweat in Cystic Fibrosis of the Pancreas. Clinical Significance and Relationship of the Disease. *Pediatrics,* 12:549–63.

di Sant'Agnese, Paul A., and Hubbard, Van S.
1984   The Pancreas. In *Cystic Fibrosis.* Edited by Lynn M. Taussig. New York: Thieme-Stratton.

Docter, Jack
1973   The Chronically Ill Child: Soma and Psyche. In *Psychosocial Aspects of Cystic Fibrosis.* Edited by Patterson, Denning, and Kutscher. New York: Columbia University Press.

Dooley, R. R.
1973   Management of the Terminal Adolescent and One Family. In *Psychosocial Aspects of Cystic Fibrosis.* Edited by Patterson, Denning, and Kutscher. New York: Columbia University Press.

Drotar, Dennis
1981   Psychological Perspectives in Chronic Childhood Illness. *Journal of Pediatric Psychology,* 6 (3):211–28.

Drotar, D., and Crawford, P.
 1985 Psychological Adaptation of Siblings of Chronically Ill Children: Research and Practice Implications. *Developmental and Behavioral Pediatrics*, 6:355–62. December.

Drotar, D.; Crawford, P.; and Bush, M.
 1984 The Family Context of Childhood Chronic Illness: Implications for Psychosocial Intervention. In *Chronic Illness and Disability Through the Life Span*. Edited by M. Eisenberg. New York: Springer.

Dunn, Judy, and Kendrick, Carol
 1982 *Siblings: Love, Envy and Understanding*. Cambridge, Mass.: Harvard University Press.

Eigen, Howard; Clark, Nouen; and Wolle, Joan
 1987 Clinical-Behavioral Aspects of Cystic Fibrosis: Directions for Future Research. In *American Review of Respiratory Disease*, 136:1509–1513.

Einstein, G., and Moss, M. S.
 1967 Some Thoughts on Sibling Relationships. *Social Case Work*, 48:549–55. November.

Fabrega, Horacio
 1974 *Disease and Social Behavior*. Cambridge, Mass.: MIT Press.

Farber, Bernard
 1964 *Family Organization and Interaction*. San Francisco: Chandler.

Farkas, Andrea
 1973 *Adaptation of Patients, Siblings, and Mothers to Cystic Fibrosis*. PhD Thesis. Michigan State University.

Farkas, A., and Schnell, R. B.
 1973 A Psychological Study of Family Adjustment to Cystic Fibrosis. In *Psychological Aspects of Cystic Fibrosis*. Edited by Patterson, Denning, and Kutscher. New York: Columbia University Press.

Farkas, A., and Shwachman, H.
 1973 Psychological Adaptation in Chronic Illness. *American Journal of Orthopsychology*, 43:259.

Featherstone, Helen
 1980 *A Difference in the Family: Life with a Disabled Child*. New York: Basic Books.

Feeman, Dorothy J.
 1987 *The Effect of Childhood Chronic Illness on Siblings of the Ill Child*. PhD Thesis. University of Michigan.

Felsenthal, Helen, and Yamamoto, K.
 1972 The Developing Self: The Parental Role. In *The Child and His Image: Self Concept in the Early Years*. Edited by K. Yamamoto. Boston: Houghton Mifflin.

Ferrari, Michael
 1982 *Chronically Ill Children and Their Siblings: Some Psychological Implications*. PhD Thesis. Rutgers University. New Brunswick.

 1984 Chronic Illness: Psychosocial Effects on Siblings: Chronically Ill Boys. *Journal of Child Psychology and Psychiatry and Allied Disciplines*, 25 (3):459–76.

Fielding, Dorothy; Moore, Bryon; Dewey, Mike; Ashley, Paula; McKendrick, Thomas; and Pinkerton, Philip

1985 Children with End-Stage Renal Failure: Psychological Effects on Patients, Siblings and Parents. *Journal of Psychosomatic Research*, 29 (5):457–65.

Findlay, Ian I.; Smith, P.; and Linton, Margerie L.
1969 Chronic Disease in Childhood: A Study of Family Reactions. *British Journal of Medical Education*, 3 (1):66–69.

Fosson, A.; D'Angelo, Sandra; Wilson, John; and Kanga, Jamshed
1991 Impact of Cystic Fibrosis and Asthma on Family Attributes. Paper Presented at the Cystic Fibrosis Meetings, Dallas. Abstract reprinted in *Pediatric Pulmonary Supplement*, 6:309.

Fosson, A.; Wilson, John; Kanga, Jamshed; and D'Angelo, Sandra
1991 *Interplay of Physical, Psychological, and Family Factors in Cystic Fibrosis: Tracking Variables in 35 Children for 24 Months.* Unpublished manuscript.

Frank, Arthur W.
1991 *At the Will of the Body.* Boston: Houghton Mifflin.

Gallimore, R.; Weisner, T. S.; Kaufman, S.; and Bernheimer, L. P.
1989 The Social Construction of Ecocultural Niches: Family Accommodation of Developmentally Delayed Children. *American Journal of Retardation*, 94 (3):216–30.

Gallo, Agatha; Breitmayer, Bonnie; Knafl, Kathleen A.; and Zoeller, Linda H.
1992 Well Siblings of Children with Chronic Illness: Parents' Reports of Their Psychologic Adjustment. In *Pediatric Nursing*. 18 (1):23–27.
1993 Mothers' Perceptions of Sibling Adjustment and Family Life in Childhood Chronic Illness. In *Journal of Pediatric Nursing*, 8 (5):318–24.

Gallo, Agatha, and Knafl, Kathleen A.
1992 *Well Siblings in Childhood Chronic Illness: A Categorical and Non-Categorical Look at Selected Literature.* Unpublished manuscript.

Gath, Ann
1972 The Mental Health of Siblings of Congenitally Abnormal Children. *Journal of Child Psychology and Psychiatry*, 13 (3):211–18.
1974 Sibling Reaction to Mental Handicap: A Comparison of Brothers and Sisters of Mongol Children. *American Journal of Child Psychology and Psychiatry*, 15 (3):187–98. July.

Gayton, William F., and Friedman, Stanford B.
1973 Psychosocial Aspects of Cystic Fibrosis. *American Journal of Diseases of Children*, 126 (6):856–59. December.

Gayton, William F.; Friedman, Stanford B.; Tavormina, Joseph F.; and Tucker, Ford
1977 Children with Cystic Fibrosis: Psychological Test Findings of Patients, Siblings, and Parents. *Pediatrics*, 59 (6):888–94.

Geertz, Clifford
1973 *The Interpretation of Cultures.* New York: Basic Books.

Gibson, Cheryl
1986 How Parents Cope with a Child with Cystic Fibrosis. *Nursing Papers*, 18 (3):31–45.

Gogan, Janice Lee; Koocher, Gerald P.; Foster, Diana; and O'Malley, John E.
1977 Impact of Childhood Cancer on Siblings. *Health and Social Work*, 2 (1):41–57.

Goldberg, I. K.; Kutscher, A. H.; and Lorin, M. I. et al.
1973 Psychological Care of the Cystic Fibrosis Patient and His Family. In *Psycho-

social Aspects of Cystic Fibrosis. Edited by Patterson, Denning, and Kutscher. New York: Columbia University Press.

Gordon, Bianca
  1974 An Interdisciplinary Approach to the Dying Child and His Family. In *Care of The Child Facing Death*. Edited by L. Burton. London: Routledge and Kegan Paul.

Gordon, Jacquie
  1988 *Give Me One Wish*. New York: W. W. Norton and Company.

Gratzick, Edward
  1973 Hospitalized Children and Young Adults with Cystic Fibrosis. In *Psychosocial Aspects of Cystic Fibrosis*. Edited by Patterson, Denning, and Kutscher. New York: Columbia University Press.

Green, Johanna
  1985 *Observations in the Waiting Room of the Cystic Fibrosis Center, St. Christopher's Hospital for Children*. Unpublished Report.

Gurwitz, Dennis; Francis, Paul; Crozier, Douglas; and Levinson, Henry
  1979 Perspectives in Cystic Fibrosis. *Pediatric Clinics of North America*, 26 (3):603–615.

Harder, Lois C.
  1981 *Siblings of Children with Cystic Fibrosis: Perceptions of the Impact of the Disease, Coping Behaviors and Psychological Adjustment*. PhD Thesis. Purdue University.

Harder, L. and Bowditch, C. E.
  1982 Siblings of Children with Cystic Fibrosis: Perceptions of the Impact of the Disease. *Children's Health Care*, 10:116–20

Henry, Jules
  1971 *Pathways to Madness*. New York: Random House.

Hewett, S.; Newson, J.; and Newson, E.
  1970 *The Family and the Handicapped Child*. Chicago: Aldine Publishing Company.

Hilbourn, John
  1973 On Disabling the Normal. *British Journal of Social Work*, 3 (4):497–507.

Hobbs, Nicholas; Perrin, James; and Ireys, Henry
  1985 *Chronically Ill Children and Their Families*. San Francisco: Jossey-Bass.

Hodson, M. E.
  1983 *Cystic Fibrosis*. London: Baillière Tindall.

Hogan, Nancy S.
  1987 *An Investigation of the Adolescent Sibling Bereavement Process and Adaptation*. PhD Thesis. Loyola University of Chicago.

Homer
  1990 *The Odyssey*. Translated by Robert Fitzgerald. New York: Random House.

Huang, Nancy
  1980 Conversations and Personal Communication as Director of Cystic Fibrosis Center at St. Christopher's Hospital for Children, Philadelphia, Pennsylvania.

Hymovich, Debra P., and Dillon Baker, Cindy
  1985 The Needs, Concerns, and Coping of Parents of Children with Cystic Fibrosis. *Family Relations*, 34:91–97.

Iles, J. Penny
  1979 Children with Cancer: Healthy Siblings' Perceptions During the Illness Experience. *Cancer Nursing*, 2 (5):371–77.

Irish, Donald P.
 1964 Sibling Interaction: A Neglected Aspect of Family Life Research. *Social Forces*, 42:279–88.
James, Allison, and Prout, Alan
 1990 *Constructing and Reconstructing Childhood*. London: Falmer Press.
Johnson, F. Leonard; Rudolph, Laura A.; and Hartmann, John R.
 1979 Helping Families Cope with Childhood Cancer. *Psychosomatics*, 20 (4):241, 245–47, 251. April.
Johnson, Mark C.; Muyskens, Martha; Palmer, Judith; Bryce, Marguerite; and Rodman, Joan
 1985 A Comparison of Family Adaptations to Having a Child with Cystic Fibrosis. *Journal of Marital and Family Therapy*, 11 (3):305–312. July.
Kalnins, I. V.
 1977 The Dying Child: A New Perspective. *Journal of Pediatric Psychology*, 2 (2):39–41.
Kashani, Javad H.; Barbero, Giulio; Wilfley, Denise E.; Morris, Debra A.; and Shepperd, James A.
 1988 Psychological Concomitants of Cystic Fibrosis in Children and adolescents. *Adolescence*, 23 (92):873–80.
Kastenbaum, Robert
 1988 Exit with Thunder. In *Qualitative Gerontology*. Edited by Shulamit Reinharz and Graham D. Rowles. New York: Springer Publishing Co.
Kellerman, Jonathan
 1980 *Psychological Aspects of Childhood Cancer*. Springfield, Ill.: Charles C. Thomas.
Kerner, John; Harvey, Bert,; and Lewiston, Norman
 1979 The Impact of Grief: A Retrospective Study of Family Function Following Loss of a Child with Cystic Fibrosis. *Journal of Chronic Disease*, 32 (3):221–25.
Klein, Susan D.
 1976 Measuring the Outcome of the Impact of Chronic Childhood Illness on the Family. In *Chronic Childhood Illness: Assessment of Outcome*. Edited by G. Grave and I. Pless. Washington, D.C.: Dept. of HEW (76–877).
Kleinman, Arthur
 1980 *Patients and Healers in the Context of Culture*. Berkeley: University of California Press.
 1988 *The Illness Narratives: Suffering Healing and Human Condition*. New York: Basic Books.
Knafl, Kathleen Astin
 1982 Parents' Views of the Response of Siblings to a Pediatric Hospitalization. *Research in Nursing and Health*, 5 (1):13–20.
 1985 How Families Manage a Pediatric Hospitalization. *Western Journal of Nursing Research*, 7 (2):151–76.
Knafl, Kathleen Astin, and Deatrick, J. A.
 1986 How Families Manage Chronic Conditions: An Analysis of the Concept of Normalization. In *Research in Nursing and Health*. 9 (3):215–22.
Koch, Alberta
 1981 *"If Only it Could be Me": The Siblings of Pediatric Cancer Patients*. PhD Thesis. University of Southern California.

Koenig, Barbara
1988   *Technological Imperative in Medical Practice*. PhD Thesis. Berkeley, University of California.
Kramer, Robin F.
1981   Living with Childhood Cancer: Healthy Siblings' Perspective. *Issues in Comprehensive Pediatric Nursing*, 5 (3):155–165.
1984   Living with Childhood Cancer: Impact on the Healthy Siblings. *Oncological Nursing Forum*, 11 (1):44–51.
Kruger, S.; Shawver, M.; and Jones, L.
1980   Reactions of Families to the Child with Cystic Fibrosis. In *Image*. 12:67–72.
Krulik, T.
1980   Successfully "Normalizing" Tactics of Parents of Chronically Ill Children. *Journal of Advanced Nursing*, 5 (1)573–578.
1987   Loneliness and Social Isolation in School-Age Children with Chronic Life-Threatening Illness. In *The Child and the Family Facing Life-Threatening Illness*. Edited by Tamar Krulik et al. Philadelphia: J. B. Lippincott.
Kucia, Carol; Drotar, Dennis; Doershuk, Carl F.; Stern, Robert C.; Boat, Thomas T.; and Mathews, LeRoy
1979   Home Observation of Family Interaction and Childhood Adjustment to Cystic Fibrosis. *Journal of Pediatric Psychology*, 4 (2):189–95.
Kulczycki, L. L.; Regal, D. A.; and Tantisunthorn, C.
1973   The Impact of Cystic Fibrosis on the Parents and Patients. In *Psychosocial Aspects of Cystic Fibrosis*. Edited by Patterson, Denning, and Kutscher. New York: Columbia University Press.
Kung, Faith H.
1981   From Diagnosis to Survival. In *Living With Childhood Cancer*. Edited by J. J. Spinetta. St. Louis: C. V. Mosby.
Kupst, M. J.
1986   Death of a Child from a Serious Illness. In *Parental Loss of a Child*. Edited by T. A. Rando. Champaign, Ill.: Research Press.
Kupst M. J., and Schulman, J. L.
1986   Coping in Siblings of Children with Serious Illness. In *Crisis Intervention with Children and Families*. Edited by S. M. Aurebach and A. L. Stalherg. Washington, D.C.: Hemisphere. 173–88.
Lamb, M., and Sutton-Smith, B.
1982   *Sibling Relationships: Their Nature and Significance Across the Life Span*. Hillsdale: Erlbaum Association.
Landon, Christopher; Rosenfield, Ronald; Northcraft, Gregory; and Lewiston, Norman
1980   Self-Image of Adolescents with Cystic Fibrosis. *Journal of Youth and Adolescence*, 9 (6):521–28.
Lask, Bryan
1995   Psychological Aspects of Cystic Fibrosis. In *Cystic Fibrosis*. Edited by Margaret Hodson and Duncan Geddes. London: Chapman and Hall.
Lask, Bryan, and Fosson, A.
1989   *Childhood Illness: The Psychosomatic Approach*. New York: Wiley.
Lavigne, J. V., and Ryan, M.
1979   Psychologic Adjustment of Siblings of Children with Chronic Illness. *Pediatrics*, 63 (4):616–27. April.

Lawler, Robert H.; Nakielny, Wladyslaw; and Wright, Nancy A.
1966   Psychological Implications of Cystic Fibrosis. *Canadian Medical Association Journal*, 94:1043–46. May 14.

Lazarus, Richard S.
1981   The Costs and Benefits of Denial. In *Living With Childhood Cancer*. Edited by J. J. Spinetta. St. Louis: C. V. Mosby.

Leiken, S. J., and Hassakis, P.
1973   Psychological Study of Parents of Children with Cystic Fibrosis. In *The Child in His Family*. Edited by E. J. Anthony and C. Koupernick. New York: John Wiley and Sons, Inc.

Leonard, Barbara
1983   *Psychosocial Consequences on Siblings of Children with Chronic Illness*. PhD Thesis. University of Minnesota. *Dissertation Abstracts International*, 44 (11):3360B.

Lesser, R. M.
1978   Sibling Transference and Countertransference. *Journal of the American Academy of Psychoanalysis*, 6 (1):37–49. January.

Lewis, Brian L.
1981   *Factors Affecting Psychosocial Adjustment in Chronically Ill Children and in Their Parents*. PhD Thesis. University of Florida. *Dissertation Abstracts International*, 42 (6). Dec.

Lewis, B., and Khaw, K. T.
1982   Family Functioning as a Mediating Variable Affecting Psychosocial Adjustment of Children with Cystic Fibrosis. *Journal of Pediatrics*, 101 (4):636–40. Oct.

Lewis, Oscar
1959   *Five Families*. New York: Basic Books.

Lewis, S., and Armstrong, S. H.
1977–78   Children with Terminal Illness: A Selected Review. *International Journal of Psychiatry in Medicine*, 8 (1):73–82.

Lewis, S.; Horton, F. T.; and Armstrong, S.
1987   Distress in Fatally and Chronically Ill Children. In *The Child and Family Facing Life-Threatening Illness*. Edited by Tamar Krulik, Bonnie Holaday, and Ida Martinson. Philadelphia: J. B. Lippincott.

Lewiston, Norman J.
1985   Cystic Fibrosis. In *Issues in the Care of Chronic Illness*. Edited by Nicholas Hobbs. San Francisco: Jossey-Bass.

Lindsay, Mary, and MacCarthy, Dermod
1974   Caring for the Brother and Sister of a Dying Child. In *Care of the Child Facing Death*. Edited by Lindy Burton. London: Routledge and Kegan Paul.

Littlefield, Christine H.
1984   *When a Child Dies: A Sociobiological Perspective*. PhD Thesis. York University, Canada. *Dissertation Abstracts International*, 45 (8):85. Feb.

Lloyd-Still, John D.
1983   *Textbook of Cystic Fibrosis*. Boston, Mass.: Wright Publishing Company.

Lobato, Debra J.
1983   Siblings of Handicapped Children: A Review. In *Journal of Autism and Developmental Disorders*. 13 (4):347–64.

Lobato, D.; Faust, D.; and Spirito, A.

1988   Examining the Effects of Chronic Disease and Disability on Children's Sibling Relationships. *Journal of Pediatric* Psychology, 13 (3):389–407.

Lorin, Martin

1973   The Twilight Hours. In *The Psychosocial Aspects of Cystic Fibrosis.* Edited by Patterson, Denning, and Kutscher. New York: Columbia University Press.

Magrab, Phyllis R.

1985   Psychological Development of Chronically Ill Children. In *Issues in the Care of Children with Chronic Illness.* Edited by Nicholas Hobbs. San Francisco: Jossey-Bass.

Marky, I.

1982   Children with Malignant Disorders and Their Families: A Study of the Implications of the Disease and Its Treatment on Everyday Life. *Acta Paediatrica Scandinavica,* 303:1–82.

Massie, Robert K., Jr.

1985   The Constant Shadow: Reflections on the Life of a Chronically Ill Child. In *Issues in the Care of Children with Chronic Illness.* Edited by N. Hobbs and J. Perrin. San Francisco: Jossey-Bass.

McCubbin, M.

1984   Nursing Assessment of Parental Coping with Cystic Fibrosis. In *Western Journal of Nursing Research,* 6 (4):407–422.

Meuwissen, H.

1971   Family Adaptation to Child with Cystic Fibrosis. *Journal of Pediatrics,* 78 (3):548. March.

Meyerowitz, Joseph H., and Kaplan, Howard B.

1967   Familial Responses to Stress: The Case of Cystic Fibrosis. *Social Science and Medicine,* 1 (3):249–66.

Meyerowitz, Joseph H., and Kaplan, Howard B.

1973   Cystic Fibrosis and Family Functioning. In *Psychosocial Aspects of Cystic Fibrosis.* Edited by Patterson, Denning, and Kutscher. New York: Columbia University Press.

Michelson, Lee Ann Simons

1985   *The Effects of Chronic Childhood Illness on Healthy Siblings.* PhD Thesis. University of Massachusetts.

Miller, Nan

1986   *The Question of Anticipatory Mourning in Latency: A Child's Reactions to Her Sibling's Life-Threatening Illness.* D.S.W. Thesis. New York University. *Dissertation Abstracts International,* 47 (8). Feb.

Miller, N. B., and Cantwell, D. P.

1976   Siblings as Therapists: A Behavioral Approach. *American Journal of Psychiatry,* 133 (4):447–50. April.

Morganstern, M.

1964   *Maternal Attitudes and Reactions of Normal Siblings in Families with a Cerebral Palsied Child.* PhD Thesis. New York University.

Mulder, H. C., and Suvrmeijer, T.P.B.M.

1977   Families with a Child with Epilepsy: A Sociological Contribution. *Journal of Biosocial Science,* 9 (1):13–24. January.

Munson, Stephen
1978   Family Structure and the Family's General Adaptation to Loss: Helping Families Deal with the Death of a Child. In *The Child and Death*. Edited by O. J. Sahler. St Louis: C. V. Mosby.

McBride, Mary M.
1987   *The Well Child's Concept of Death During a Sibling's Life-Threatening Illness*. PhD Thesis. Case Western Reserve University. Health Sciences Nursing. *Dissertation Abstracts International*, 48 (6):1642B. Dec.

McCollum, Audrey T.
1971   Cystic Fibrosis: Economic Impact on the Family. *American Journal of Public Health*, 61 (7):1335–40. July.

McCollum, A. T., and Gibson, L. E.
1970   Family Adaptation to the Child with Cystic Fibrosis. *Journal of Pediatrics*, 77 (4):571–78.

McCown, Darlene E.
1982   *Selected Factors Related to Childrens' Adjustment Following Sibling Death*. PhD Thesis. Oregon State University.

McCrae, W. M.; Cull, A. M.; Burton, L.; and Dodge, J.
1973   Cystic Fibrosis: Parents' Response to the Genetic Basis of the Disease. *The Lancet*, 2 (821):141–43. July.

McKey, Robert
1973   Coping with a Family Shattering Disease. In *Psychosocial Aspects of Cystic Fibrosis*. Edited by Patterson, Denning, and Kutscher. New York: Columbia University Press.

McMichael, Joan
1971   *Handicap: A Study of Physically Handicapped Children and Their Families*. Pittsburgh: University of Pittsburgh Press.

Nadler, Henry L., and Ben-Yoseph, Yoav
1984   Genetics. In *Cystic Fibrosis*. Edited by L. M.Taussig. New York: Thieme-Stratton.

National Cystic Fibrosis Research Foundation
1972   *Educational and Vocational Counseling for the Young Adult with Cystic Fibrosis*.

Nolan, T.; Desmond, Katherine; Herlich, R.; and Hardy S.
1986   Knowledge of Cystic Fibrosis in Patients and Their Parents. *Pediatrics*, 77 (2):229–235. February.

Norman, A. P., and Hodson, M. E.
1983   Emotional and Social Aspects of Treatment. In *Cystic Fibrosis*. London: Baillère Tindall.

Obetz, W. S., et al.
1980   Children who Survive Malignant Disease: Emotional Adaptation of the Children and Families. In *The Child with Cancer*. Edited by J. L. Schulman and M. J. Kupst. Springfield, Ill.: Charles C. Thomas.

O'Brien, Eileen Liscik
1987   *Living with Chronically Ill Siblings: A Developmental Study*. PhD Thesis. Catholic University of America.

Parsons, T., and Fox, R.
1952   Illness, Therapy, and the Modern Urban American Family. *Journal of Social Issues*, 8 (4):31–44.

Patterson, Paul; Denning, Carolyn; and Kutscher, Austin, eds.
1973   *Psychosocial Aspects of Cystic Fibrosis.* New York: Columbia University Press.

Pauly, M. V.
1983   The Economics of Cystic Fibrosis. In *Textbook of Cystic Fibrosis.* Edited by J. D. Lloyd-Still. Boston: John Wright Publishing Company.

Peshkin, M. M.
1964   The Role of Emotions in Children with Intractable Bronchial Asthma. *Journal of Asthma Research,* 2 (2):143–146. December.

Pettle, Michael S. A., and Lansdown, R. G.
1986   Adjustment to the Death of a Sibling. *Archives of Disease in Childhood,* 61 (3):278–283. March.

Pfouts, J. H.
1976   The Sibling Relationship: A Forgotten Dimension. *Social Work,* 21 (3):200–204. May.

Pilling, Doria
1973   *The Child with a Chronic Medical Problem: Cardiac Disorders, Diabetes, Hemophilia: Social, Emotional and Educational Adjustment.* New York: Humanities Press.

Pless, I. B., and Perrin, J. M.
1985   Issues Common to a Variety of Illnesses. In *Issues in the Care of Children with Chronic Illness.* Edited by N. Hobbs and J. M. Perrin. San Francisco: Jossey-Bass.

Pollack, G. H.
1962   Childhood Parent and Sibling Loss in Adult Patients. *Archives of General Psychiatry,* 7 (4):295–305. Oct.

Prout A., and James A.
1990   A New Paradigm for the Sociology of Childhood Provenance, Promise and Problems. In *Constructing and Reconstructing Childhood.* New York: Falmer Press.

Quinton, Paul M.
1984   Exocrine Glands In *Cystic Fibrosis.* Edited by L. M. Taussig. New York: Thieme-Stratton.

Quittner, A.; DiGirolamo, A. M.; Jacobsen, J.; and Eigen, H.
1991   *A Contextual Model of Parenting Problems and Outcomes for Newly Diagnosed Families.* Paper presented at the Cystic Fibrosis Foundation meetings, Dallas.

Quittner, A.; DiGirolama, A.; Michel, M.; and Eigen, H.
1992   Parental Response to Cystic Fibrosis: A Contextual Analysis of One Phase. *Journal of Pediatric Psychology,* 17 (6):683–704.

Ratjen, Bjorn
1989   *Communication Between Children with Cancer and Their Caretakers.* PhD Thesis. University of British Columbia.

Richards, Martin, and Light, Paul
1986   *Children of Social Worlds.* Cambridge: Polity Press.

Richmond, Sharon Lynn
1985   *Factors Influencing Sibling Reaction to Childhood Cancer.* PhD Thesis. Johns Hopkins University. *Dissertation Abstracts International,* 46 (6). Dec.

Robinson, Carole
1993   Managing Life with a Chronic Condition: The Story of Normalization. In *Qualitative Health Research,* 3 (1):6–28.

Rosen, Helen
1986 *Unspoken Grief: Coping with Childhood Sibling Loss*. Lexington, Mass.: Lexington Books.

Rosenberg, Charles and Golden, Janet
1992 *Framing Disease: Studies in Cultural History*. New Brunswick, N.J.: Rutgers University Press.

Rosenstein, B. J.
1970 Cystic Fibrosis of the Pancreas: Impact on Family Functioning. In *The Chronically Ill Child and His Family*. Edited by M. Debuskey. Springfield, Ill.: Charles C. Thomas.

Rosenstein, Beryl J., and Langbaum, Terry S.
1984 Diagnosis. In *Cystic Fibrosis*. Edited by L. M. Taussig. New York: Thieme-Stratton.

Sanjek, Roger
1990 *Fieldnotes: The Makings of Anthropology*. Ithaca, N.Y.: Cornell University Press.

San Martino, M., and Newman, M. B.
1974 Siblings of Retarded Children: A Population at Risk. *Child Psychiatry and Human Development*, 4 (3):168–77. Spring.

Scheper-Hughes, Nancy
1992 *Death without Weeping: The Violence of Everyday Life in Brazil*. Berkeley: University of California Press.

Schildkrout, Enid
1991 Ambiguous Messages and Ironic Twists: Into the Heart of Africa and the Other Museum. In *Museum Anthropology*, 15 (2):16–23.

Schvaneveldt, Jay D., and Ihinger, Marilyn
1979 Sibling Relationships in the Family. In *Contemporary Theories about the Family*. Vol. 1. Edited by W. Burr et al. London: The Free Press.

Schwirian, P. M.
1976 Effects of the Presence of a Hearing Impaired Preschool Child in the Family on Behavior Patterns of Older Normal Siblings. *American Annals of the Deaf*, 121 (4):373–80.

Sibinga, Maaten; Friedman, Jack C.; and Huang Nancy
1973 The Family of the Cystic Fibrosis Patient. *Psychosocial Aspects of Cystic Fibrosis*. Edited by Patterson, Denning and Kutscher. New York: Columbia University Press.

Siemon, M.
1984 Siblings of the Chronically Ill or Disabled Child: Meeting Their Needs. *Nursing Clinics of North America*, 19 (2):295–307. June.

Sourkes, Barbara
1980 Siblings of the Pediatric Cancer Patient. In *Psychological Aspects of Childhood Cancer*. Edited by J. Kellerman. Springfield, Ill.: Charles C. Thomas. 47–69.

Speece, Mark W., and Brent, Sandor B.
1984 Children's Understanding of Death: A Review of Three Components of a Death Concept. *Child Development*, 55 (5):1671–86.

Spinetta, John J.
1978 Communication Patterns in Families Dealing with Life-Threatening Illness. In *The Child and Death*. Edited by O. J. Sahler. St. Louis: C. V. Mosby.

Spinetta, J. J., and Deasey-Spinetta, P.
 1981　Talking with Children That Have a Life-Threatening Illness. In *Living with Childhood Cancer*. Edited by J. J. Spinetta. St. Louis: C. V. Mosby.

Spinetta, J. J., and Deasey-Spinetta, P.
 1981　*Living with Childhood Cancer*. St. Louis: C. V. Mosby.

Spinetta, John J.; McLaren, Helen; Fox, Robert; and Sparta, Steven.
 1981　The Kinetic Family Drawing in Childhood Cancer: A Revised Application of an Age-Dependent Measure. In *Living With Childhood Cancer*. Edited by J. J. Spinetta. St. Louis: C. V. Mosby.

Stadnyk, S.
 1973　The Team Approach to Death and Dying. In *Psychosocial Aspects of Cystic Fibrosis*. Edited by Patterson, Denning, and Kutscher. New York: Columbia University Press.

Starfield, Barbara
 1985　The State of Research on Chronically Ill Children. In *Issues in the Care of Children with Chronic Illness*. Edited by N. Hobbs and J. M. Perrin. San Francisco: Jossey-Bass.

Stehbens, J. A. et al.
 1974　Psychological Follow-up of Families with Childhood Leukemia. *Journal of the Annual of Psychology*, 30 (3):394–97. July.

Straker, G., and Kuttner, M.
 1980　Psychological Compensation in the Individual with a Life-Threatening Illness: A Study of Adolescents with Cystic Fibrosis. *South African Medical Journal*, 57 (2):61–62. Jan.

Strauss, Anselm L.
 1984　A Basic Strategy: Normalizing. In *Chronic Illness and the Quality of Life*. Edited by A. L. Strauss. St. Louis: Mosby. Chap. 7, pp. 79–87.

 1984　Management of Regimens. In *Chronic Illness and Quality of Life*. Edited by A. L. Strauss. St. Louis: Mosby. Chap. 2, pp. 34–48.

 1984　Reordering of Time. In *Chronic Illness and Quality of Life*. Edited by A. L. Strauss. St. Louis: Mosby. Chap. 4, pp. 60–63.

 1984　Managing and Shaping the Trajectory. In *Chronic Illness and Quality of Life*. Edited by A. L. Strauss St. Louis: Mosby. Chap. 5, pp. 64–74.

Strauss, A. L., and Glasser, B. G.
 1984　*Chronic Illness and the Quality of Life*. St. Louis: C. V. Mosby.

Stubblefield, R. L., and Coltharp, F.
 1963　Psychiatric Observations on Asthmatic Children. *Texas Journal of Medicine*, 59:89–92. Feb.

Sutton-Smith, B.
 1982　Birth Order and Sibling Status Effects. In *Sibling Relationships: Their Nature and Significance Across the Life Span*. Edited by M. Lamb and B. Sutton-Smith. Hillsdale: Erlbaum. Chap. 7 :133–65

 1982　Epilogue: Framing the Problem. In *Sibling Relationships: Their Nature and Significance Across the Life Span*. Edited by M. Lamb and B. Sutton-Smith. Hillsdale: Erlbaum.

Sutton-Smith, B., and Rosenberg, B. G.
 1970　*The Sibling*. New York: Holt, Rinehart and Winston.

Switzer, Vicki A.
 1984   *The Psychosocial Adjustment of Siblings of Children with Diabetes*. PhD Thesis. George Peabody College For Teachers of Vanderbilt University. *Dissertation Abstracts International*, 45 (6):1926. Dec.

Talamo, Richard C., and Schwartz, Robert H.
 1984   Immunologic and Allergic Manifestations. In *Cystic Fibrosis*. Edited by L. M.Taussig. New York: Thieme-Stratton.

Taussig, Lynn M.
 1984   *Cystic Fibrosis*. New York: Thieme-Stratton.

Tavormina, J. F.; Kastner, L. S.; Slater, P. M.; and Watt, S. L.
 1976   Chronically Ill Children: A Psychologically and Emotionally Deviant Population? In *Journal of Abnormal Child Psychology*, 4 (2):99–110.

Tew, B. J., and Laurence, K. M.
 1973   Mothers, Brothers, and Sisters of Patients with Spina Bifida. *Developmental Medicine and Child Neurology*, suppl. 29:69–76.

Thomas, Clayton L.
 1980   *Taber's Cyclopedic Medical Dictionary*. Philadelphia: F. A. Davis.

Tiller, J.W.G.; Ekert, H.; and Rickards, W. S.
 1977   Family Reactions in Childhood Acute Lymphoblastic Leukemia in Remission. *Australian Pediatric Journal*, 13 (3):176–81.

Tluczek, A.; Bowers, B.; Morris, M.; and Peterson, N.
 1991   *Diagnosing Cystic Fibrosis: Parents' and Providers' Perspectives*. Paper presented at the Cystic Fibrosis Foundation meetings, Dallas.

Tooley, K.
 1975   The Choice of Surviving Siblings as a "Scapegoat" in Some Cases of Maternal Bereavement: A Case Report. *Journal of Child Psychology and Psychiatry*, 16 (4):331–39.

Townes, B., and Wold, D.
 1977   Childhood Leukemia. In *The Experience of Dying*. Edited by E. Pattison. Englewood Cliffs: Prentice-Hall.

Treiber, F.; Mabe, P. A.; and Wilson, G.
 1987   Psychological Adjustments of Sickle Cell Children and Their Siblings. In *Children's Health Care*. 16:82–88.

Tritt, S. G., and Esses, L. M.
 1988   Psychosocial Adaptation of Siblings of Children With Chronic Medical Illnesses. *American Journal of Orthopsychiatry*, 58 (2):211–20. April.

Tropauer, A.; Franz, M. N.; and Dilgard, V. W.
 1970   Psychological Aspects of the Care of Children with Cystic Fibrosis. *American Journal of Diseases of Children*, 119 (5):424–32. May.

Turk, J.
 1964   Impact of Cystic Fibrosis on Family Functioning. *Pediatrics*, 34:67–71. July.

Waechter, Eugenia
 1987   Concomitants of Death Imagery in Stories Told by Chronically Ill Children Undergoing Intrusive Procedures. In *The Child and Family Facing Life-Threatening Illness*. Edited by Tamar Krulik, Bonnie Holaday, and Ida Martinsen. Philadelphia: J. B. Lippincott.

Walker, Caroline Louise

1990   Siblings of Children with Cancer. In *Oncology Nursing Forum*, 17 (3):355–60.

1986   *Stress and Coping in the Siblings of Children with Cancer*. PhD Thesis. University of Utah. *Dissertation Abstracts International*, 47 (7):1987

Walker, Lynn
1991   *Maternal Distress, Illness Severity and Child Adjustment in Cystic Fibrosis*. Paper presented at Cystic Fibrosis Foundation meetings, Dallas.

Weisner, Thomas, and Gallimore, Ronald
1977   My Brother's Keeper: Child and Sibling Caretaking. *Current Anthropology*, 18 (2):169–90. June.

Weisner, Thomas
1991   *Siblings in Cultural Place: Ethnographic and Ecocultural Perspectives*. NICHD conference paper. Rockville, Md.

Weyhing, Mary
1983   Parental Reactions to Handicapped Children and Familial Adjustments to Routines of Care. In *Parent-Professional Partnerships in Developmental Disability Services*. Cambridge, Mass.: Academic Guild. 125–37

Wilson, J.; Fosson, A.; Kanga, J.; and D'Angelo, S.
1990   *Longitudinal Relationships Between Family Environment and Clinically Significant Deterioration of Pulmonary Function*. Paper presented at Cystic Fibrosis Foundation meetings, Arlington, Va.

Wing, L.
1969   A Handicapped Child in the Family. *Developmental Medicine and Child Neurology*, 11 (5):643–44. October.

Wood, Robert E.
1984   Prognosis. In *Cystic Fibrosis*. Edited by L. M. Taussig. New York: Thieme-Stratton.

Yamamoto, K. ed.
1972   *The Child and His Image: Self-Concept in the Early Years*. Boston: Houghton Mifflin Company.

Zeltzer, L. K.
1978   Chronic Illness in the Adolescent. In *Adolescent Medicine*. Edited by I. R. Shenker. New York: Thieme-Stratton Intercontinental Medical Book Corp.

Zeltzer, L.; Kellerman, J.; Ellenberg, L.; Dash, J.; and Rigler, D.
1980   Psychologic Effects of Illness in Adolescence. II. Impact of Illness in Adolescents—Crucial Issues and Coping Styles. *Journal of Pediatrics*, 97 (1):132–38. July.

Zirinsky, Linda, and Black, Dora
1990   *Psychological Functioning in Siblings of Children With End-Stage Renal Failure*. Paper presented at the International Congress, International Association Child and Adolescent Psychiatry and Allied Professions. Royal Free Hospital, London.

Index